Body Contouring

Editor

J. PETER RUBIN

CLINICS IN
PLASTIC SURGERY

www.plasticsurgery.theclinics.com

October 2014 • Volume 41 • Number 4

ELSEVIER

1600 John F. Kennedy Boulevard ● Suite 1800 ● Philadelphia, Pennsylvania, 19103-2899

http://www.theclinics.com

CLINICS IN PLASTIC SURGERY Volume 41, Number 4
October 2014 ISSN 0094-1298, ISBN-13: 978-0-323-32628-5

Editor: Joanne Husovski
Developmental Editor: Donald Mumford

Clinics in Plastic Surgery (ISSN 0094-1298) is published quarterly by Elsevier Inc., 360 Park Avenue South, New York, NY 10010-1710. Months of issue are January, April, July, and October. Business and Editorial Offices: 1600 John F. Kennedy Blvd., Suite 1800, Philadelphia, PA 19103-2899. Periodicals postage paid at New York, NY and additional mailing offices. Subscription prices are $490.00 per year for US individuals, $716.00 per year for US institutions, $240.00 per year for US students and residents, $555.00 per year for Canadian individuals, $853.00 per year for Canadian institutions, $630.00 per year for international individuals, $853.00 per year for international institutions, and $305.00 per year for Canadian and foreign students/residents. To receive student/resident rate, orders must be accompanied by name of affiliated institution, date of term, and the *signature* of program/residency coordinator on institution letterhead. Orders will be billed at individual rate until proof of status is received. Foreign air speed delivery is included in all *Clinics* subscription prices. All prices are subject to change without notice. **POSTMASTER:** Send address changes to *Clinics in Plastic Surgery*, Elsevier Health Sciences Division, Subscription Customer Service, 3251 Riverport Lane, Maryland Heights, MO 63043. **Customer Service: 1-800-654-2452 (US and Canada). From outside of the United States and Canada, call 314-447-8871. Fax: 314-447-8029. E-mail: JournalsCustomerService-usa@elsevier.com (for print support); JournalsOnlineSupport-usa@elsevier.com (for online support).**

Reprints. For copies of 100 or more of articles in this publication, please contact the Commercial Reprints Department, Elsevier Inc., 360 Park Avenue South, New York, New York 10010-1710. Tel.: +1-212-633-3874; Fax: +1-212-633-3820; E-mail: reprints@elsevier.com.

Clinics in Plastic Surgery is covered in *Current Contents, EMBASE/Excerpta Medica, Science Citation Index, MEDLINE/PubMed (Index Medicus), ASCA,* and *ISI/BIOMED.*

Contributors

EDITOR

J. PETER RUBIN, MD, FACS
Chair, Department of Plastic Surgery;
Director, Life After Weight Loss Surgical Body
Contouring Program;
UPMC Endowed Professor of Plastic Surgery,
Professor of Bioengineering,
University of Pittsburgh,
Pittsburgh, Pennsylvania

AUTHORS

PAUL N. AFROOZ, MD
Resident, Department of Plastic Surgery,
University of Pittsburgh Medical Center,
Pittsburgh, Pennsylvania

AL ALY, MD, FACS
President-Aesthetic Surgery Education &
Research Foundation; Editor-in-Chief, Plastic
Surgery Education Network; Professor of
Plastic Surgery, Consultant Plastic Surgeon,
Cleveland Clinic Abu Dhabi, Abu Dhabi

STEFAN J. CANO, PhD
Clinical Neurology Research Group, Plymouth
University Peninsula Schools of Medicine and
Dentistry, Plymouth, Devon, United Kingdom

JOSEPH F. CAPELLA, MD
Chief, Post-Bariatric Body Contouring, Division
of Plastic Surgery, Capella Plastic Surgery,
Ramsey, New Jersey; Division of Plastic
Surgery, Hackensack University Medical
Center, Hackensack, New Jersey

BARRY E. DiBERNARDO, MD, FACS
Clinical Associate Professor, Division of Plastic
Surgery, Department of Surgery, University of
Medicine and Dentistry of New Jersey,
Newark, New Jersey; Director, New Jersey
Plastic Surgery, Montclair, New Jersey

JEFFREY A. GUSENOFF, MD
Co-Director, Life After Weight Loss Program;
Associate Professor of Plastic Surgery,
Department of Plastic Surgery, UPMC Plastic
Surgery Center, University of Pittsburgh,
Pittsburgh, Pennsylvania

JOSEPH P. HUNSTAD, MD, FACS
Section Head, Plastic Surgery Carolinas
Medical Center, University Hospital, Charlotte,
North Carolina; Associate Consulting
Professor, Division of Plastic Surgery,
University of North Carolina, Chapel Hill, North
Carolina; President, Hunstad-Kortesis Centers
and Medical Spa, Huntersville and Charlotte,
North Carolina

DENNIS HURWITZ, MD
Director, Hurwitz Center for Plastic Surgery;
Professor of Plastic Surgery, Department of
Plastic Surgery, University of Pittsburgh
Medical Center, Pittsburgh, Pennsylvania

PHILLIP D. KHAN, MD
Aesthetic Plastic Surgery Fellow, Hunstad-
Kortesis Center for Cosmetic Plastic Surgery
and Medspa, Charlotte, North Carolina

ANNE F. KLASSEN, DPhil
Department of Pediatrics, McMaster
University, Hamilton, Ontario, Canada

ALAN MATARASSO, MD
Manhattan Eye, Ear & Throat Hospital, Lenox
Hill Hospital, North Shore-Long Island Jewish
Hospital System, New York, New York

DANA MOORE MATARASSO
Alan Matarasso MD, Private Practice,
New York, New York

EMMA JAMES MATARASSO
Alan Matarasso MD, Private Practice,
New York, New York

**RYAN TAYLOR MARSHALL MITCHELL,
MD, FRCSC**
The Bengtson Center for Aesthetics and
Plastic Surgery, Grand Rapids, Michigan

MELISSA MUELLER, MD
Resident, Department of Plastic Surgery,
University of California Irvine, Orange,
California

NIMA NAGHSHINEH, MD, MSc
Resident, Department of Plastic Surgery,
University of Pittsburgh Medical Center,
Pittsburgh, Pennsylvania

JASON N. POZNER, MD, FACS
Adjunct Clinical Faculty, Department of Plastic
Surgery, Cleveland Clinic Florida, Weston,
Florida

ANDREA L. PUSIC, MD, MHS
Department of Surgery, Memorial Sloan-
Kettering Cancer Center, New York, New York

LAWRENCE S. REED, MD
Clinical Assistant Professor of Surgery
(Plastic Surgery), Weill Cornel Medical College,
New York, New York

DIRK F. RICHTER, MD, PhD
Department for Plastic and Reconstructive
Surgery, Dreifaltigkeits-Hospital, Wesseling,
Germany

J. PETER RUBIN, MD, FACS
Chair, Department of Plastic Surgery;
Director, Life After Weight Loss Surgical Body
Contouring Program;
UPMC Endowed Professor of Plastic Surgery,
Professor of Bioengineering,
University of Pittsburgh,
Pittsburgh, Pennsylvania

RENATO SALTZ, MD, FACS
Owner and Medical Director, Saltz Plastic
Surgery & Spa Vitória, Salt Lake City and
Park City, Utah

AMIE SCOTT, MSc
Department of Surgery, Memorial
Sloan-Kettering Cancer Center, New York,
New York

KENNETH C. SHESTAK, MD
Professor, Department of Plastic Surgery,
University of Pittsburgh School of Medicine;
Chief of Plastic Surgery, Plastic Surgery
Service, Magee Womens Hospital, Pittsburgh,
Pennsylvania

ALEXANDER STOFF, MD, PhD
Department for Plastic and Reconstructive
Surgery, Dreifaltigkeits-Hospital, Wesseling,
Germany

ELENA TSANGARIS, MSc
Department of Clinical Epidemiology and
Biostatistics, McMaster University, Hamilton,
Ontario, Canada

Contents

The obesity pandemic has resulted in increasing cases of bariatric surgery and subsequent issues related to excess skin and laxity for patients. This patient population requires unique insight and consideration as part of the preoperative evaluation. Nutritional derangements are common and psychosocial issues prevalent. These factors, together with the sequelae of past and present medical conditions, can all affect surgical planning and outcomes. This article familiarizes the plastic surgeon with the issues of the body contouring candidate and provides tools that may assist in surgical planning.

Patient-reported outcome (PRO) instruments are questionnaires designed to measure outcomes of importance to patients from their perspective. This article describes the methods used to develop a new PRO instrument for obese patients and patients having bariatric and cosmetic body contouring surgery. The BODY-Q is composed of 19 newly designed scales that measure: (1) appearance; (2) health-related quality of life; and (3) process of care. Recommended guidelines for PRO instrument development were followed to ensure that the BODY-Q meets requirements of regulatory bodies. The BODY-Q is currently being field-tested in an international study.

Examination of abdominal contour surgery candidates permits categorization of patients (the abdominolipoplasty system of classification and treatment) according to their treatable soft tissue layers of skin, fat, and muscle into the appropriate treatment level. Typically, postpartum abdominal wall changes are most thoroughly addressed by abdominoplasty surgery. The indications and goals for abdominoplasty with liposuction (lipoadminoplasty) or without liposuction are presented. Surgical markings, technique, pain management, and postoperative care are described.

Vertical abdominoplasty is a safe and effective procedure to correct abdominal contour abnormalities in individuals with excessive soft tissue in both the vertical and transverse orientation. It is a powerful procedure for addressing epigastric skin laxity after massive weight loss. The literature, although limited, supports the effectiveness of this procedure in addressing this clinical scenario. Further, the complication rates are comparable to a standard transverse abdominoplasty. Patient selection, preoperative planning, and technique are described.

postbrachioplasty aesthetic deformity is introduced. These aesthetic shortcomings are best avoided, because they are difficult to correct. The L brachioplasty with liposuction is described and applied to a variety of deformities to show the range of applicability and quality of results. The role of liposuction in arm reshaping is examined. The aesthetic advantages and low complication rate of the L brachioplasty are contrasted with other currently popular brachioplasty techniques.

Brachioplasty with Limited Scar   753

Lawrence S. Reed

There is a growing interest in upper arm aesthetic surgery but many patients do not accept the visible inner arm scar. Minimal incision brachioplasty using a shorter scar, concealed in the axilla, produces results equal to that of the traditional approach in comparable cases. Patients with massive weight loss may not meet the criteria for surgery. Patient selection and careful preoperative markings are critical to the success of the procedure. The author describes the technique he has been using for more than 30 years along with refinements. Minimal incision brachioplasty is an alternative to the traditional long scar approach in selected patients. It is a less involved procedure, with a low complication rate and high patient satisfaction.

Circumferential Truncal Contouring: The Belt Lipectomy   765

Al Aly and Melissa Mueller

The primary goal of belt lipectomy surgery is to improve the contour of the inferior truncal circumferential unit and to place the resultant scar in natural junctions. Excessive intra-abdominal content is a contraindication for belt lipectomy. The higher the presenting patient's body mass index (BMI), the higher the risk of postoperative complications and the less impressive the results. The converse is also true: the lower the BMI, the lower the risk of complications and the better the results. The most common complications are small wound separations and seromas.

Circumferential Body Contouring: The Lower Body Lift   775

Dirk F. Richter and Alexander Stoff

A 2-position circumferential approach for body contouring of the lower trunk is presented. Mostly indicated in patients after massive weight loss, this approach allows the simultaneous skin resection and reshaping in the abdominal, flank, lateral thigh, back, and gluteal region in the same operation, with only one position change during surgery. Reconstruction of the abdominal wall and gluteal restoration allow volume and shape enhancement with autologous tissue transpositioning. This article explains the required preconditions, assessment of gluteal deformities, and perioperative management of this procedure, and presents common complications.

Noninvasive and Minimally Invasive Techniques in Body Contouring   789

Paul N. Afrooz, Jason N. Pozner, and Barry E. DiBernardo

Major surgical body contouring procedures have several inherent drawbacks, including hospitalization, anesthetic use, pain, swelling, and prolonged recovery. It is for these reasons that body contouring through noninvasive and minimally invasive methods has become one of the most alluring areas in aesthetic surgery. Patient expectations and demands have driven the field toward safer, less-invasive procedures with less discomfort, fewer complications, and a shorter recovery. In this article, the current minimally invasive and noninvasive modalities for body contouring are reviewed.

CLINICS IN PLASTIC SURGERY

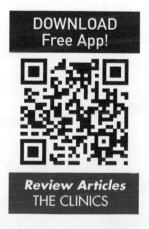

Preface
Body Contouring

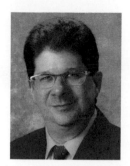

J. Peter Rubin, MD, FACS
Editor

Body contouring is a wonderfully diverse and complex discipline that has incredible impact on the lives of our patients. Changes due to aging, pregnancy, and weight loss are corrected through thoughtful planning and execution of procedures designed to address each patient's unique deformities and anatomic considerations. The rise of bariatric surgery has, in particular, led to an entirely new population of body-contouring patients with deformities spanning all regions of the body.

Body contouring is a constantly evolving field rich in innovation. Improved understanding of anatomy and aesthetic goals give rise to new patterns of excision and scar placement. Concepts of repositioning tissue and integrating liposuction with excision, as well as fat grafting, provide more power for achieving superior outcomes.

This issue covers the latest approaches for reshaping the trunk and extremities safely and effectively. Principles of patient safety, patient selection, assessing outcomes, and avoiding complications are presented. Expert perspectives on specific procedures for brachioplasty, abdominoplasty, lower body lift, upper trunk contouring, and thigh contouring are highlighted in this issue of *Clinics in Plastic Surgery*. Multiple surgical approaches for different regions are also highlighted. In addition, we present an article on the latest energy based technologies for fat reduction.

I wish to express my sincere gratitude to all of the authors who have given their time and expertise to compose the articles that comprise this outstanding reference. It is a privilege to work with these respected leaders. Their dedication and leadership propel the dynamic field of body contouring forward to the benefit of our patients.

J. Peter Rubin, MD, FACS
Department of Plastic Surgery
Life After Weight Loss Surgical Body
Contouring Program
University of Pittsburgh
Scaife Hall
3550 Terrace Street
Pittsburgh, PA 15261, USA

E-mail address:
rubinjp@upmc.edu

Clin Plastic Surg 41 (2014) xi
http://dx.doi.org/10.1016/j.cps.2014.08.001
0094-1298/14/$ – see front matter © 2014 Published by Elsevier Inc.

Preoperative Evaluation of the Body Contouring Patient
The Cornerstone of Patient Safety

Nima Naghshineh, MD, MSc, J. Peter Rubin, MD*

KEYWORDS

• Body contouring • Bariatric surgery • Skin laxity • Weight loss • Skin excess • Nutritional evaluation

KEY POINTS

- Body contouring after massive weight loss is often the final phase of a long and positive journey for the bariatric patient.
- As the prevalence of obesity increases and many more continue to seek bariatric and subsequently body contouring surgery, it is critical that plastic surgeons become well versed in not only techniques that address skin laxity, but also more familiar with the unique set of issues that the postbariatric patient presents.
- A careful and comprehensive approach like the one presented in this article allows for safe and effective treatment of these patients.

INTRODUCTION

As a result of the obesity pandemic, more and more individuals are seeking bariatric surgery for weight loss and resolution of conditions related to obesity. As the numbers have risen to greater than 200,000 cases per year, the number of post-bariatric massive weight loss patients presenting to the plastic surgeon for body contouring to address excess skin laxity is increasing.[1] However, this patient population requires unique insight and consideration as part of the preoperative evaluation. Nutritional derangements are common, psychosocial issues are prevalent, and the sequelae of past and present medical conditions can all affect surgical planning and outcomes. This article familiarizes the plastic surgeon with the body contouring candidate and provides tools that may assist in surgical planning.

We have identified six key assessment points as part of a comprehensive evaluation of the massive weight loss patient presenting for potential body contouring surgery: (1) time from gastric bypass to body contouring procedures; (2) body mass index (BMI) at presentation; (3) evaluation of medical comorbidities; (4) nutritional assessment; (5) psychosocial status; and (6) physical deformities and potential for combined procedures. An overview of these points is presented in **Box 1**.

PREOPERATIVE EVALUATION AND PROCEDURE TIMING

Initial preoperative history should focus on age of onset of obesity, family history of obesity, type and date of bariatric surgery performed, and course of weight loss since surgery. Anthropometric measures should include height, weight (highest, lowest, and current), and BMI. Determination regarding patient's weight stability should be made because many patients have a 12- to 18-month period of continued weight loss after

Department of Plastic Surgery, University of Pittsburgh Medical Center, 6B Scaife Hall, Suite 690, 3550 Terrace Street, Pittsburgh, PA 15261, USA
* Corresponding author.
E-mail address: rubinjp@upmc.edu

Clin Plastic Surg 41 (2014) 637–643
http://dx.doi.org/10.1016/j.cps.2014.07.002
0094-1298/14/$ – see front matter © 2014 Published by Elsevier Inc

their bariatric surgery. Inquiry into weight changes over the past 1 and 3 months before presentation should be made as part of the patient's history. We define weight stability as no more than an average of 5 lb/month loss over 3 months. A patient still undergoing significant weight loss may be in a state of protein-calorie deficiency and consequently may be at risk of suboptimal wound healing. Those deemed not stable are delayed and reevaluated in 3 months. An overview of our timing of surgical planning is provided in **Box 2**.

PATIENT BMI

Provided the patient has achieved weight stability, evaluation of BMI can be an indicator of potential complications and aesthetic outcomes. We consider patients with BMI less than 30 kg/m^2 to be the best candidates for a wide range of procedures and combinations thereof.[2] A prospective study of 511 postbariatric body contouring cases revealed that higher prebariatric maximum BMI and BMI at time of presentation were associated with increased complications in patients undergoing single procedures.[3] Similarly, the degree of change between these two measures (maximum BMI and BMI at time of presentation) was found to be correlated with overall complications in patients undergoing multiple procedures.[3] Other studies have also shown similar findings related to complication rates and higher BMI.[2,4] Those presenting with BMI between 30 and 35 kg/m^2 should be considered based on their individual body fat distribution. For example, a patient with BMI 35 and a gynecoid body type is likely to have a better aesthetic outcome from abdominal body contouring compared with an individual with the same BMI but an android body type. Patients presenting with BMI between 35 and 40 kg/m^2 are poorer aesthetic candidates because they typically have thicker subcutaneous tissue and intra-abdominal fat content. Surgery performed in these patients is often single procedure or staged and focuses on functional improvements (ie, panniculectomy and reduction mammoplasty) so that the patient can improve exercise tolerance and further reduce weight for future aesthetic body contouring. Unless, there is a significant medical indication, patients with BMI greater than 40 are deferred for further weight reduction.

MEDICAL COMORBIDITIES

The resultant weight loss from bariatric surgery often improves or resolves active health issues, such as diabetes and hypertension. In fact, this effect can typically be seen within the first 6 months

Box 2
Timing of surgical planning

2-3 months before surgery

Initial evaluation

Weight loss history, evaluation of BMI (maximum, current, and change)

Medical and surgical history

Evaluation of medical comorbidities

Social history evaluation

Nutritional analysis

Psychological evaluation

Physical examination

Delineation of patient goals and management of expectations

Photographs are taken

Follow-up visit 2-3 mo if further weight loss/weight stability is needed

1 month before surgery

Formal preoperative visit

Surgical plan reviewed

Questions answered

Informed consent obtained

Preoperative laboratory blood specimens are drawn

Preoperative medical evaluations should be performed as necessary

2 weeks before surgery

Antiplatelet medicines (e.g. aspirin, NSAIDs) are discontinued

Laboratory tests and medical clearances are reviewed

Nutrition is optimized

Day before surgery

Light bowel preparation (1/2 bottle of magnesium citrate at noon, followed by clear liquids) is administered for all abdominal procedures

Transportation in confirmed

Surgical plan and photographs are reviewed by the surgical team

From Bossert RP, Rubin JP. Evaluation of the weight loss patient presenting for plastic surgery consultation. Plast Reconstr Surg 2012;130(6):1363; with permission.

after surgery.[5] However, complete resolution of disease states may not occur and the plastic surgeon must be aware of the most common medical comorbidities with which the weight loss patient

may present. Prospective evaluation of weight loss patients presenting to the body contouring plastic surgeon has shown comorbidities of high prevalence of arthritis (41%), depression (53%), anxiety (27%), and anemia (24%).[1]

Although up to 82% of obese patients may show some degree of diabetes resolution,[6] many have persistent insulin resistance of varying severity. Monitoring of fasting glucose and hemoglobin A_{1C} provides immediate and long-term evidence of glucose control. Preoperatively, oral hypoglycemics are held and insulin dosages are adjusted for fasting state. Intraoperatively and postoperatively, glucose levels are checked every 6 hours and the patient is placed on a sliding scale insulin dosing.

Cardiac disease is prevalent in the obese population, and although weight loss may reduce immediate cardiac risk, long-term effects of obesity cannot be ignored. Therefore, careful preoperative screening is recommended, including assessment of exercise tolerance and other cardiac screening tests as determined by the patient's primary care physician or cardiologist. Likewise, hypertension is common among the obese. Although 50% to 60% of patients become normotensive after bariatric surgery,[7,8] optimization of blood pressure in the preoperative, intraoperative, and postoperative period decreases the risk of complications related to poor blood pressure control, such as hematoma and stroke.

Obstructive sleep apnea is another common comorbidity among the obese that may persist after weight loss. Patient interview should inquire about sleep studies and input from the patient's spouse or partner may reveal evidence toward persistent obstruction. Evaluation from a pulmonologist or internist may be indicated and those with known obstructive sleep apnea should bring their continuous positive airway pressure machines with them for use after surgery, or at the minimum be familiar with their customized settings.

Venous thromboembolism (VTE) is a significant risk for body contouring patients with contributing risk factors, such as current obesity, immobility, increasing age, and venous varicosities.[9] Thorough history taking may reveal evidence for hereditary coagulopathy, such as spontaneous abortions and family history of clotting disorders.[10] Those with a history of prior VTE should be referred to a hematologist for a complete hypercoagulable state work-up, whereas consultation with vascular surgery or interventional radiology may be necessary for those with the indications for inferior vena cava filters. The body contouring population has an overall risk for VTE of 2.9%, which increases to 8.9% for those with BMI greater than 35.[11] Although there are no clear guidelines for VTE chemoprophylaxis for plastic surgery, we recommend sequential compression devices before induction, early ambulation, and consideration of preoperative and postoperative chemoprophylaxis.

Screening for other coagulopathies and platelet dysfunction may reduce risk of bleeding and hematoma, and may be evident by easy bruising during history taking. Cessation of aspirin-containing products, certain herbal products, and nonsteroidal anti-inflammatory agents before surgery is also recommended.

Tobacco and nicotine use may also adversely affect outcomes and can be considered a modifiable risk. We recommend smoking cessation at least 1 month before surgery. This is often confirmed by urine cotinine tests. If the patient fails, surgery may be delayed.

NUTRITIONAL STATUS

It is important to gauge the nutritional status of the body contouring candidate because surgery can increase the caloric and protein demand by 25% from normal baseline.[12] Unfortunately, a significant number of body contouring patients have some type of nutritional derangement.

Assessment should include review of past surgical history, which may include restrictive procedures (gastric banding or vertical banded gastroplasty), Roux-en-Y gastric bypass (restrictive and malabsorptive), or older malabsorptive procedures (biliopancreatic diversion or duodenal switch). These patients may experience persistent nausea, vomiting, constipation, and diarrhea. If so, these may be signs of mechanical obstruction. Dumping syndrome, which nearly half of all patient experience after bariatric surgery, has similar symptoms and can be an independent risk factor for malnutrition.[1]

Because surgery increases the nutritional demand on the body, we recommend our patients increase their protein intake to 70 to 100 g/day. This may be difficult because many experience food aversions. Often, high-protein, low-fat, and carbohydrate whey supplements can be a solution. Nevertheless, it has been shown that 13.8% of preoperative patients have low albumin and 6.5% have low prealbumin in laboratory measures. Interestingly, these two measures did not correlate in this population, nor did they correlate with the reported protein intake. Therefore, we recommend both a thorough nutritional interview and laboratory studies to fully elucidate the nutritional state of the preoperative body contouring candidate.[1]

In addition to protein-calorie deficiency, a multitude of micronutrient deficiencies also exists in the postbariatric population.[13–15] Our study shows an iron deficiency prevalence of nearly 40%.[1] Other nutrient deficiencies often related to bariatric surgery include low calcium, vitamin B_{12}, folate, and thiamine levels. As a result, history and physical examination should look for signs and symptoms of anemia, muscle, reflex, and balance dysfunction, which may then warrant laboratory evaluation of micronutrient levels.

PSYCHOLOGICAL CONSIDERATIONS AND MANAGING PATIENT EXPECTATION

Psychological issues are widely prevalent in the obese population. Those with a BMI of greater than 40 have a five-fold increased prevalence of major depression.[16] Even after weight loss, depression, anxiety, low self-esteem, poor eating habits, and poor body image persist.[1,13,17–19] Although excess skin and laxity may contribute to these issues, often patients find shedding their former body image difficult and still consider themselves as being obese. Untreated anxiety, depression, bipolar disorder, and schizophrenia warrant evaluation from a mental health provider.

Patients recover best when they have optimal mental and physical health and have an adequate support system at home. Dramatic weight loss can be life altering, and many patients report changes in interpersonal relationships, including separation, divorce, or new relationships. The plastic surgeon should ensure that the patient has adequate support in the postoperative period to assist in activities of daily living and provide needed mental and emotional support.

As with all aesthetic cases, patient motivations, goals, and expectations need to be clearly explored and delineated before surgery. What may be the most obvious areas of anatomic deformity to the surgeon may not be the most concerning to the patient. Therefore, areas of greatest priority to the patient should be noted. Many patients approach body contouring as part of a long transformation that started with weight loss surgery, and many are well informed and have realistic expectations. Regardless, the preoperative discussion should outline the significant scars and recovery associated with surgery with the ultimate goal of improvements (not perfection) in shape and contour. Standardized preoperative photography is critical in surgical planning and documentation and provides a reminder to patients about their significant improvements achieved. Those individuals who perseverate on or attribute personal issues, such as lack of career advancement, to their skin laxity, expect perfection, or have questionable motivations are likely to be dissatisfied with any surgical outcome and should be deferred or require preoperative psychological evaluation.[17,20,21]

The informed consent process should discuss general risks of surgery, such as bleeding and infection, but should address potential risk and benefits specific to each procedure. We recommend procedure-specific written consents. Massive weight loss skin differs from unstretched skin and the potential for recurrent laxity after surgery should be noted. Body contouring offers a multitude of procedures designed to address specific anatomic issues.

What can and cannot be accomplished by the procedures elected must be clearly explained. The power of many of these procedures comes from the design of the resections and involves significant scars. Patients must be willing to accept these scars (and their recovery) and understand that procedures that offer minimal scars are likely to yield minimal results.

COMBINING AND STAGING PROCEDURES

Because skin laxity often involves multiple anatomic areas, patients often present with multiple regions they would like to have addressed through body contouring. Tackling these regions in order of the patient's priority likely yields higher satisfaction. All preoperative considerations for single procedures may have even greater importance with combined procedures (ie, comorbidities, nutritional status, and so forth). However, additional factors, such as surgeon experience, facilities, operative team, and the financial burden placed on the patient, must also be considered. Longer combined cases may be more appropriate in the setting of a hospital with inpatient capabilities and in patients with low cardiac and preoperative risks. A larger operative team that may include physician extenders, residents, or a second surgeon expedites cases and reduces surgeon fatigue.

When conditions are not optimal or the patient may be at higher risk for complications, opting for staged procedures reduces complication rates and allows for necessary revision surgery for recurrent skin laxity. When staging is planned, we prefer a minimum of 3 months between procedures.[21] We also prefer to avoid combining procedures with opposite vectors of pull, those that may significantly impact blood supply to skin flaps, or those that displace the intended location of scars. General guidelines for selecting procedure combinations are found in **Box 3**. Pros and cons of staging and combining procedures are noted in **Table 1**.

Intraoperative monitoring of blood pressure, fluid balances, body temperature, and blood loss

---

Box 3
General guidelines for selecting procedure combinations

Generally favorable combinations
- Brachioplasty and mastopexy
- Vertical thigh lift and mastopexy
- Vertical thigh lift and brachioplasty
- Upper body lift and mastopexy
- Circumferential lower body lift and mastopexy
- Circumferential lower body lift and brachioplasty
- Abdominoplasty and mastopexy
- Abdominoplasty and brachioplasty

Important considerations
- Markings and planned scars may move as a result of combining procedures. For example, inframammary folds may displace during abdominoplasty.
- Combining upper and lower body procedures may limit patient's mobility and ambulation needed in the early postoperative phase

Combinations that require more careful consideration
- Transverse upper body lift and brachioplasty
  - Avoid joining brachioplasty and upper body lift scars along the lateral chest wall to a high tension T-point, which can be prone to breakdown
- Circumferential lower body lift and vertical thigh lift
  - In addition to opposing vectors of tension, we find that this combination of procedures requires significantly longer recovery time
- Circumferential lower body lift and transverse upper body lift
  - Opposing vectors of tension

Adapted from Rubin JP. Principles of plastic surgery after massive weight loss. In: Thorne CH, editor. Grabb and Smith's plastic surgery. 7th edition. Philadelphia: Lippincott Williams & Wilkins; 2014. p. 717; with permission.

---

is critical in combined cases. During the consent process, patients should be aware that the number of procedures performed might be truncated if factors indicate increased risk to the patient. Overall, combining procedures can be done in a safe manner in the appropriate patient population. Using the guidelines in this article, it has been shown that complication rates in combined versus

Table 1
Pros and cons of staging and combining procedures

Advantages	Disadvantages
Staging procedures	
• Faster patient recovery • Provides greater opportunity for revisions • Decreased operative time and surgeon fatigue • Avoidance of opposing pulling forces	• Greater number of work/life disruptions • Increased number of operations • Increased cost to the patient
Combining procedures	
• Lower financial burden for patient • Potentially less overall recovery time • Decreased number of operations	• Longer recovery period • Longer operative time and greater surgeon fatigue • Greater potential for blood loss • Revision surgery cannot be performed in combination with a second planned procedure and may lead to unplanned cost and recovery

Adapted from Rubin JP. Principles of plastic surgery after massive weight loss. In: Thorne CH, editor. Grabb and Smith's plastic surgery. 7th edition. Philadelphia: Lippincott Williams & Wilkins; 2014. p. 717; with permission.

single body contouring cases are similar on a per procedure basis.[22]

SUMMARY

Body contouring after massive weight loss is often the final phase of a long but positive journey for the bariatric patient. As the prevalence of obesity increases and many more continue to seek bariatric and subsequently body contouring surgery, it is critical that plastic surgeons become well versed in not only techniques that address skin laxity, but also more familiar with the unique set of issues that the postbariatric patient presents. A careful and comprehensive approach like the one presented in this article allows for safe and effective treatment of these patients.

REFERENCES

1. Naghshineh N, O'Brien Coon D, McTigue K, et al. Nutritional assessment of bariatric surgery patients presenting for plastic surgery: a prospective analysis. Plast Reconstr Surg 2010;126(2):602–10.
2. Nemerofsky RB, Oliak DA, Capella JF. Body lift: an account of 200 consecutive cases in the massive weight loss patient. Plast Reconstr Surg 2006; 117(2):414–30.
3. Coon D, Gusenoff JA, Kannan N, et al. Body mass and surgical complications in the postbariatric reconstructive patient: analysis of 511 cases. Ann Surg 2009;249(3):397–401.
4. Au K, Hazard SW III, Dyer AM, et al. Correlation of complications of body contouring surgery with increasing body mass index. Aesthet Surg J 2008; 28(4):425–9.
5. Buchwald H. Consensus conference statement bariatric surgery for morbid obesity: health implications for patients, health professionals, and third-party payers. Surg Obes Relat Dis 2005;1(3):371–81.
6. Pories WJ, Swanson MS, MacDonald KG, et al. Who would have thought it? An operation proves to be the most effective therapy for adult-onset diabetes mellitus. Ann Surg 1995;222(3):339–50 [discussion: 350–2].
7. Carson JL, Ruddy ME, Duff AE, et al. The effect of gastric bypass surgery on hypertension in morbidly obese patients. Arch Intern Med 1994;154(2):193–200.
8. Benotti PN, Bistrain B, Benotti JR, et al. Heart disease and hypertension in severe obesity: the benefits of weight reduction. Am J Clin Nutr 1992; 55(Suppl 2):586S–90S.
9. Geerts WH, Pineo GF, Heit JA, et al. Prevention of venous thromboembolism: the Seventh ACCP Conference on Antithrombotic and Thrombolytic Therapy. Chest 2004;126(Suppl 3):338S–400S.
10. Friedman T, O'Brien Coon D, Michaels VJ, et al. Hereditary coagulopathies: practical diagnosis and management for the plastic surgeon. Plast Reconstr Surg 2010;125(5):1544–52.
11. Shermak MA, Chang DC, Heller J. Factors impacting thromboembolism after bariatric body contouring surgery. Plast Reconstr Surg 2007;119(5): 1590–6 [discussion: 1597–8].
12. Van Way C. Nutritional support in the injured patient. Surg Clin North Am 1991;71:537–48.
13. Song A, Fernstrom MH. Nutritional and psychological considerations after bariatric surgery. Aesthet Surg J 2008;28(2):195–9.
14. Sebastian JL. Bariatric surgery and work-up of the massive weight loss patient. Clin Plast Surg 2008; 35(1):11–26.
15. Agha-Mohammadi S, Hurwitz DJ. Potential impacts of nutritional deficiency of postbariatric patients on body contouring surgery. Plast Reconstr Surg 2008;122(6):1901–14.
16. Onyike CU, Crum RM, Lee HB, et al. Is obesity associated with major depression? Results from the Third

National Health and Nutrition Examination Survey. Am J Epidemiol 2003;158(12):1139–47.

17. Sarwer DB, Fabricatore AN. Psychiatric considerations of the massive weight loss patient. Clin Plast Surg 2008;35(1):1–10.

18. Sarwer DB, Thompson JK, Cash TF. Body image and obesity in adulthood. Psychiatr Clin North Am 2005;28(1):69–87, viii.

19. Sarwer DB, Thompson JK, Mitchell JE, et al. Psychological considerations of the bariatric surgery patient undergoing body contouring surgery. Plast Reconstr Surg 2008;121(6):423e–34e.

20. Rubin JP, O'Toole JE. Evaluation of the massive weight loss patient who presents for body contouring surgery. In: Rubin JP, Matarasso A, editors. Aesthetic surgery after massive weight loss. London: Elsevier; 2007. p. 13–20.

21. Song AY, Rubin JP, Thomas V, et al. Body image and quality of life in post massive weight loss body contouring patients. Obesity (Silver Spring) 2006;14(9): 1626–36.

22. Coon D, Michaels J, Gusenoff JA, et al. Multiple procedures and staging in the massive weight loss population. Plast Reconstr Surg 2010;125(2):691–8.

National Health and Nutrition Examination Survey. Am J Epidemiol 2003;158(12):1139-47.

17. Sarwer DA, Fabricatore AN. Psychiatric considerations of the massive weight loss patient. Clin Plast Surg 2008;35(1):1-10.

18. Sarwer DB, Thompson JK, Cash TF. Body image and obesity in adulthood. Psychiatr Clin North Am 2005;28(1):69-87, viii.

19. Sarwer DB, Thompson JK, Mitchell JE, et al. Psychological considerations of the bariatric surgery patient undergoing body contouring surgery. Plast Reconstr Surg 2008;131(6):423e-34e.

20. Rubin JP, O'Toole JP. Evaluation of the massive weight loss patient who presents for body contouring surgery. In: Rubin JP, Matarasso A, editors. Aesthetic surgery after massive weight loss. London: Elsevier 2007. p. 13-20.

21. Song AY, Rubin JP, Thomas V, et al. Body image and quality of life in post massive weight loss body contouring patients. Obesity (Silver Spring) 2006;14(9):1626-36.

22. Coon D, Michaels J, Gusenoff JA, et al. Multiple procedures and staging in the massive weight loss population. Plast Reconstr Surg 2010;125(2):691-8.

Assessing Outcomes in Body Contouring

Anne F. Klassen, DPhil[a],*, Stefan J. Cano, PhD[b],
Amie Scott, MSc[c], Elena Tsangaris, MSc[d],
Andrea L. Pusic, MD, MHS[c]

KEYWORDS

- Bariatric surgery ● Body contouring ● Aesthetic surgery ● Obesity ● Outcomes ● Quality of life
- Psychometrics ● BODY-Q

KEY POINTS

- Weight loss following bariatric surgery leaves many patients with unsightly excesses of skin.
- Body contouring procedures have the potential to improve appearance and health-related quality of life.
- Patient-reported outcome (PRO) instruments are questionnaires designed to measure outcomes from the point of view of the patient.
- The BODY-Q is a new PRO instrument designed for obese patients and patients having bariatric and cosmetic body contouring surgery.
- BODY-Q scales measure appearance, health-related quality of life, and process of care.
- The BODY-Q can be used to measure change over the entire weight loss journey, starting at obesity and ending after body contouring surgery is performed.
- The BODY-Q is being designed using modern psychometric methods (ie, Rasch Measurement Theory analysis).

INTRODUCTION

Increasing rates of obesity, coupled with the growing pursuit of a slender physique, have resulted in an increasing number of people seeking both bariatric and body contouring surgery. Although bariatric surgery and subsequent weight loss may have a positive impact on medical conditions such as diabetes and heart disease, many patients seek such procedures primarily to improve quality of life and body image. This trend is also true for many normal-weight patients, who increasingly pursue cosmetic body contour surgery to address so-called problem areas and to improve satisfaction with their appearance.

Bariatric Surgery

Bariatric surgery has been shown to be the most effective therapy available for weight loss in moderately and severely obese people.[1–3] In addition to reducing body weight, such surgery can improve or resolve a range of obesity-related conditions, such as type 2 diabetes, heart disease,

Disclosure: This study received funding from the National Endowment for Plastic Surgery and the Canadian Institutes of Health Research. In addition, A.F. Klassen holds a CIHR Mid-Career Award in Women's Health.
[a] Department of Pediatrics, McMaster University, 3N27, 1200 Main Street West, Hamilton, Ontario L8N 3Z5, Canada; [b] Clinical Neurology Research Group, Plymouth University Peninsula Schools of Medicine and Dentistry, Tamar Science Park, Davy Road, Plymouth, Devon PL6 8BX, UK; [c] Department of Surgery, Memorial Sloan-Kettering Cancer Center, 1275 York Avenue, New York, NY 10065, USA; [d] Department of Clinical Epidemiology and Biostatistics, McMaster University, 3N27, 1200 Main Street West, Hamilton, Ontario L8N 3Z5, Canada
* Corresponding author.
E-mail address: aklass@mcmaster.ca

Clin Plastic Surg 41 (2014) 645–654
http://dx.doi.org/10.1016/j.cps.2014.06.004
0094-1298/14/$ – see front matter © 2014 Elsevier Inc. All rights reserved.

sleep apnea, hypertension, and high cholesterol. The large amount of weight loss that can be achieved through bariatric surgery leaves many patients with excess skin that is cosmetically unsightly as well as detrimental to their body image and physical, psychological, and social function; that is, their health-related quality of life (HR-QOL).[4]

Research measuring the HR-QOL impact of bariatric surgery requires urgent attention. After reviewing 26 publications in a National Institutes of Health Research (United Kingdom) clinical and cost-effectiveness study of bariatric surgery,[2] the investigators called for further research to provide detailed data on patient HR-QOL because of conflicting findings. More recently, a systematic search by Tayyem and colleagues,[5] who looked for HR-QOL instruments used in bariatric research, identified that 112 studies used 42 HR-QOL instruments (8 generic, 9 obesity specific, and 25 other condition-specific instruments). The content (items and scales) of these 42 questionnaires varies substantially, suggesting a lack of consensus about which questionnaires should be used to measure patient outcomes. The most frequently used generic patient-reported outcome (PRO) instrument was the Short Form 36 (SF-36),[6] which was used in 28 studies. Although generic instruments are helpful for making comparisons with population norms and other patient groups, the use of such an instrument in research with patients having bariatric surgery and/or body contouring would miss important health concepts and underestimate the HR-QOL impact of their condition.[7]

The most frequently used condition-specific instruments included the Moorehead-Ardelt Quality of Life Instrument (MAQOL),[8] Impact of Weight on Quality of Life–Lite (IWQOL-Lite) instrument,[9] and the Swedish Obese Subjects Obesity Psychosocial Problem (OSQOL) module.[10] The most common of these, used in 29 studies, was the MAQOL,[8] created to accompany the Bariatric Analysis and Reporting Outcome System (BAROS),[11] which measures bariatric surgery clinical outcomes. This short HR-QOL instrument is composed of only 6 items that cover self-esteem and physical, social, work, sexual, and eating behavior. The MAQOL does not ask about appearance even though bariatric patients are usually left with excess hanging skin, which has a negative impact on their HR-QOL.

Two additional measures that are specific to bariatric patients and are not covered in the Tayyem and colleagues[5] review are the Bariatric Quality of Life (BQL) Index[12] and the Treatment Related Impact Measure of Weight (TRIM-Weight).[13] The BQL assesses HR-QOL in terms of 14 items (eg, exercise, social activities, feeling under pressure, depression, life satisfaction, restrictions, self-confidence). The TRIM-Weight is a new 22-item questionnaire developed to measure the key HR-QOL impact of bariatric medicine. This instrument was developed by carefully following internationally recommended guidelines for item generation, item reduction, and psychometric evaluation.

Body Contouring

Body contouring is a growing area in plastic surgery. According to the 2013 American Society of Plastic Surgery procedural statistics, 436,006 body contouring procedures were performed in the United States and included liposuction (199,817), abdominoplasty (111,986), upper arm lift (15,769), breast lift (mastopexy) (90,006), thigh lift (8709), lower body lift (7281), and buttock lift (2438).[14] Together, these procedures made up 26.1% of total cosmetic surgical procedures in 2013. Although body contouring for cosmetic reasons is common, body contouring following massive weight loss is less common. In 2012, a total of 45,534 body contouring procedures were performed on patients after massive weight loss.[15] Whether performed purely for cosmetic reasons or as a component of the post–bariatric surgery treatment plan, body contouring surgery has the potential to improve or restore a patient's body image and HR-QOL.

Our team published a systematic review of HR-QOL instruments in patients having body contouring surgery.[16] MEDLINE, EMBASE, PsychINFO, CINAHL, HAPI, Science Citation Index/Social Sciences Citation Index, and Ovid Evidence Based Medicine databases were searched from the inception of each database to August 2010. Articles included in the study described the development and/or psychometric evaluation of a PRO instrument for patients having body contouring. From 1504 articles 5 such instruments were found, including a liposuction questionnaire (Freiburg Questionnaire on Aesthetic Dermatology and Cosmetic Surgery[17]), a general plastic surgery questionnaire (Derriford Appearance Scale[18–20]), and 3 breast reduction instruments: Breast Reduction Assessed Severity Scale Questionnaire (BRASSQ),[21,22] Breast Related Symptoms questionnaire,[23] and the BREAST-Q.[24] Detailed examination by our team revealed that the first 3 instruments are limited in terms of content range and psychometric properties, leaving only 2 breast surgery–specific instruments that have strong psychometric properties and could be recommended for use. Although the BREAST-Q and

BRASSQ could be used with patients having breast reduction, there is a lack of adequately developed instruments for other body contouring procedures.

Need for a New PRO Instrument: The BODY-Q

An important oversight in the literature to date is the lack of evidence about how HR-QOL and other important patient outcomes, such as body image and satisfaction with appearance, change over the weight loss journey (ie, starting at obesity and ending after body contouring surgery is performed). A limitation in the pursuit of such evidence is the lack of availability of an instrument designed specifically to cover concerns that are common across patients having cosmetic body contouring surgery as well as obese patients and patients after massive weight loss. To address this oversight, our team set out to develop a new PRO instrument called the BODY-Q. We followed recommended guidelines for PRO instrument development[25–29] to ensure that the BODY-Q meets requirements of regulatory bodies. In the first phase, a conceptual model to be measured is formally defined, and a pool of items is generated and developed into scales. In the second phase, the scales are field-tested in a large sample of target subjects. In the field test, items for the refined scales are retained based on their performance against a set of psychometric criteria and the new scales are evaluated with respect to their psychometric properties (ie, reliability, validity, responsiveness). In the third phase, psychometric evaluation of the item-reduced scales is performed in various samples of participants to further explore, report, and improve the scientific soundness of the instrument. This article describes the steps we have taken to date to develop the BODY-Q scales, and what remains to be accomplished to refine these scales for future use in research and clinical practice.

METHODS AND RESULTS
Phase 1

Theoretic approach
We started our research by developing a conceptual framework and preliminary set of scales using an approach called interpretive description, which is an applied health services qualitative method.[30] Interpretive description presumes that there is theoretic knowledge, clinical knowledge, and a scientific basis informing a study.[30]

Literature review
As described briefly earlier, we conducted a systematic literature review to identify published

PRO instruments for patients having body contouring surgery.[16] The 2 objectives for the review were to identify instruments designed to measure patient satisfaction, body image, and/or quality of life issues of patients having body contouring surgery; and to evaluate these instruments with respect to their development process, content, and psychometric properties. We searched multiple databases from their inception to August 2010. In each database, we used search terms that enabled us to find relevant articles for the following topics: obesity or overall body image, plastic surgery in general or specific body contouring surgical procedures, and quality of life outcomes in general or as assessed with questionnaires. From articles that used a PRO instrument, we evaluated the content to identify preoperative and postoperative issues likely to be relevant to the body contouring population. Five PRO instruments were found that were specifically developed for patients having body contouring. The content covered in these instruments helped our team in the development of an initial interview guide (**Box 1** for example questions).

Qualitative interviews
We conducted qualitative interviews with 14 patients having cosmetic body contouring and 49 postbariatric patients (37 had undergone body contouring and 12 were waiting for body contouring). Participants were recruited between September 2009 and February 2012 from the offices of 5 plastic surgeons located in the United States and Canada. We interviewed patients aged 18 years or older who had undergone bariatric surgery and were at any point along their weight loss journey and/or patients who had undergone any form of body contouring surgery within the past 7 years. Patient characteristics are shown in **Table 1**. Interviews were used to explore the impact that obesity, weight loss, and body contouring surgery had on participants' appearance and HR-QOL (eg, physical, psychological, sexual, and social function), and process of care (eg, relationship with health care providers, expectations, information needs). The interviews were digitally recorded and transcribed verbatim with any identifiable information excluded from interview transcripts.

Data were coded using a line-by-line approach with the application of codes to text within NVivo 8 software.[31] Constant comparison was used to examine relationships within and across codes in order to develop themes and subthemes.[32] In an earlier qualitative article, we described a range of important health and aesthetic concerns of obese patients, patients after massive weight loss, and

Box 1
Topics included in the interview guide for weight loss and cosmetic patients

Why did you decide to have weight loss and/or body contouring surgery?

What methods of weight loss you have used in the past?

Tell me about the weight loss and/or body contouring surgery you had or are planning to have.

Describe any postoperative issues you experienced after weight loss and/or body contouring surgery (eg, pain, complications).

What was it like going back to work or your normal routine after body contouring surgery?

How have weight loss and/or body contouring changed the way you look?

How satisfied are you with how your body looked before/now?

How satisfied are you with how specific areas of your body looked before/now (eg, arms, abdomen, buttocks, hips, legs, skin)?

Can you describe how your body contouring scars look/feel (eg, redness, swelling, size)?

How did weight loss/excess skin and/or body contouring affect how you look (eg, in clothes, naked, in mirror, photos, age)?

Describe any physical problems caused by your weight/excess skin after weight loss/any changes following body contouring surgery.

Describe any activity limitations caused by your weight/excess skin after weight loss/any changes following body contouring surgery.

Describe how your weight/excess skin after weight loss affected your emotional health and any changes following body contouring surgery.

Describe how your weight/excess skin after weight loss affected how you feel about your body and any changes following body contouring surgery.

Describe how your weight/excess skin after weight loss affected your sexual life and any changes following body contouring surgery.

Describe how your weight/excess skin after weight loss affected social relationships and any changes following body contouring surgery.

Describe how your weight/excess skin after weight loss interfered with your usual social roles and any changes following body contouring surgery (eg, work, family life, friends).

How satisfied are you with the weight loss and/or body contouring health care you received?

How did you feel about the information you received regarding weight loss and/or body contouring?

How did you feel about your weight loss and/or body contouring physician, team, and office staff?

Are you pleased with the results of your weight loss and/or body contouring surgery?

Would you do it again?

Note: these questions are examples of the types of questions asked during interviews. Depending on the treatment history of a participant, questions were tailored to fit their experiences.

patients having body contouring surgery.[4] Note that we described that body contouring played an instrumental role in the completion of the weight loss process for formerly obese patients.

The qualitative findings were used to develop a conceptual framework composed of 3 major themes: appearance, HR-QOL, and process of care. Within each theme were a varying number of subthemes. For example, the subthemes under the HR-QOL theme included body image and psychological, social, sexual, and physical function and physical symptoms.

Development of preliminary items and scales
The next step involved developing a comprehensive set of preliminary items from the qualitative data. This step necessitated creating coding reports within NVivo 8 software in order to extract all the data (coded text) associated with each of the subthemes. For each subtheme, the patient quotes for coded text were cut and pasted into Excel spreadsheets. Then, each code text was considered in turn and 1 or more preliminary items generated. To provide an example, one participant said the following about the appearance of her

Table 1
Patient characteristics

	Qualitative Interviews	Cognitive Interviews	
		Round 1	Round 2
Number of Participants	63	19	3
Age (y)			
Mean (SD)	48 (12)	47 (11)	42 (3)
Range	23–71	28–63	39–44
Gender, N (%)			
Female	60 (95)	16 (84)	3 (100)
Male	3 (5)	3 (16)	0 (0)
Marital Status, N (%)			
Married/common law	32 (51)	10 (53)	1 (33)
Other	31 (49)	8 (42)	2 (67)
Missing	0	1 (5)	0
Highest Level of Education, N (%)			
High school	8 (13)	2 (11)	1 (33)
College/university diploma	50 (79)	11 (58)	2 (67)
Other	0	5 (26)	0
Missing	5 (8)	1 (5)	0
Employment Status, N (%)			
Employed	38 (60)	13 (68)	2 (67)
Other	22 (35)	5 (26)	1 (33)
Missing	3 (5)	1 (5)	0
Household Income, N (%)			
<$40,000	10 (16)	3 (16)	1 (33)
$40,000–100,000	30 (48)	7 (37)	2 (67)
>$100,000	14 (22)	7 (37)	0
Missing	9 (14)	2 (10)	0
Type of Patient, N (%)			
Cosmetic body contouring	14 (22)	11 (58)	0
Before weight loss body contouring	12 (19)	6 (32)	3 (100)
After weight loss body contouring	37 (59)	2 (10)	0
Body Contouring Procedures, N (%)			
Abdominoplasty	43 (68)	10 (53)	0
Liposuction	27 (43)	4 (21)	0
Upper arm lift	15 (24)	0	0
Breast lift	12 (19)	3 (16)	0
Thigh lift	9 (14)	0	0
Buttock lift	6 (10)	0	0
Breast reduction	9 (14)	2 (11)	0
Lower body lift	5 (8)	0	0

Abbreviation: SD, standard deviation.

body after weight loss and before body contouring surgery: "I looked very old. My whole body was like my mother's [body] who was 90 with all the skin hanging." This quote was similar to another participant, who said: "You're, like, older because of that hanging skin there." These patient's quotes had been coded as Appearance (theme) as well as Skin (subtheme) in NVivo8. We developed preliminary items from the patient data, which are reflected in the following 2 items that appear in the final version of the Skin scale: "Your excess skin making you look older than you are" and "How much your excess skin hangs."

Once we had developed a comprehensive list of items, we used the item pool to populate a set of scales. At this stage we also examined other published obesity/bariatric[5] and body contouring–specific[16] PRO instruments to assess whether we had missed any important issues. In creating the wording of items for our scales, our intention was to retain the words of patients as much as possible to ensure that the items would resonate with patients, we used positive or neutral language, and we used simple wording to ensure comprehension.

For each scale, we developed Likert scale scoring options. The response options were limited to 4 labeled options to keep our scales simple and in line with guidelines published by Khadka and colleagues.[33] This research team showed that rating scales with complicated question formats, a large number of response categories, or unlabeled categories tended to be problematic and recommended that PRO instruments should have simple question formats, only a few (4–5 at most) response options, and that all response options should be labeled using words (eg, strongly agree, agree, disagree, strongly disagree).

Cognitive interviews

The BODY-Q scales (**Table 2**) were shown to 22 patients in a series of one-on-one cognitive interviews. Qualitative methods, such as cognitive interviews, are valuable for identifying new items as well as tailoring existing item wording, item format, and presentation to ensure that they are optimally understood by respondents.[28] Cognitive interviews often lead to modifications to instrument content (eg, item deletion, addition, rewording).[28]

In the first round of interviews, 19 participants were asked to provide feedback on the instructions, response options, and items. A total of 258 items were tested in this first round. All 19 participants found the instructions and response options acceptable and easy to understand, thus these were left unchanged. Based on participant feedback, 212 items were kept without revision, 26 items were revised, 20 items were rejected, and 39 new items were added.

To give an example, it was common for participants in the qualitative interviews to talk about not looking normal because of either their size before weight loss or their excess skin after weight loss. One participant expressed it this way: "I felt before that I was just abnormal, I was just large and not normal, not the norm." Comments about not looking normal were made with regard to the

body as a whole, as well as different parts of the body such as the upper arms. For example, one participant said about her arms: "… you know, you have flapping wings [laughs] … not normal." We thus went on to develop a set of items (1 in each appearance scale) using the word normal (eg, "How normal your body looks"). However, we found that 10 out of 19 participants in the cognitive interviews expressed a concern about at least 1 of these items. Comments such as the following were made: "Don't know what normal means." "Is that with clothes or without clothes?" "Everyone will have a different normal." "Normal is too personal." Based on this patient feedback, we removed the items asking about normal from the appearance scales.

In the second round, 3 patients were interviewed to obtain feedback on the revised and new items. Based on patient input, 175 items were kept without revision, 64 items were revised, 38 items were rejected, and 21 new items added.

Expert input

Our preliminary scales were shown to 9 plastic surgeons who were asked to examine thoroughly and provide written feedback to members of our research team. Expert opinion was used to ensure that the scales we developed would be useful to clinicians, and that all clinically relevant aspects of each concept were captured in the scales. Feedback received was used to revise the scales. In addition, expert input identified the need for a scale to measure appearance of stretch marks, given that this is a clinically important concern for body contouring patients but overlooked by our team. To create this scale, we went back to the qualitative dataset in order to develop items that measure patients concerns using their words as much as possible. The field-test version of the BODY-Q consists of 20 newly created independently functioning scales composed of a total of 262 items (see **Table 2**).

Phase 2

Field test

The field test is currently underway in multiple bariatric and plastic surgery clinics in Canada, the United States, and the United Kingdom. We are testing 2 modes of administration (ie, electronic and paper). Participants are asked to complete the BODY-Q either directly into an iPad for online data collection using REDCap software[34] or by completing a paper version. REDCap is a secure Web application for building and managing online surveys and databases.

Each scale represents a stand-alone instrument because they were developed to measure

Table 2
BODY-Q scales following cognitive interviews and expert input

Name of Scale	Items	Example Item	Response Option Format	Time Frame (wk)	Flesch-Kincaid Grade Level Average (Range)
Appearance					
Body	11	The size (ie, weight) of your body	Dissatisfied/satisfied	Past 2	2.1 (0.5–3.7)
Abdomen	13	How your abdomen looks when you are naked	Dissatisfied/satisfied	Past 2	2.5 (0.0–4.8)
Upper arms	10	How your upper arms look in long-sleeved shirts	Dissatisfied/satisfied	Past 2	1.5 (0.5–5.2)
Back	8	How the skin on your back looks	Dissatisfied/satisfied	Past 2	0.0 (0.0–3.9)
Buttocks	9	How your clothes fit your buttocks	Dissatisfied/satisfied	Past 2	0.9 (0.5–3.6)
Inner thighs	9	How similar (ie, the same) your inner thighs look	Dissatisfied/satisfied	Past 2	1.2 (0.5–4.9)
Hips and outer thighs	10	The shape of your hips and outer thighs	Dissatisfied/satisfied	Past 2	1.3 (0.8–2.6)
Excess skin	14	Having to dress in a way to hide your excess skin	Not at all/extremely bothered	Past 2	4.0 (0.5–7.6)
Stretch marks	13	The color of your stretch marks	Not at all/extremely bothered	Past 2	1.3 (0–4.4)
Body contouring scars	12	How noticeable your scars are	Not at all/extremely bothered	Past 2	1.6 (0.0–5.2)
Quality of Life					
Body image	12	My body is not perfect but I like it	Agree/disagree	Past 2	2.8 (0.5–6.4)
Psychological Function	16	I feel good about myself	Agree/disagree	Past 2	3.7 (0.5–9.5)
Social function	15	I feel included in social situations	Agree/disagree	Past 2	4.3 (1.0–8.3)
Sexual function[a]	13/11	I am comfortable having the lights on during sex	Agree/disagree	N/A	4.5 (0.5–7.5)
Physical function	13	Putting on or taking off clothes	All the time/never	Past 2	3.4 (0.5–12.3)
Physical symptoms	15	Skin rash or infection	All the time/never	Past 2	3.0 (0.0–9.1)
Process of Care					
Information[b]	20/19	The kinds of complications that could happen	Dissatisfied/satisfied	N/A	4.4 (0.8–11.1)
Doctor	17	Talked to you in a way that was easy to understand	Agree/disagree	N/A	3.9 (0.5–14.6)
Medical team	15	Treated you with respect	Agree/disagree	N/A	4.2 (0.5–14.6)
Office staff	17	Were available when you had concerns	Agree/disagree	N/A	5.1 (0.5–14.6)

Abbreviation: N/A, not applicable.
[a] Obesity version = 13 items; cosmetic version = 11 items.
[b] Obesity version = 20 items; cosmetic version = 19 items.

unidimensional constructs. **Table 2** shows characteristics for each scale, including number of items, an example item, response option format, and time period addressed (eg, past 2 weeks). Also shown is the Flesh-Kincaid grade reading level[35] (mean and range), which indicates comprehensibility. The average Flesh-Kincaid grade reading level for BODY-Q scales is below a grade 6 level (range 0–5.1). **Table 3** shows, as an example, a subset of items from the BODY-Q scale entitled Satisfaction with Back scale.

The field-test data are used to perform item reduction. We keep the items that represent the best indicators of outcome based on their performance against a standardized set of psychometric criteria. Rasch measurement theory[36] is performed, which involves a set of statistical and graphical tests that were described in 2009 in detail by Hobart and Cano.[37] These tests are used to evaluate each item in a scale. The evidence is then used to make a judgment about the overall quality of the scale. Assessment of validity involves examination of thresholds for item response options, item fit statistics, targeting, and differential item functioning. Assessment of reliability involves examination of the Person Separation Index. In addition, unidimensionality of a scale is a requirement of the Rasch model and is examined using a method proposed by Smith using independent t-tests.[38] Once completed, each scale provides a stand-alone score from 0 to 100, with higher scores indicating a better outcome.

DISCUSSION

Jabir[39] searched multiple databases through to March 2013, and found 11 studies that used PRO instruments in patients having massive weight loss body contouring surgery. None were developed specifically for patients having body contouring surgery. Jabir[39] states that there is an urgent need to develop specific and well-constructed PRO instruments in order to obtain reliable information regarding quality of life and patient satisfaction following body contouring surgery in patients after massive weight loss.

The BODY-Q differs from other PRO instruments in that we have developed a set of independently functioning scales to measure not only HR-QOL but also appearance-related concerns and the patient experience of health care. Although the themes in our HR-QOL scales (psychological, social and sexual function, body image, physical function) are covered to some extent by other obesity-specific[5] and body contouring[16]–specific PRO instruments, the BODY-Q is considerably more comprehensive, composed of a set of unidimensional scales (no total scores) that retain as much as possible the wording of obese patients and patients having body contouring and bariatric surgery. Furthermore, our scales were designed for use over the entire weight loss journey rather than just 1 phase in the process. We also have scales that are specific to patient concerns relevant at certain junctures (eg, Appraisal of Skin scale for patients after bariatric weight loss and patients having body contouring; Appraisal of Scar scale for patients having body contouring), and scales to evaluate process of care subthemes (eg, satisfaction with information and physician).

In addition, the use of modern psychometric methods[37] to develop and validate the BODY-Q scales will ensure that our scales are appropriate for use in clinical practice with individual patients; no other PRO instrument for this patient population has been developed using modern psychometric methods. Advantages of using Rasch have been summarized elsewhere[37] and include (1) that they provide measurements of people that are independent of the sampling distribution of the items used, and locate items in each scale

Table 3
Example items from the BODY-Q Satisfaction with back scale

With your BACK in mind, in the past 2 weeks, how dissatisfied or satisfied have you been with:

	Very Dissatisfied	Somewhat Dissatisfied	Somewhat Satisfied	Very Satisfied
How your back looks when you are <u>dressed</u>?	1	2	3	4
The <u>shape</u> of your back?	1	2	3	4
How <u>toned</u> your back looks?	1	2	3	4
How your <u>clothes fit</u> your back?	1	2	3	4
How your back looks when you are <u>naked</u>?	1	2	3	4

independent of the sampling distribution of the people in whom they are derived; (2) as such, they allow for more accurate individual person measurements on fixed rulers; and (3) the more accurate measurement improves the potential for PRO instruments to measure clinically meaningful change. PRO instruments developed using Rasch are well suited for use in both research and clinical practice.[37]

SUMMARY

Although PRO instruments were initially developed for use in research, they are now also used to improve care by assisting clinicians to provide better and more patient-centered care, assess and compare the quality of providers, and provide data for evaluating practices and policies.[40] For example, in the United Kingdom, our team's BREAST-Q[24,41] was the primary outcome measure in a voluntary audit of approximately 8000 women having mastectomy and/or breast reconstruction in 2008.[42] Reports that are publicly available compare the performance of National Health Service Hospital Trust for each BREAST-Q scale, showing poor performers and suggesting benchmarks as targets to be achieved for quality improvement. Also in the United Kingdom, a mandatory audit using PRO instruments to evaluate the patient perspective of 4 common elective procedures (hip and knee replacement, groin hernia repair, and varicose veins surgery) was implemented in 2009, with results used to evaluate quality of care through public comparisons of providers' performance.[43]

Our research team has developed a comprehensive set of PRO scales to measure outcomes important to obese patients bariatric and patients having cosmetic body contouring. Once development is completed, the BODY-Q could be used to support patient advocacy; patient education; and provincial, national, and international research efforts. Furthermore, using BODY-Q scales in clinical practice, patients are able to report and then discuss their key health concerns and expectations directly with their health care provider, who can use this to inform treatment decisions and improve patients' satisfaction and HR-QOL.

REFERENCES

1. Colquitt JL, Picot J, Loveman E, et al. Surgery for obesity. Cochrane Database Syst Rev 2009;(2): CD003641.
2. Picot J, Jones J, Colquitt JL, et al. The clinical effectiveness and cost-effectiveness of bariatric (weight loss) surgery for obesity: a systematic review and economic evaluation. Health Technol Assess 2009; 13(41):1–190, 215–357, iii–iv.
3. Buchwald H, Avidor Y, Braunwald E, et al. Bariatric surgery: a systematic review and meta-analysis. JAMA 2004;292(14):1724–37.
4. Klassen AF, Cano SJ, Scott A, et al. Satisfaction and quality-of-life issues in body contouring surgery patients: a qualitative study. Obes Surg 2012;22(10): 1527–34.
5. Tayyem R, Ali A, Atkinson J, et al. Analysis of health-related quality-of-life instruments measuring the impact of bariatric surgery: systematic review of the instruments used and their content validity. Patient 2011;4(2):73–87.
6. Available at: http://www.qualitymetric.com/. Accessed March 10, 2014.
7. Fayers PM, Machin D. Quality of life: the assessment, analysis, and interpretation of patient-reported outcomes. 2nd edition. Chichester (United Kingdom), Hoboken (NJ): J Wiley; 2007.
8. Moorehead MK, Ardelt-Gattinger E, Lechner H, et al. The validation of the Moorehead-Ardelt quality of life questionnaire II. Obes Surg 2003;13(5):684–92.
9. Kolotkin RL, Crosby RD, Kosloski KD, et al. Development of a brief measure to assess quality of life in obesity. Obes Res 2001;9(2):102–11.
10. Karlsson J, Taft C, Sjöström L, et al. Psychosocial functioning in the obese before and after weight reduction: construct validity and responsiveness of the obesity-related problems scale. Int J Obes Relat Metab Disord 2003;27(5):617–30.
11. Oria HE, Moorehead MK. Bariatric analysis and reporting outcome system (BAROS). Obes Surg 1998;8(5):487–99.
12. Weiner S, Sauerland S, Fein M, et al. The bariatric quality of life index: a measure of well-being in obesity surgery patients. Obes Surg 2005;15(4): 538–45.
13. Brod M, Hammer M, Kragh N, et al. Development and validation of the treatment related impact measure of weight (TRIM-Weight). Health Qual Life Outcomes 2010;8:19.
14. Available at: http://www.plasticsurgery.org/Documents/news-resources/statistics/2013-statistics/cosmetic-procedures-national-trends-2013.pdf. Accessed March 10, 2014.
15. Available at: http://www.plasticsurgery.org/Documents/news-resources/statistics/2012-Plastic-Surgery-Statistics/body-contouring-after-massive-weight-loss.pdf. Accessed March 10, 2014.
16. Reavey PL, Klassen AF, Cano SJ, et al. Measuring quality of life and patient satisfaction after body contouring: a systematic review of patient-reported outcome measures. Aesthet Surg J 2011;31(7): 807–13.
17. Augustin M, Zschocke I, Sommer B, et al. Sociodemographic profile and satisfaction with treatment of

patients undergoing liposuction in tumescent local anesthesia. Dermatol Surg 1999;25(6):480–3.

18. Carr T, Harris D, James C. The Derriford Appearance Scale (DAS-59): a new scale to measure individual responses to living with problems of appearance. Br J Health Psychol 2000;5:201–15.

19. Carr T, Moss T, Harris D. The DAS24: a short form of the Derriford Appearance Scale DAS59 to measure individual responses to living with problems of appearance. Br J Health Psychol 2005;10(Pt 2): 285–98.

20. Harris DL, Carr AT. The Derriford Appearance Scale (DAS59): a new psychometric scale for the evaluation of patients with disfigurements and aesthetic problems of appearance. Br J Plast Surg 2001; 54(3):216–22.

21. Sigurdson L, Kirkland SA, Mykhalovskiy E. Validation of a questionnaire for measuring morbidity in breast hypertrophy. Plast Reconstr Surg 2007; 120(5):1108–14.

22. Sigurdson L, Mykhalovskiy E, Kirkland SA, et al. Symptoms and related severity experienced by women with breast hypertrophy. Plast Reconstr Surg 2007;119(2):481–6.

23. Kerrigan CL, Collins ED, Striplin D, et al. The health burden of breast hypertrophy. Plast Reconstr Surg 2001;108(6):1591–9.

24. Pusic AL, Klassen AF, Scott AM, et al. Development of a new patient-reported outcome measure for breast surgery: the BREAST-Q. Plast Reconstr Surg 2009;124(2):345–53.

25. Available at: http://www.ispor.org/workpaper/FDA %20PRO%20Guidance.pdf. Accessed March 10, 2014.

26. Lasch KE, Marquis P, Vigneux M, et al. PRO development: rigorous qualitative research as the crucial foundation. Qual Life Res 2010;19(8):1087–96.

27. Patrick DL, Burke LB, Gwaltney CJ, et al. Content validity–establishing and reporting the evidence in newly developed patient-reported outcomes (PRO) instruments for medical product evaluation: ISPOR PRO good research practices task force report: part 1–eliciting concepts for a new PRO instrument. Value Health 2011;14(8):967–77.

28. Patrick DL, Burke LB, Gwaltney CJ, et al. Content validity–establishing and reporting the evidence in newly developed patient-reported outcomes (PRO) instruments for medical product evaluation: ISPOR PRO good research practices task force report: part 2–assessing respondent understanding. Value Health 2011;14(8):978–88.

29. Scientific Advisory Committee of the Medical Outcomes Trust. Assessing health status and quality-of-life instruments: attributes and review criteria. Qual Life Res 2002;11(3):193–205.

30. Thorne SE. Interpretive description. Developing qualitative inquiry. Walnut Creek (CA): Left Coast Press; 2008. p. 272.

31. QSR International. NVivo 8. Australia: QSR International; 2008.

32. Charmaz K. Constructing grounded theory. London, Thousand Oaks (CA): Sage Publications; 2006. p. 208, xiii.

33. Khadka J, Gothwal VK, McAlinden C, et al. The importance of rating scales in measuring patient-reported outcomes. Health Qual Life Outcomes 2012;10:80.

34. Available at: http://www.project-redcap.org. Accessed March 10, 2014.

35. Available at: http://office.microsoft.com/en-ca/word-help/ test-your-document-s-readability-HP010148506.aspx. Accessed March 10, 2014.

36. Rasch G. Probabilistic models for some intelligence and attainment tests. Studies in mathematical psychology. Chicago, IL: University of Chicago Press; 1980. p. xiii, 184.

37. Hobart J, Cano S. Improving the evaluation of therapeutic interventions in multiple sclerosis: the role of new psychometric methods. Health Technol Assess 2009;13(12):iii, ix–x, 1–177.

38. Smith EV Jr. Detecting and evaluating the impact of multidimensionality using item fit statistics and principal component analysis of residuals. J Appl Meas 2002;3(2):205–31.

39. Jabir S. Assessing improvement in quality of life and patient satisfaction following body contouring surgery in patients with massive weight loss: a critical review of outcome measures employed. Plast Surg Int 2013;2013:515737.

40. Black N. Patient reported outcome measures could help transform healthcare. BMJ 2013;346:f167.

41. Cano SJ, Klassen AF, Scott AM, et al. The BREAST-Q: further validation in independent clinical samples. Plast Reconstr Surg 2012;129(2):293–302.

42. Jeevan R, Cromwell D, Browne J. Annual national mastectomy and breast reconstruction audit 2011. Leeds (United Kingdom): The NHS Information Centre for Health and Social Care; 2011.

43. Available at: http://webarchive.nationalarchives. gov.uk/20130107105354/http://www.dh.gov.uk/en/ Publicationsandstatistics/Publications/Publications PolicyAndGuidance/DH_092647. Accessed March 10, 2014.

Abdominoplasty
Classic Principles and Technique

Alan Matarasso, MD[a],*, Dana Moore Matarasso[b], Emma James Matarasso[b]

KEYWORDS

- Abdominal contour surgery • Abdominolipoplasty system of classification & treatment • Liposuction
- Mini abdominoplasty • Abdominoplasty • Lipoabdominoplasty
- Pregnancy and postpartum abdomen

KEY POINTS

- Examination of the treatable layers of the abdominal wall (skin, fat, and muscle) and the nontreatable conditions in order to classify patients into the appropriate abdominal contour surgery procedure.
- Reconcile patients' anatomic findings and their tolerance for the level of procedures, risks, recovery, and expected outcome.
- Recognize that downstaging patients from their appropriate anatomic level of treatment based on the examination to less invasive options do not yield equivalent results as more invasive options.
- Abdominoplasty in appropriate circumstances can be combined with other procedures. Length of surgery is an important consideration in determining the number of procedures that can be safely performed simultaneously.
- Abdominoplasty is the aesthetic surgical procedure associated with the greatest risk for systemic complications.

INTRODUCTION

Abdominoplasty is a commonly requested procedure for many reasons, including the concerns of an aging population determined to maintain a youthful physique, women intent on restoring their prepregnancy appearance, the rise in massive weight loss patients who are seeking to remove the stigmata of residual excess skin from weight loss. The goal of abdominal contour surgery is the aesthetic improvement of the affected soft tissue layers of skin, fat, and muscle through the least conspicuous incision feasible. Depending on the anatomic nature of the "disagreeable biologic condition," the goal can be achieved through a range of procedures referred to as the abdominolipoplasty system of classification and treatment. These operations include liposuction alone (type I), the limited abdominoplasties (type II, mini abdominoplasty; type III, modified abdominoplasty), and a full standard abdominoplasty (type IV) with liposuction (lipoabdominoplasty) or without liposuction of the flap (**Fig. 1, Table 1**).[1–4]

If additional abdominal, flank, or posterior skin needs to be resected, an abdominoplasty can be extended to address those regions (eg, Fleur di Lis, flankplasty, or extended–circumferential abdominoplasty).[5]

The modern history of abdominal contour surgery and abdominoplasty can be traced back to the late 1960s and the contributions of several surgeons. Those procedures have evolved into present day abdominal contour surgery owing to advances in technique (eg, incision design, muscle treatment), technology (eg, liposuction), changing patient population (eg, massive weight loss), a

Disclosures: The authors have nothing to disclose.
[a] Manhattan Eye, Ear & Throat Hospital, Lenox Hill Hospital, North Shore-Long Island Jewish Hospital System, 1009 Park Avenue, New York, NY 10028, USA; [b] 1009 Park Avenue, New York, NY 10028, USA
* Corresponding author.
E-mail address: dam@drmatarasso.com

Clin Plastic Surg 41 (2014) 655–672
http://dx.doi.org/10.1016/j.cps.2014.07.005
0094-1298/14/$ – see front matter © 2014 Published by Elsevier Inc.

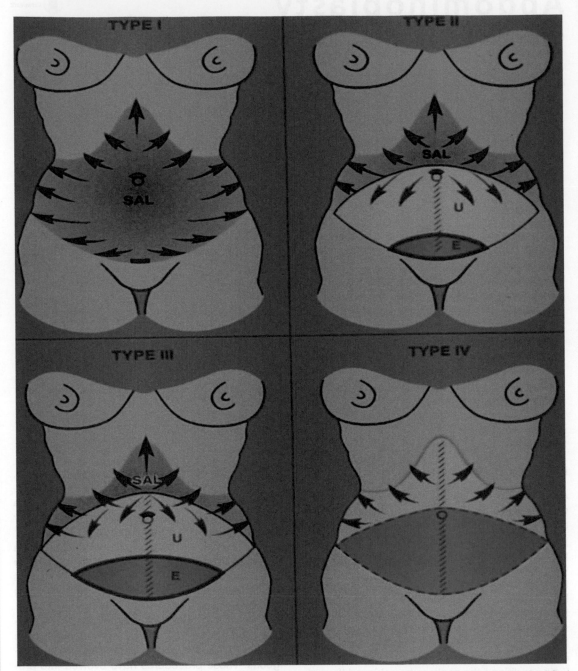

Fig. 1. The 4 common abdominal procedures: Type I, liposuction; type II, mini abdominoplasty; type III, modified abdominoplasty; type IV, full abdominoplasty with liposuction (lipoabdominoplasty) or without liposuction. E, excision; SAL, suction assisted lipectomy; U, undermining. (*From* Matarasso A. Traditional abdominoplasty. Clin Plast Surg 2010;37(3):415–37; with permission.)

better understanding of physiology (eg, wetting solutions), and anatomy (the ability to do combined procedures and flap liposuction). Similar to many scientific advances, in abdominoplasty these strides have been incremental. Numerous surgeons have provided varying degrees of contributions to present-day abdominoplasty surgery.

Table 2 offers a brief, incomplete overview of milestones in abdominoplasty evolution.[6–9]

This article focuses on abdominoplasty with liposuction (lipoabdominoplasty) or abdominoplasty without concomitant liposuction, in the most commonly encountered scenario of abdominoplasty, the postpartum abdomen.

Table 1
Abdominolipoplasty system of classification and treatment for abdominal contour surgery. This is based on the treatable soft tissue layers of skin, fat and muscle

Type	Skin	Fat	Musculofacial System	Treatment
I	Minimal laxity	Variable	Minimal diastasis	Suction-assisted lipectomy
II	Mild laxity	Variable	Lower diastasis	Mini abdominoplasty
III	Moderate laxity	Variable	Lower ± upper diastasis	Modified abdominoplasty
IV	Severe laxity	Variable	Complete diastasis	Standard abdominoplasty with or without suction lipectomy

PATIENT SELECTION AND SCREENING

Females undergo the inevitable consequences everyone does: aging, weight fluctuations, and sun damage, in addition to the profound changes that accompany pregnancy. These issues manifest themselves as loose, damaged, and excess skin, rectus muscle diastosis and stretching, lipodystrophy, widened bony pelvic girth, potentially umbilical hernias and umbilical skin damage, and finally mons pubis alteration with distortion, widening, and ptosis. A full abdominoplasty is the procedure that most comprehensively addresses these changes. It can be supplemented with additional flap liposuction[10] with hernia repair, additional skin removal (flankplasty)[5] with hernia repair[11], or adjacent liposuction[10,12–30] as well as other unrelated procedures.

Patients are examined and classified based on their anatomy to the appropriate abdominoplipoplasty level of treatment. Their physical concerns are addressed and this information is reconciled with their tolerance for incisions, discomfort, healing time, and so on. They are then offered the abdominal contour procedure most suitable to their needs. It cannot be overemphasized that less invasive procedures (downstaging), although associated with less operative time, faster recovery, and lower costs, do not provide the same outcome as a full abdominoplasty.

Anatomic conditions that can be identified and cannot be improved with abdominoplasty, such as intraabdominal fat, spinal disfigurements, uterine malposition, and "bloating," are clearly communicated to the patient.

PREOPERATIVE PLANNING AND PREPARATION

Preoperative preparation begins from the time of the initial consultation and is a multidimensional process based on a series of conversations with

Table 2
Milestones in the evolution of abdominoplasty and abdominolipoplasty

Time	Milestone
1960s–1970s	Pitanguy, Regnault, Grazar: Classic abdominoplasty
1982	Introduction of S.A.L.: Illouz
1987	Greminger, Noone, Wilkinson, and Hakme: Mini abdominoplasty with Liposuction
1988	Matarasso, Psilakis: Abdominoplasty system classification and treatment
1991	Matarasso: Liposuction as an adjunct to full abdominoplasty
1992	Illouz: Abdominoplasty 'mesh undermining,' marriage abdominoplasty (Shestak- 1999)
1995	Lockwood: HLT abdominoplasty
1995	Matarasso: SA 1-4 goes based on Huger zones
2001	Survey of c/o ABD: Only 54% of board-certified plastic surgeons perform liposuction of abdominoplasty flap
2001	Hakme, Avelar, Saldahina, De Souza Pinto, Saltz: Lipo
2000s	Rise in bariatric plastic surgery
Late 2010s	Persing/others: Validation studies of lipoabdominoplasty and measures to improve safety and including research and recommendation regarding DVT/PE
2012	Pannuci, et al, ASPS VTE Task force, Eric Swanson etc.: VTE prophylaxis

Abbreviations: ABD, abdominoplasties; DVT, deep venous thrombosis; HLT, high lateral tension; PE, pulmonary embolism; SA, suction assisted; SAL, suction assisted lipectomy; VTE, venous thromboembolism.

the physician, their staff, the anesthesiologist, ancillary personnel, and the patient.

Patients receive an extensive informational brochure package at the time of the consultation. Before surgery, they receive a detailed package outlining their anticipated preparations and care, which includes a copious list of products that adversely affect coagulation. For all abdominal contour surgery procedures, patients are instructed to cease nicotine-containing products and compounds that affect clotting before the procedure. All patients are evaluated by an internist and undergo appropriate blood and diagnostic testing. Consideration is given to "special" hematology testing for genetic prothrombogenic factors because patients who have these factors are at an increased risk for blood clots (a history of miscarriages can be a marker for these hypercoagulable risk factor situations). Abdominoplasty, in general, has the highest incidence of venous thromboembolism of all aesthetic procedures and one half or more of abdominal fatalities are owing to thromboembolism. Thromboembolism deterrent stockings and Venodyne compression devices are always used. The use of pharmacologic intervention for venous thromboembolism prophylaxis (eg, enoxaparin sodium [Lovenox, Sanofi Aventis US, Bridgewater, NJ] 40 mg subcutaneously every 12 hours from onset of surgery) is an unresolved and evolving concept. Many surgeons who advocate anticoagulation utilize a risk base model such as the Venturi modification of the Davision-Caprini system to determine the need for anticoagulation.

Patients begin antimicrobial skin washes, including the area above and beyond the surgical site, 3 days preoperatively. No shaving of body hair is done. Broad-spectrum perioperative antibiotics are employed and may be continued until any drains that are used are removed. However, evidence-based information, which confirms that antibiotics may reduce surgical site infections in abdominoplasty, suggests that a single preoperative antibiotic is as effective as preoperative and postoperative doses.

The arms are symmetrically placed on arm boards while avoiding pressure points and secured with Kerlix wraps. Preoperatively, the operating room table is checked to verify that it can reach a maximum beach chair position, which is necessary for wound closure and removing the old umbilical site (**Fig. 2**). A Foley catheter is inserted for all open abdominal contour procedures. Abdominoplasty is generally performed as an outpatient procedure and it is usually the last procedure in a multisurgical operation (eg, breasts, or liposuction, or face).

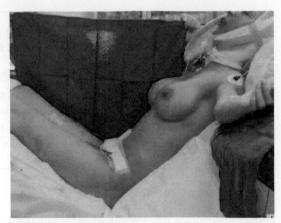

Fig. 2. The Miami Beach chair position. Significant operating room bed flexion is often necessary to ensure removal of all the lower abdominal skin including the old umbilical site.

SURGICAL MARKINGS

Surgical markings are made in conjunction with the patient so that stab wound incisions for liposuction are well hidden and abdominoplasty incisions are confined to their undergarments. The abdominal excision is essentially an ellipse of tissue removal between the umbilicus and mons pubis (**Fig. 3**).

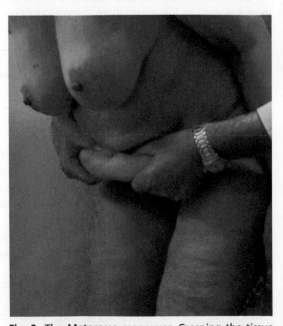

Fig. 3. The Matarasso maneuver. Grasping the tissue from umbilicus to pubis ensures that with the proper flap undermining and operating room bed positioning (see **Fig. 2**) the lower half of abdominal skin and old umbilical site can be resected.

Markings begin with the patient comfortably fitted in their preferred undergarments. The upper and lower edges of the garment are marked, and it is then removed. While the patient is in a bent over, sitting position, the length of the abdominoplasty incisions is then determined by locating the ends of the pannus' skin creases, and by placing a mark on either side. After this marking, the patient gently elevates their pannus while the surgeon joins these lateral marks, with the midline position, approximately 6 to 8 cm above the vulva cleft. We try to incorporate the removal of any old scars, such as cesarean sections, in our excision. The upward pull helps to avoid a scar that is too high by accounting for eventual upward scar contraction or migration.

A flexible ruler can then be used on the lower incision and reversed to demarcate the upper limb of the ellipse as a mirror image of the lower incision. The upper incision is then drawn across the top of the umbilicus from hip-point to hip-point, joining the lower incision and completing the ellipse. The ability to remove the lower abdominal skin pannus from umbilicus to pubis is then re-verified by the surgeon grasping the skin and confirming that the upper and lower incision meet and therefore can be closed (see **Fig. 3**). In an abdominoplasty, it is preferable to remove enough tissue so that the old umbilicus site is removed with it. In the operating room, the markings are verified by placing long silk sutures (after any liposuction is performed) in the midline at the xyphoid and pubis and overlapping them at multiple points on the upper and lower incision to ascertain symmetry between sides of the incision (**Fig. 4**).

SURGICAL TECHNIQUE

All procedures are undertaken with systemic anesthesia (spontaneous ventilation general anesthesia, or spinal/epidural) administered by an anesthesiologist. The operative field is injected with approximately 1 L of superwet anesthesia (1 L of Ringer's lactate, 20 mL of 1% lidocaine, 1 mL of 1:1000 epinephrine). Limiting the volume of wetting solution to the abdomen provides a margin of safety to allow infiltration of additional operative sites, by avoiding potentially toxic doses of lidocaine or epinephrine (the toxic dose is 0.07 mg/kg of 1:1000 epinephrine). Moreover, excess injectate would ultimately encumber electrocauterization during surgery.

The operation begins by liposuctioning as indicated (**Fig. 5**). The surgeon then changes gloves and rechecks the abdominal excision markings. The umbilicus is again cleansed with betadine. The abdominoplasty proceeds by incising and freeing the umbilicus. The pannus is then prepared for preexcision in a vest-over-pants fashion (after Jaime Plannas). This maneuver is accomplished by incising the upper limb of the ellipse to the level of the rectus fascia while beveling the cut inwards at approximately a 45° angle. The upper abdominal flap is then completely undermined in a narrow tunnel resembling an inverted "v" corresponding with the zone of complete undermining (**Fig. 6**), maintaining the

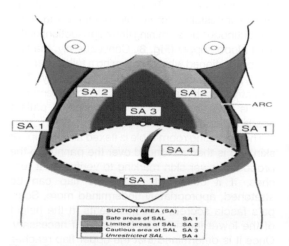

Fig. 5. Suction areas 1 through 4. Suction area 4 is the pannus that is excised. Suction area 1 is the region where the lateral intercostal blood supply that perfuses the abdominoplasty flap originates from. Suction areas 2 and 3 are the undermined flap. These are random pattern perfused areas from suction area 1. Suction area 3 is the "terrible abdominoplasty triangle" where, if ischemia occurs, is most likely at this location.

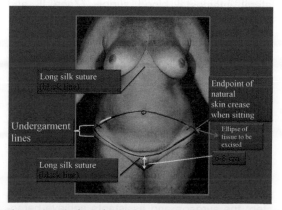

Fig. 4. Surgical markings are made confining the incisions to reasonable undergarments (paired hashmarks at either side of skin fold). This is verified intraoperatively with underlying crisscrossed silk sutures. The black line ellipse is marked for excision.

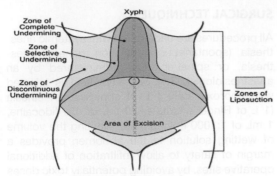

Fig. 6. The upper flap is undermined in an inverted 'v' pattern (zone of complete undermining) enough to allow rectus fascia plication. Then additional selective undermining and discontinuous undermining is done to reduce any excessive skin bunching that occurs after muscle plication. (*From* Matarasso A. Traditional abdominoplasty. Clin Plast Surg 2010;37(3):415–37; with permission.)

intercostal blood supply (Huger zone III, **Figure 7**) sufficiently to achieve rectus muscle repair and anterior sheath plication. Preservation of the blood supply in this manner allows for appropriate liposuction of the flap. Dissection is done by scalpel and electrocautery. Moreover the inverted 'V' undermining may actually preserve Zone 1 DSEA (Huger Zone 1, **Figure 7**) the preoperative predominant blood supply.

An intact zone surrounding this tunnel or zone of selective undermining is undermined as needed to diminish the inevitable skin bunching that occurs after muscle closure. This action maintains a broad intact subcostal perforator blood supply (**Fig. 7**) by discontinuous undermining (from liposuction) of the axial blood supply (**Fig. 8**). Consequently, the flap can be suctioned when performing a full abdominoplasty, hence the term lipoabdominoplasty. This operative technique serves as a standard template and is adjusted according to individual patient needs unless they do not require liposuction.

The operating room table is flexed and the upper skin flap is then advanced over the pannus to the proposed lower skin marking to verify that it reaches. If it does not reach, the flap can be stretched, appropriately undermined more, Scarpa's fascia scored, or adjustments in the height of the lower incision can be made, if necessary. Once it is determined that the upper flap reaches the lower skin incision, the skin island is grasped with Allis clamps on the side of the surgeon and excised en bloc from side to side. This vest-over-pants preexcision of the pannus has the following advantages: leaving the pannus that will later be resected in place preserves heat and blood, it is faster than elevating a flap that will ultimately be excised, and it avoids the tendency of wide upper

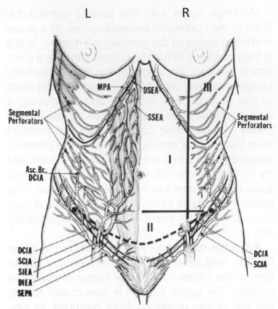

Fig. 7. (*Left*) The Huger zones I through III blood supply to the abdominal wall. In the unoperated abdomen zone I deep superior epigastric artery is the predominant blood supply. (*Right*) After the skin flap is elevated zone III (segmental or lateral intercostal perforators) and a minor contribution from zone II perfuse the flap. Asc. Br., ascending branch; DCIA, deep circumflex iliac artery; DIEA, deep inferior epigastric artery; DSEA, deep superior epigastric artery; MPA, main pulmonary artery; SCIA, superficial circumflex iliac artery; SEPA, superficial external pudendal artery; SIEA, superficial inferior epigastric artery; SSEA, superficial superior epigastric artery. (*From* Matarasso A. Traditional abdominoplasty. Clin Plast Surg 2010;37(3):415–37; with permission.)

flap undermining ensuring upper flap tunneling in an inverted "v" fashion, thereby maintaining the lateral intercostal blood supply (Zone III and possibly Zone I).

Some authors recommend leaving a thin layer of fibro-fatty tissue on top of the fascia (and/or quilting sutures when closing), which may reduce the incidence of seromas. In massive weight loss patients, a large pannus can distort the anatomy and bring the spermatochord into the surgical field, therefore, care must be taken as the incision proceeds down to the rectus fascia.

A plastic button (ocular conformer) is sutured to the umbilicus to be used for subsequent identification by palpation through the skin and removed when the umbilicus is later exteriorized. At each step, the surgeon and assistants achieve hemostasis with electrocautery, and particularly before perforators retract below the fascia.

The rectus muscle diastasis, which begins as early the second trimester of pregnancy, is marked

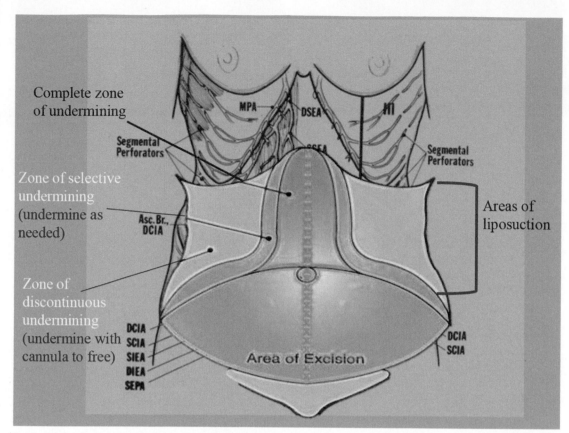

Fig. 8. Abdominal wall blood supply superimposed on the areas of undermining. Asc. Br., ascending branch; DCIA, deep circumflex iliac artery; DIEA, deep inferior epigastric artery; DSEA, deep superior epigastric artery; MPA, main pulmonary artery; SCIA, superficial circumflex iliac artery; SEPA, superficial external pudendal artery; SIEA, superficial inferior epigastric artery; SSEA, superficial superior epigastric artery. Note undermining goes to xyphoid. (*From* Matarasso A. Traditional abdominoplasty. Clin Plast Surg 2010;37(3):415–37; with permission.)

so that it closes without excessive tension while in the supine position, with ink in a long vertical ellipse from xyphoid to pubis. The section above and then below the umbilicus is closed in layers with running 0-loop nylon suture. A second layer of buried interrupted 2-0 Neurolon sutures is used to further imbricate and reinforce the first layer. In thin patients with minimal intraabdominal adiposity, additional waistline narrowing can be performed by placing one or two 2-0 Neurolon sutures horizontal to the umbilicus (Ian Jackson). No further fascial muscle tightening is necessary or desirable. Once appropriately closed, the amount of flattening achieved with rectus plication cannot be predicted or increased.[31,32] Furthermore, some relaxation and stretching of the fascial repair is likely to occur over time. Certain sites along the rectus fascia plication from xyphoid to pubis warrant consideration (**Fig. 9**).

Puckering that develops in the upper skin flap, where it is still adherent to the underlying muscle subsequent to fascial closure, is gently freed by blunt and sharp selective dissection (zone of discontinuous undermining). Small amounts of bunching are tolerated and indeed desirable, because intact skin maintains its blood supply. This condition resolves in the early postoperative period. The cavity is irrigated with saline, and final inspection and hemostasis is performed. Ten milliliters of Exaparel (Pacira Pharmaceuticals, San Diego, CA) 0.25% Marcaine with epinephrine mixed with 80 mL of normal saline is linearly injected by threading technique into various points in the rectus sheath and open wound for analgesia.

The table is returned to the degree of beach chair position required to achieve wound closure, which begins by placing a deep 2-0 Vicryl suture and approximating the midline. The wound edges are temporarily aligned with staples to minimize dog-ear formation. A 2-0 polydioxanone bidirectional barbed suture (Quill SRS, Angiotech, Vancouver, Canada) is used in the deep layers incorporating the Scarpas fascia up to the dermis on either side of the midline in a running fashion. While in the flexed position and with most of the

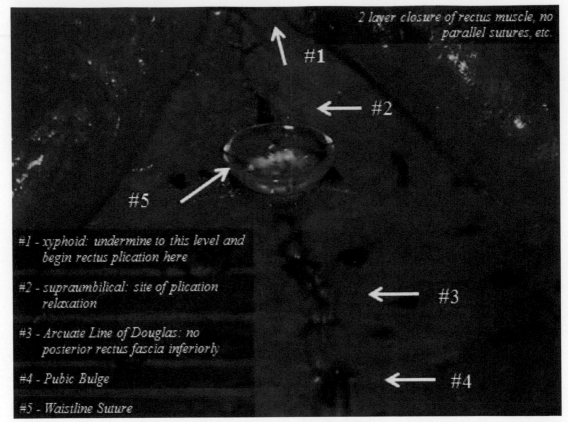

2 layer closure of rectus muscle, no parallel sutures, etc.

#1

#2

#5

#1 - xyphoid: undermine to this level and begin rectus plication here

#2 - supraumbilical: site of plication relaxation

#3 - Arcuate Line of Douglas: no posterior rectus fascia inferiorly

#4 - Pubic Bulge

#5 - Waistline Suture

#3

#4

Fig. 9. Vertical rectus muscle fascia closure in 2 layers from xyphoid to pubis. An eyelid conformer is temporarily sewn to umbilicus. Five key points along closure.

wound closed, the umbilical button is palpated and marked on the skin in the midline slightly higher than its naturally occurring position. The dimensions of the abdomen—vertical, horizontal, and so forth—can be expected to change (shorten) after abdominoplasty (**Fig. 10**). A second layer of 3-0 monoderm Quill sutures is used in the subcuticular layer. Two Jackson Pratt drains (4 are used in massive weight loss patients) exit the mid to lateral aspect of the wound. They are secured with 3-0 nylon sutures. Drains remain in place for several days until wound drainage subsides and fluid color becomes less red. Initial drainage may be greater in patients who have had tumescent fluid injected for adjacent areas of liposuction.

When preparing to exteriorize the umbilicus, the patient's midline is verified with the silk marking sutures and by observing the midline position using the vulva cleft as a reference. The umbilical site is determined and a 2.5-cm inverted V-type incision is made in the midline of the skin. The upper and (more so) lower skin edges of the umbilical opening are defatted. The author no

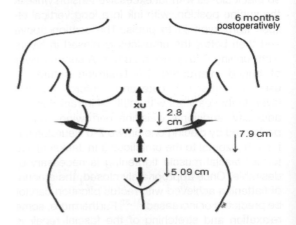

6 months postoperatively

XU
2.8 cm
W
7.9 cm
UV
5.09 cm

(postoperatively)

Fig. 10. On the right is the average reduction in dimensions after an abdominoplasty. UV, umbilicus to vulva reduces 5.09 cm; W, waistline reduces 7.9 cm; XU, xyphoid to umbilicus reduces 2.8 cm. (*From* Matarasso A. Traditional abdominoplasty. Clin Plast Surg 2010;37(3):415–37; with permission.)

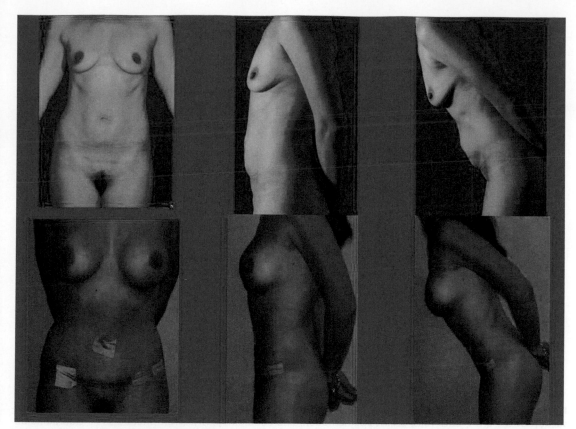

Fig. 11. *Top row,* preoperative. *Bottom row,* postoperative. A 31-year-old gravid 2, para 2 undergoing breast augmentation and abdominoplasty. (*From* Matarasso A. Traditional abdominoplasty. Clin Plast Surg 2010;37(3):415–37; with permission.)

longer tacks the umbilicus to the fascia because, if any site pulls free from it, this can change its midline appearance. The umbilicus is exteriorized and the button removed. Deep absorbable sutures are placed from umbilicus to skin flap, and the umbilical skin is then closed with interrupted 3-0 and 4-0 nylon sutures. The umbilicus is packed with a strip of 2 × 6-cm xeroform gauze. Antibiotic ointment is placed on the wound and it is covered with a Telfa dressing or prineo dressing (Dermabond, San Lorenzo, Puerto Rico). A binder can be used. The patient is transferred to a special stretcher that mimics the beach chair operating room bed in the same maximally flexed position. Patients should ambulate that day as if they are using a walker, and over the next few days progressively begin to fully straighten out (**Figs. 11–13**).

In most cases, the skin between the umbilicus and the pubis is excised, including the old umbilicus site, which is a significant patient preference as first identified by Grazer and Goldwyn.[6] This maneuver necessitates maximal flexion (see **Fig. 2**) of the operating room table and can result in tension of the undermined flap. Flap tension,

and the degree of flap undermining and liposuction should be reconciled to help avoid wound ischemia. Indeed, the equation of collateral blood supply over wound tension and degree of extent of liposuction defines flaps safety in lipoabdominoplasty.

Concerns about the appearance of a circumscribed umbilicus have been among the reasons that have motivated patients and surgeons to perform alternative procedures that do not require an umbilical incision, such as lower abdominoplasty or panniculectomy with extensive liposuction. These procedures yield different results than a full abdominoplasty, often with a similar length of lower skin incision, albeit without an umbilical scar (**Fig. 14**). The appearance of a circumscribed umbilicus is part of the discussion and decision-making process in selecting the appropriate abdominal contour operative procedure that the patient and surgeon have (**Fig. 15**).

POTENTIAL COMPLICATIONS

Traditionally, pulmonary issues (eg, atelectasis) were considered the most common complication

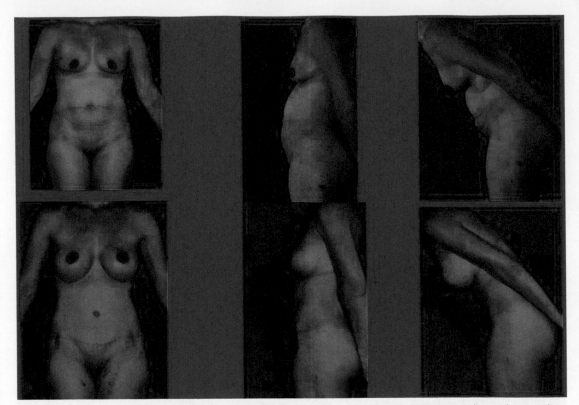

Fig. 12. *Top row,* preoperative. *Bottom row,* postoperative. A 35-year-old gravid 4, para 4 who underwent liposuction of the arms, back rolls, breast augmentation, and abdominoplasty. (*From* Matarasso A. Traditional abdominoplasty. Clin Plast Surg 2010;37(3):415–37; with permission.)

of abdominoplasty. However, data on complications, which are now available from many different reporting agencies and most report seroma as the most common (**Box 1**).[33–38] In the final analysis, it is absolutely essential to bear in mind that, because of the way data are captured, the complications and risk factors that are generated from various databases will have an inherent bias and differ based on their capture universe. For example, the Doctors Insurance Company database yields data from lawsuits. Cosmet Assure's database has data from patients who have insurance to cover surgery, should they need to return to the operating room within 30 days of surgery (**Table 3**). Their most recent data on abdominoplasty reveals that (1) age over 40, (2) female gender, and (3) body mass index over 25 kg/m² were risk factors for complications. Moreover, males have a statistically significantly greater chance of hematoma formation. Interestingly, in their cohort, seromas generally now considered the most frequent complication are not captured as a complication, and smoking does not represent a risk. This is likely owing to the fact that ischemia and limited wound healing problems or seromas may be managed in an office and Cosmet Assure does not look at complications treated in

an office. Finally, abdominoplasty with another cosmetic procedure performed concurrently, in contrast with other reporting agencies (eg, American Association for the Accreditation of Ambulatory Surgical Facilities) in Cosmet Assure's data did not result in more complications. They speculate that this may be owing to surgeons' improved ability to select appropriate patients for combined surgery. Finally, Cosmet Assure's database is listed in **Tables 4–6**. In their data, about one half of the suspected deep venous thromboses (DVTs) turned out to actually be DVTs and almost all of the suspected pulmonary embolisms (PEs) were in fact PEs. They also state an overall complication rate of 4.7%, which is more than double (1.57%) the rate from other cosmetic procedures. Thirty-seven percent underwent abdominoplasty alone and 63% had multiple procedures. Their average age was 44 years, with an average body mass index of 27 kg/m². In the patients having complications, 12 of 163 (7%) were smokers and 7 of the 163 (4%) were diabetic; single complications occurred in 155 of 163 (95%) and multiple 8 of 163 (5%). Cosmet Assure data confirm that abdominoplasty carries the highest risk of complications of all aesthetic plastic surgery. Indeed, body contour surgery is more risky.

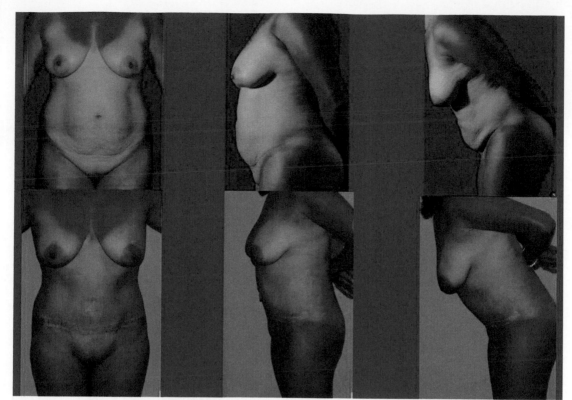

Fig. 13. *Top row,* preoperative. *Bottom row,* postoperative. A 39-year-old, gravida 3, para 2 who underwent lipoabdominoplasty and liposuction of the thighs and back rolls. The total amount liposuctioned was 2750 g. (*From* Matarasso A. Traditional abdominoplasty. Clin Plast Surg 2010;37(3):415–37; with permission.)

The American Association for the Accreditation of Ambulatory Surgical Facilities has large number of patients that had office-based surgery yielding data on procedure's complications, morbidity, and so on, for aesthetic surgery.

Maintenance of Certification data reports the most common complications from abdominoplasty to be infection, seromas, and DVT/PE. Tracking Operations and Outcomes for Plastic Surgery data report the most common adverse event recorded by American Society of Plastic Surgeons members as infection (3.5%).

Maintenance of Certification data advise a single dose of antibiotics to reduce infections. For reducing seromas, which are generally considered the most frequent complication (15%–40%), they suggest modifying the level of dissection to leave a loose areola plane of tissue on the muscle fascia, or progressive tension sutures, or drains, or both. The author has published a protocol to treat chronic seromas in an attempt to reduce the disturbing sequel (eg, infection) of pseudobursa formation.

Thromboembolism is the most dreaded complication and accounts for approximately one half of all fatalities in abdominoplasty. With regard to DVT/PE, the Maintenance of Certification implications for practice state to consider the patient's risk for bleeding and consider enoxaparin postoperatively. Some suggest using heparin or low-molecular-weight heparin preoperatively, whereas others consider its use, which are extrapolated from other surgical subspecialties' experiences, to be inappropriate for abdominoplasty. Ideally, patients should begin ambulating on the day of surgery.[35,39–53]

POSTPROCEDURAL CARE

A frequent trifecta "of patient concerns" in abdominoplasty are scars, drains, and pain.

SCARS

When planning patient's surgical markings, incisions can be designed to be located below the limits of their undergarment so that they are covered. All abdominal excisional procedures require an incision/scar whose length is commensurate with the amount of skin to be resected. The old umbilical site should also be removed if appropriate. Determining whether all of the infraumbilical

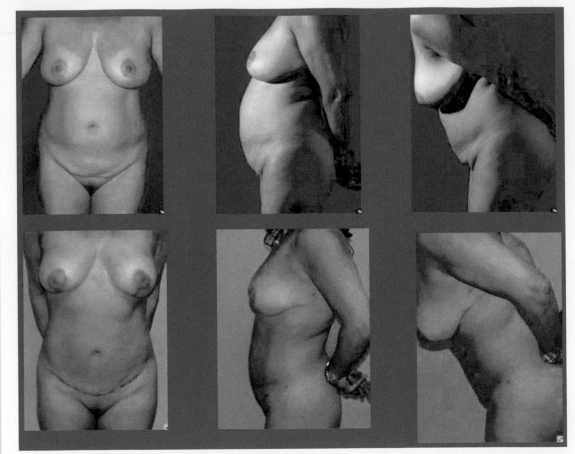

Fig. 14. *Top row,* preoperative. *Bottom row,* postoperative. A 39-year old female, gravida 2, para 2, undergoing modified (lower abdominoplasty) with 2175 mL of liposuction. No Umbilical circumscription was performed. This was an alternative to a full abdominoplasty to avoid a periumbilical scar.

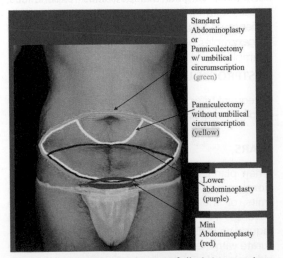

Standard Abdominoplasty or Panniculectomy w/ umbilical circumscription (green)

Panniculectomy without umbilical circumscription (yellow)

Lower abdominoplasty (purple)

Mini Abdominoplasty (red)

Fig. 15. Various alternatives to a full abdominoplasty that avoid umbilical circumscription and scarring.

skin can be removed can be done by testing preoperatively (Matarasso maneuver; see **Fig. 3**). This ensures that intraoperatively a preexcision (upper incision made first) of the pannus can be performed. To achieve this maximal operative table flexion (Miami Beach chair position) to ensure wound closure is frequently necessary (see **Fig. 2**).

Patients, in an attempt to reassure themselves about their tolerance for the scar, may inquire about seeing before and after photographs of other patients. The only thing that other patient photographs will teach a prospective patient with certainty about a scar is the approximate location of their scar, not what theirs will necessarily heal like.

Loose upper abdominal or periumbilical skin are also frequent concerns of prospective patients. Although procedures such as reverse abdominoplasty or applying noninvasive technology to the skin may have some benefit for these conditions,

Box 1
Various sources provide databases for complications in abdominoplasty

1. *Case series* of a surgeon.

2. *Surveys* of groups of plastic surgeons (eg, American Society of Plastic Surgeons, American Society for Aesthetic Plastic Surgery).

3. *TOPS*[TM] (Tracking Operations and Outcomes for Plastic Surgery): National database of plastic surgery procedures and outcomes self-reported by members of American Society of Plastic Surgeons.

4. *Cosmet Assure*: A medical insurance program covering 17 elective cosmetic procedures performed by active or candidate members of the American Society of Plastic Surgeons. Coverage includes complications treated in an emergency room, those requiring hospital admission, or intervention in an accredited surgical center within 30 days of the procedure. It does not include complications treated on an outpatient basis, such as seroma drainage, wound care, or oral antibiotics, which TOPS should include.

5. *The Doctors Insurance Company*: Databased on claims that the insured physician's medical malpractice covers.

6. *Maintenance of Certification* (MOC): Data collected by the American Board of Plastic Surgeons for board certification.

7. *American Association for the Accreditation of Ambulatory Surgical Facilities*: Data collected from outpatient accredited surgery centers.

Table 3
Cosmet-Assure database of complications based on their insured patients who returned to the operating room within 30 days of their abdominoplasty

Complication	%
Infection	1.63
Hemorrhage	1.17
Fluid overload	0.33
R/O DVT[a]	0.30
Hypoxia	0.24
Pulmonary dysfunction	0.22
R/O PE[a]	0.22
PE	0.19
Severe hypertension	0.16
DVT	0.16
Overall r/o rate of abdominoplasties %	4.7
Versus other cosmetic procedures	1.37
Abdominoplasty alone	37
Abdominoplasty with multiple procedures	63

Abbreviations: DVT, deep venous thrombosis; PE, pulmonary embolism; R/O, reportable occurrence.
[a] About half of suspected ruled out DVTs were DVTs. Almost all suspected PEs were positive.

in this author's experiences these respond best to a full abdominoplasty.

PEREGRINATIONS ON THE UMBILICUS

A full abdominoplasty requires circumscription around the umbilicus and hence a scar around the new umbilical site. Because the lower abdominoplasty incision is usually hidden by clothing and the "new umbilicus" is likely to be exposed, it is the umbilical scar that often concerns patients the most. As stated I routinely remove the old umbilical site in order to avoid the additional scar from its wound closure, if the old site is not removed. Various modification such as a lower abdominoplasty, mini-abdominoplasty, reverse abdominoplasty, or panniculectomy (see **Fig 14**) can be designed to avoid the periumbilical scar. However none of these options will result in the same amount of skin removal and the same outcome that a full abdominoplasty would.[64]

Moreover despite what patients may believe the umbilicus is not "removed". Its skin can be severely damaged from pregnancy, hernias, etc. and abdominoplasty will not ameliorate this. Indeed the damage may be more apparent postoperatively due to the attention brought to it by the scar and improvement rendered to the surrounding skin by the results of the abdominoplasty. Postoperatively the umbilicus no longer blends as gently into the surrounding tissue, tantamount to how a circumscribed areolar will appear following a breast reduction. Inevitably then the umbilicus looks different postoperatively. Also an "outtie" umbilicus is generally an umbilical hernia that may resolve or be repaired with abdominoplasty. To ensure its resolution separate attention must be paid to treating the hernia, which may or may not be feasible at the time of the abdominoplasty.

An umbilicus starts out as a scar, hence doesn't appear as vital as normal skin, and its difference from normal skin is exacerbated by the effects of pregnancy. Special awareness about severely damaged umbilical skin or "postage stamp" appearing umbilicus warrants discussion. These patients are often thin with little subcutaneous fat and damaged (loss of elasticity) surrounding

Table 4
Local abdominal contour surgery complications

Complications	Liposuction (%)	Limited Abdominoplasties (%)	Full Abdominoplasties (%)
Contour irregularity	9.20	4.90	5
Major skin necrosis (requiring reoperation)	0	1	1
Minor skin necrosis (healed spontaneously)	0	4	4.40
Scar revision	0.03	2.40	4.90
Hematoma	0.04	0.08	1.40
Wound infection	1	0.02	1.10
Wound dehiscence	0	1	1
Umbilical abnormality (requiring reoperation)	0	0.05	1.20
Dissatisfied patients (unfulfilled expectations)	3.30	2.90	2.20
Need for second surgery	3.50	2.40	3.40

Data from the author national survey of American Society of Plastic Surgeons member on complications in abdominoplasty. Matarasso A, Swift R, Rankin M. Abdominoplasty and abdominal contour surgery: a national plastic surgery survey. Plast Reconstr Surg 2006;117(6):1797–808.

abdominal skin. The appearance of their umbilicus is manifested by: cutaneous hyperpigmentation, a short umbilical stalk, (making it almost flush with the surrounding skin), thinned skin of the umbilicus, and possibly worsened by an underlying hernia exerting forward pressure on it. Consequently the umbilicus' final postoperative appearance after closure, looks flattened, stretched and wider than normal, and almost flush (not having the depth of an unoperated umbilicus) to the surrounding abdominal skin (**Fig. 14**). The inevitable

postoperative appearance of these pregnancy damaged umbilici are a source of frustration to patient and surgeon.

We use scar modifiers on incisions as indicated (**Fig. 16**).

DRAINS

Abdominoplasty carries a high risk of seroma formation. Seromas are multifaceted in etiology and can range from a trivial nuisance, to an untoward

Table 5
Systemic abdominal contour surgery complications

Complications	Liposuction (%)	Limited Abdominoplasties (%)	Full Abdominoplasties (%)
Local anesthesia (ie, wetting solution)	0	0	0
Major anesthesia	0	0	0
Malpractice action	0	0	0.01
Blood transfusion	0	0	0.04
Deep vein thrombophlebitis	0	0.01	0.04
Pulmonary embolism	0	0	0.02
Pulmonary fat embolism	0	0	0
Intra-abdominal perforation	0	0	0
Death	0	0	0
Readmission to hospital	0.01	0.01	0.05

Data from the author national survey of American Society of Plastic Surgeons member on complications in abdominoplasty. Matarasso A, Swift R, Rankin M. Abdominoplasty and abdominal contour surgery: a national plastic surgery survey. Plast Reconstr Surg 2006;117(6):1797–808.

Table 6
Comparison of results of abdominoplasty complications

Complication	Matarasso et al	Hester et al,[18] 1989	Grazar & Goldwyn	Pitanguy	Teimourian & Rogers,[20] 1989
No. of procedures	11,016	563	10,490	539	25,562
Local (%)					
Necrosis minor	4.4	0.9 (minimal slough)	5.4 (wound dehiscence)	1.4	
Necrosis major	1.0			0.3	
Seroma		2.5		5.8	8.58
Infection	1.1	1.1	7.3		
Blood loss	<1.0	14.2			
Hypertrophic scars	<1.0			3.7	
Hematoma	1.4		6		
Wound infection	1				
Dehiscence	1			0.3	
Umbilical abnormality	1.2			0.3	
Dissatisfied patient	2.2				
Need for second operation	3.4				
Scar revision	4.9				
Contour irregularity	5.0				
Systemic (%)					
Deep vein thrombosis	0.04		1.1		0.29
Pulmonary embolism	0.02	1.1	0.8		0.25
Pulmonary fat embolism	0				0.02
Blood transfusion	0.04				0.04
Death	0		0.16		0.04
Anesthesia complications	0				0.01
Readmission to hospital	0.05				
Malpractice action	0.01		0.18		

Data from the author national survey of American Society of Plastic Surgeons member on complications in abdominoplasty. Matarasso A, Swift R, Rankin M. Abdominoplasty and abdominal contour surgery: a national plastic surgery survey. Plast Reconstr Surg 2006;117(6):1797–808.

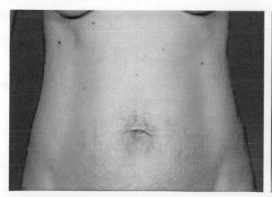 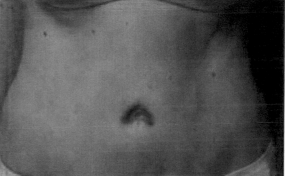

Fig. 16. The early appearance of a severe "postage stamp" umbilicus in a 38-year old female G2/P2 patient.

sequelae, to a complication resulting in psuedo-bursa formation. Consequently, methods to reduce seroma formation should be considered. Drains, quilting sutures, or both are the most popular methods to reduce fluid collection and the sequelae of seromas. Drains do not prevent seromas or hematomas.

Other surgeons advise leaving a loose areola layer over the fascia to decrease seroma formation. Some surgeons advocate pressure dressings to diminish fluid collections. Others advise for or against binders as preventing or inciting seromas. Recently a tissue glue received FDA approval to eliminate the use of drains and decrease seroma rates.

Attention has also focused on the role electrocautery versus scalpel dissection can play in seroma formation.[54–63]

PAIN

A frequent concern of abdominoplasty patients is what they have been told about the pain associated with abdominoplasty. In this author's experience, most patients who have had a caesarean section and can accurately recall those events associated with it report a caesarean section to be more uncomfortable than an abdominoplasty. Various strategies preoperatively, intraoperatively, and postoperatively are incorporated to reduce any discomfort of abdominoplasty.

In addition to enhancing the "experience" of the operation, reducing pain prevents a cascade of problems that can result in hematoma or even paralytic illness from the effects of surgery and opioid use. A detailed description of our pain management protocol can be found in the authors' papers in the journal *Plastic and Reconstructive Surgery*.[64,65]

REHABILITATION AND RECOVERY

Patients are discharged to a hotel-like facility accompanied by an experienced registered nurse, who monitors them for 24 to 48 hours. A defined protocol, including blood pressure control, pain management, fluids and food intake, movement, ambulation, hygiene, and pulmonary management, are followed.

Preoperatively, we offer patients testing for prothrombogenic blood clotting factors that, if present, would dramatically increase their risk for venous thromboembolism. Postoperatively, venous Doppler testing is done if there is any suspicion of DVT or at the patient's request.

SUMMARY

Abdominoplasty is the most common 'open' operative procedure (in males or females) in a spectrum of procedures available for abdominal contouring (the abdominolipoplasty system of classifation and treatment. Abdominoplsty with liposuction (abdominolipoplasty) or without liposuction is an effective operation for treating the majority of sequelae that pregnancy causes on the postpartum abdomen. In more than one half the cases, abdominoplasty is performed in conjunction with other aesthetic operations, such as liposuction, breast surgery, or facial surgery. Combined surgery may increase surgical risk and should be performed with specific guidelines and in an appropriate albeit arbitrary time frame (such as <4 hours).

Males account for approximately 11% to 16% of all abdominoplasty contour surgery patients.[64,66,67] They most commonly and overwhelmingly undergo liposuction of the abdomen and flanks as the treatment of choice, unless they are massive weight loss patients. Then, depending on their concerns, some form of an abdominoplasty may be considered.

Statistically, a secondary complete abdominal contour operation occurs in approximately 13% to 15% of all procedures.

REFERENCES

1. Matarasso A. Abdominolipoplasty: a system of classification and treatment for combined abdominoplasty and suction-assisted lipectomy. Aesthetic Plast Surg 1991;15:111–21.
2. Matarasso A. Abdominolipoplasty. Clin Plast Surg 1989;16:2. Philadelphia: WB Saunders and Company; (cited in Selected Readings in Plastic Surgery, 1992).
3. Matarasso A. Abdominplasty. In: Achaner BM, Eriksson E, Guyuron B, et al, editors. Plastic surgery. Indications, operations and outcomes. Aesthetic surgery, vol. 5. St Louis (MO): Mosby; 2000. p. 2783–821.
4. Shestak KC. Short scar abdominoplasty update. Clin Plast Surg 2010;37(3):505–13.
5. Matarasso A. Traditional abdominoplasty. Clin Plast Surg 2010;37:415–37.
6. Grazer FM, Goldwyn RM. Abdominoplasty assessed by survey, with emphasis on complications. Plast Reconstr Surg 1977;59:513–7.
7. Pitanguy I, Ceravolo MP. Our experience with combined procedures in aesthetic plastic surgery. Plast Reconstr Surg 1983;71:64–5.
8. Matarasso A. Abdominoplasty and abdominolipoplasty. In: Cohen M, editor. Mastery in plastic surgery, vol. 3. Boston: Little Brown & Company; 1994. p. 1385.
9. Jackson IT, Downie PA. Abdominoplasty–the waistline stitch and other refinements. Plast Reconstr Surg 1978;61:180–3.

10. Matarasso A. Liposuction as an adjunct to a full abdominoplasty. Plast Reconstr Surg 1995;95: 829–36.

11. Matarasso A, Abramson D, Ninestein R. Umbilical hernia repair in conjunction with abdominoplasty using the ventralex hernia patch. Plast Reconstr Surg.

12. Matarasso A, Smith DM. Combined breast surgery and abdominoplasty: strategies for success. Plast Reconstr Surg, in press.

13. Matarasso A (1993) Abdominoplasty: Evaluation and techniques in abdominal contour surgery. In: Newman MH (ed) Plastic Surgery Education Foundation Instructional course. Vol 6. Mosby, Chicago, IL. P 1–17.

14. Matarasso A, Wallach SG. Abdominal contour surgery: treating all aesthetic units, including the mons pubis. Aesthet Surg J 2001;21:111–9.

15. Saldanha OR, Azevedo SF, Delboni PS, et al. Lipoabdominoplasty: the Saldanha technique. Clin Plast Surg 2010;37(3):469–81.

16. Dillerud E. Abdominoplasty combined with suction lipoplasty. A study of complications, revisions, and risk factors in 487 cases. Ann Plast Surg 1990;25: 333–43.

17. Matarasso A, Smith D. (Invited Article). Strategies for aesthetic reshaping of the post-partum patient. Plast Reconstr Surg.

18. Hester TR, Baird W, Bostwick J III, et al. Abdominoplasty combined with other major surgical procedures: safe or sorry? Plast Reconstr Surg 1989; 83:997–1004.

19. Stevens WG, Cohen R, Vath SD, et al. Is it safe to combine abdominoplasty with elective breast surgery? A review of 151 consecutive cases. Plast Reconstr Surg 2006;118(1):207–12 [discussion: 213–4].

20. Teimourian B, Rogers BW III. A national survey of complications associated with suction lipectomy: a comparative study. Plast Reconstr Surg 1989; 84:628–31.

21. Stokes RB, Williams S. Does concomitant breast surgery add morbidity to abdominoplasty? Aesthet Surg J 2007;27:612–5.

22. Simon S, Thaller SR, Nathan N. Abdominoplasty combined with additional surgery: a safety issue. Aesthet Surg J 2006;26:413–6.

23. Wall S Jr. SAFE circumferential liposuction with abdominoplasty. Clin Plast Surg 2010;37:485–501.

24. Nahai FR. Anatomic considerations in abdominoplasty. Clin Plast Surg 2010;37(3):407–14.

25. Chin SH, Marin WJ, Matarasso A. Do waistline and umbilical position really change after abdominoplasty? Plast Reconstr Surg 2010;125(1):27e–8e.

26. Beran SJ. Combination procedures: balancing risk and reward. Aesthet Surg J 2006;26:443.

27. Stevens WG, Vath SD, Stoker DA. "Extreme" cosmetic surgery: a retrospective study of morbidity in patients undergoing combined procedures. Aesthet Surg J 2004;24:314–8.

28. Stevens WG, Repta R, Pacella SJ, et al. Safe and consistent outcomes of successfully combining breast surgery and abdominplasty: an update. Aesthet Surg J 2009;29:129–34.

29. Goldwyn RM. Abdominoplasty as a combined procedure: added benefit or double trouble? Plast Reconstr Surg 1986;78:383.

30. de Castro C, Cupella AM. Analysis of 60 cases of simultaneous mammoplasty and abdominoplasty. Aesthetic Plast Surg 1990;14:35–41.

31. Gutowski KA, Warner JP. Incorporating barbed sutures in abdominoplasty. Aesthet Surg J 2013; 33(3 Suppl):76s–81s.

32. Nahas FX, Ferreira LM. Concepts on correction of the musculoaponeurotic layer in abdominoplasty. Clin Plast Surg 2010;37(3):527–38.

33. Matarasso A. Awareness and avoidance of abdominoplasty complications. Aesthet Surg J 1997;17:256–61.

34. Velasco MG, Arizti P, Toca RG. Surgical correction of the "small" postpartum ptotic breast. Aesthet Surg J 2004;24:199–205.

35. Keyes GR, Singer R, Iverson RE, et al. Mortality in outpatient surgery. Plast Reconstr Surg 2008;122: 245–50.

36. Buck DW 2nd, Mustoe TA. An evidence-based approach to abdominoplsty. Plast Reconstr Surg 2010;126(6):2189–95.

37. Matarasso A, Levine SM. (Invited MOC Article). Liposuction; evidence based leading edge MOC. Plast Reconstr Surg 132(6):1697–705.

38. Hatef DA, Kenkel JM, Nguyen MQ, et al. Thromboembolic risk assessment and the efficacy of enoxaparin prophylaxis in excisional body contouring surgery. Plast Reconstr Surg 2008;122: 269–79.

39. Caprini JA, Arcelus JI, Reyna J. Effective risk stratification of surgical and nonsurgical patients for venous thromboembolic disease. Semin Hematol 2001;38:12–9.

40. Davison SP, Venturi ML, Attinger CE, et al. Prevention of venous thromboembolism in the plastic surgery patient. Plast Reconstr Surg 2004;114: 43e–51e.

41. Geerts WH, Pineo GF, Heit JA, et al. Prevention of venous thromboembolism the Seventh ACCP Conference on Antithrombotic and Thrombolytic Therapy. Chest 2004;126:338S–400S.

42. Broughton G II, Rios JL, Rohrich RJ, et al. Deep venous thrombosis prophylaxis practice and treatment strategies among plastic surgeons: survey results. Plast Reconstr Surg 2007;119:157–74.

43. Gravante G, Araco A, Sorge R, et al. Pulmonary embolism after combined abdominoplasty and flank liposuction: a correlation with the amount of fat removed. Ann Plast Surg 2008;60:604–8.

44. Murphy RX Jr, Alderman A, Gutowski K, et al. Evidence-based practices for thromboembolism prevention: summary of the ASPS venous thromboembolism task force report. Plast Reconstr Surg 2012;130: 168e–75e.

45. Spring MA, Gutowski KA. Venous thromboembolism in plastic surgery patients: survey results of plastic surgeons. Aesthet Surg J 2006;26:522–9.

46. Howland WS, Schweizer O. Complications associated with prolonged operation and anesthesia. Clin Anesth 1972;9:1–7.

47. Scott CF. Length of operation and morbidity: is there a relationship? Plast Reconstr Surg 1982;69: 1017–21.

48. Rambachan A, Mioton LM, Saha S, et al. Increased operative time is associated with higher complication rates in plastic surgery patients. Plast Reconstr Surg 2013;132:103.

49. Chung KC, Kotsis SV. Complications in surgery: root cause analysis and preventive measures. Plast Reconstr Surg 2012;129:1421.

50. Trussler AP, Tabbal GN. Patient safety in plastic surgery. Plast Reconstr Surg 2012;130:470e–8e.

51. Hatef DA, Trussler AP, Kenkel JM. Procedural risk for venous thromboembolism in abdominal contouring surgery: a systematic review of the literature. Plast Reconstr Surg 2010;125(1):356–62.

52. Jobin S, Kalliainen L, Adebayo L, et al. Venous thromboembolism prophylaxis. Bloomington (MN): Institute for Clinical Systems Improvement (ICSI); 2012.

53. Young VL, Watson ME. Continuing medical education article-patient safety: the need for venous thromboembolism (VTE) prophylaxis in plastic surgery. Aesthet Surg J 2006;26:157–75.

54. Warner JP, Gutowski KA. Abdominoplasty with progressive tension closure using a barbed suture technique. Aesthet Surg J 2009;29:221–5.

55. Baroudi R, Ferreira CA. Seroma: how to avoid it and how to treat it. Aesthet Surg J 1998;18:439–41.

56. Bercial ME, Neto MS, Calil JA, et al. Suction drains, quilting sutures, and fibrin sealant in the prevention of seroma formation in abdominoplasty: which is the best strategy? Aesthetic Plast Surg 2012;36:370–3.

57. Khan UD. Risk of seroma with simultaneous liposuction and abdominoplasty and the role of progressive tension sutures. Aesthetic Plast Surg 2008;32:93–9.

58. Nahas FX, Ferreira LM, Ghelfond C. Does quilting suture prevent seroma in abdominoplasty? Plast Reconstr Surg 2007;119:1060–4.

59. Nahas FX, di Martino M, Ferreira LM. Fibrin glue as a substitute for quilting suture in abdominoplasty. Plast Reconstr Surg 2012;129:212e–3e.

60. Pollock H, Pollock T. Progressive tension sutures: a technique to reduce local complications in abdominoplasty. Plast Reconstr Surg 2000;105:2583–6.

61. Mangano A. Seroma in lipoabdominoplasty and abdominoplasty: a comparative study using ultrasound - a note about statistics. Plast Reconstr Surg 2011;128(2):600–1.

62. Najera RM, Ashel W, Sayeed SM, et al. Comparison of seroma formation following abdominoplasty with or without liposuction. Plast Reconstr Surg 2011; 127(1):417–22.

63. Pollock TA, Pollock H. No-drain abdominoplasty with progressive tension sutures. Clin Plast Surg 2010;37(3):515–24.

64. Matarasso A, Schneider L, Barr J. The incidence and management of secondary abdominoplasty and secondary abdominal contour surgery. Plast Reconstr Surg 2014;133(1):40–50.

65. Matarasso A. Constantine F. Pain management for plastic surgery. Plast Reconstr Surg. (In press).

66. Core GB, Grotting JC. Reoperative surgery of the abdominal wall. Reoperative Aesthetic & Reconstructive Plastic Surgery. Grotting JC, editor. Second Edition. Quality Medical Publishing, St. Louis, Missouri, 2007 (44):1741–823, Vol II.

67. Matarasso A, Wallach SG, Rankin M, et al. Secondary abdominal contour surgery: a review of early and late reoperative surgery. Plast Reconstr Surg 2005;115(2):627–32.

The Fleur-De-Lis Abdominoplasty

Ryan Taylor Marshall Mitchell, MD, FRCSC[a], J. Peter Rubin, MD, FACS[b],*

KEYWORDS

- Fleur-de-lis abdominoplasty • Vertical abdominoplasty • Abdominal contour abnormalities

KEY POINTS

- Vertical abdominoplasty is a safe and effective procedure to correct abdominal contour abnormalities in individuals with excessive soft tissue in both the vertical and transverse orientation.
- The literature, although limited, supports the effectiveness of this procedure in addressing this clinical scenario.
- The complication rates are comparable to a standard transverse abdominoplasty.

BACKGROUND

A difficult aspect of abdominal contouring is the management of patients with excessive epigastric laxity. Once a unique clinical entity, this patient presentation has been on the rise.[1–4] As more and more individuals undergo bariatric-assisted weight loss, the acuity and severity of the associated weight reduction results in patients who are burdened by a pendulous pannus, rashes in skin folds, and chronic skin irritation or breakdown.[4–7] Further, changes to skin elasticity prevent retraction of the skin envelope, often seen in individuals with less severe weight loss associated with diet and exercise.[8] Unlike the typical abdominoplasty patient who has excessive skin and fat in the vertical orientation with minimal redundancy in the transverse direction, individuals with massive weight loss have excessive laxity in both the vertical and transverse axes. A common misconception is that the excessive laxity in the transverse axis will resolve with redraping of the abdominoplasty flap in a standard procedure. However, this is often underpowered and fails to address the redundant tissue of the upper abdomen, does not improve contour to the hip and flank region or narrow the waist, and often leaves behind surgical dog-ears at the extent of the transverse incision.[2,6,9,10] Since its early description in 1967,[11] and subsequently popularized by Dellon in 1985,[12] the vertical abdominoplasty has remained a valuable tool in the armamentarium for body contour surgery. The inclusion of a vertical component to the resection pattern allows the surgeon the ability to directly excise the redundant soft tissue in the midline while simultaneously contouring the lateral hips and flank. Although there have been minor modifications to the classic description of the vertical abdominoplasty, the general principles of the procedure have stood the test of time.

To prevent both the patient and surgeon from being displeased with the outcome of an abdominal-contouring procedure, a comprehensive preoperative examination is essential to identify the degree of redundancy in the transverse axis. Further, this physical examination also identifies any preexisting abdominal scars that may potentially be excised within the vertical extension of the procedure.

PATIENT SELECTION

The ideal patient is often one who has undergone significant weight loss in a short period of time,[9]

[a] The Bengtson Center for Aesthetics and Plastic Surgery, 555 Midtowne Street NE Suite 110, Grand Rapids, Michigan 49503, USA; [b] Department of Plastic Surgery, University of Pittsburgh, Scaife Hall, 3550 Terrace Street, Pittsburgh, Pennsylvania, USA
* Corresponding author.
E-mail address: rubinjp@upmc.edu

Clin Plastic Surg 41 (2014) 673–680
http://dx.doi.org/10.1016/j.cps.2014.07.007
0094-1298/14/$ – see front matter © 2014 Elsevier Inc. All rights reserved.

manifests skin redundancy as a result of multiple pregnancies,[13] or has preexisting widened midline scars.[14] The speed and magnitude associated with massive weight loss secondary to bariatric procedures results in a moderate to severe excess of skin and epigastric laxity in the vertical and transverse axis. Further, the presence of preexisting abdominal scarring allows the surgeon an opportunity to revise (midline vertical scar) or completely remove the scar (eg, subcostal or port site).[14,15] However, as with all body-contouring procedures, the patient must be aware of the tradeoff of scar burden with effective contouring, and this procedure should be considered contraindicated in individuals who are unwilling to accept a midline vertical scar. Further, the additional scar poses concerns regarding wound healing in poor candidates. Care needs to be taken with individuals who have preexisting medical comorbidities, such as smoking, diabetes, immune compromise, and morbid obesity. The main concern regarding the vertical abdominoplasty is the potential for wound compromise at the intersection of the vertical and transverse extension of the resection margins, commonly referred to as the T-junction. In a prospective review of individuals with massive weight loss (more than 50-pound weight loss) undergoing abdominal-contouring procedures, 31% underwent a vertical component to the procedure.[3] There was a statistically significant difference ($P = .03$) in the number of men (18%) versus women (33%) who underwent this approach.

The preoperative assessment is broken down into 2 separate visits. In the initial visit, a thorough medical history and physical examination is conducted. Medical comorbidities pertinent to the procedure are documented both before and after the significant weight loss. The mechanism of weight loss is obtained, as is the highest, lowest, and current body mass index (BMI). The duration of the stability of the patient's current weight is noted, as is its deviation from the goal body weight. A physical examination noting the pattern and distribution of adipose tissue, the quality of the overlying skin, and the laxity of the surrounding soft tissue is performed. After consideration of all these factors in conjunction with the patient's own wishes and desires, a surgical recommendation is made. The patient is then given time to reflect on the surgical plan. As needed, the patient also has the opportunity to further reduce his or her BMI, trial topical therapies for persistent rashes, and stop tobacco use. The patient is brought back for a second consultation where any additional questions are answered and the informed consent is discussed at greater length. Potential complications are discussed, including

injury or loss of the umbilicus, malposition of the umbilicus, numbness in the lower and midline abdomen, wound separation, skin loss, change in pubic hair shape and/or hair loss, abdominal tightness, prolonged pain, presence of surgical "dog-ears," contour irregularity, failure to relieve symptoms of back pain or rashes, seroma formation, visible scars in the vertical and horizontal position, and extension of the scar superiorly onto the chest.

SURGICAL TECHNIQUE

The initial approach to the vertical abdominoplasty is similar to that of the traditional procedure. The inferior incision is marked 6 cm cephalad from the anterior vulvar commissure with the tissues on stretch. A midline reference mark is placed extending from the sternum to the inferior incision. The right and left lateral extent of the skin roll is identified and the lateral extent of the excision is marked. This mark is placed on the apex of the lateral hip roll to prevent dog-ear formation in the subsequent closure. The preoperative marks at the midline and lateral extents are connected to form the full extent of the inferior incision (**Fig. 1**). In the population with massive weight loss, this mark is often inferior to the inguinal ligament lateral to the mons; however, with resection of the overhanging pannus, the final position of this scar is pulled to a more superior position as a result of tensile forces from the abdominal closure. A pinch

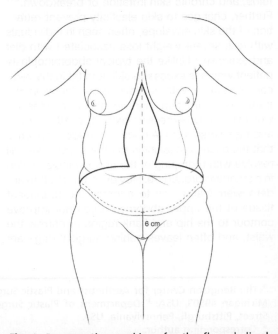

Fig. 1. Preoperative markings for the fleur-de-lis abdominoplasty. The area of resection is estimated and then confirmed during the procedure.

test in the vertical axis is marked as an estimate for soft tissue resection.

In the operative room, the patient is placed in the supine position and the abdomen is prepped and draped. 1 mg of 1/1000 epinephrine is diluted in 100 mL of saline, and 20 to 40 mL is injected along the preoperative markings. In the mons region, the incision is carried down directly down to the deep fascia. Laterally, the superficial inferior epigastric artery and superficial inferior epigastric vein vessels are identified and ligated. As the incision is carried out laterally, care must be taken in the population with massive weight loss, particularly when the preoperative marking is inferior to the inguinal ligament. In this situation, dissection is carried superficially in the cephalad direction beyond the inguinal ligament. Once this level has been reached, the plane of dissection is deepened to the muscle fascia. If plication is indicated, the dissection is carried in the fascial plane centrally. If plication is not warranted, subcutaneous fat may be preserved over the rectus fascia at the discretion of the surgeon. Lateral abdominal flap dissection is conducted to allow for adequate re-draping of the abdominal flap for an esthetic contour. Care is taken not to undermine beyond the level required to accomplish this, as it adds to the degree of surgical dead space, increases the potential for seroma formation, and increases the potential for wound complications as a result of disrupted cutaneous perforators. If further undermining is required, this can be carried out indirectly through the use of discontinuous undermining via a blunt liposuction cannula. The umbilicus is dissected free of the abdominal flap, taking care not to denude the fat from the umbilical stalk. The operative table is then placed in a flexed position and the superior extent of the resection is determined with a flap marking technique; an inverted towel clip placed on the inferior incision edge can be transposed under the flap and palpated. Final scar placement is checked for symmetry and the transverse component of the abdominoplasty is excised first. Attention is then directed to the vertical component. In order to prevent distraction of the transverse incision line while marking the final vertical resection, the transverse resection margins are closed with towel clips. Starting from a level just caudal to the xiphoid process, the estimation of the vertical resection is checked with a pinch test (**Fig. 2**). At the inferior margin of the vertical pattern, the marking is biased back toward the midline to preserve tissue at the T-junction. The pattern can be viewed as a true "fleur-de-lis" in its orientation. The intended incision lines are then injected with the epinephrine solution and incised with the plane of resection

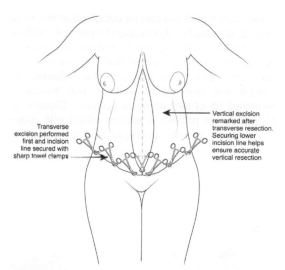

Fig. 2. The transverse resection is performed first and closed temporarily with sharp towel clips. The location of the T-junction is set and secured with a towel clip. With the horizontal suture line secured, a pinch test will estimate the vertical extension resection margins.

directed cautiously so as to not undermine the abdominal flaps outside of the area of resection. Unnecessary undermining of the abdominal flaps disrupts the direct cutaneous perforators and increases the risk of wound complications (**Fig. 3**).

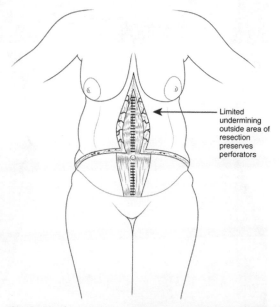

Fig. 3. Final resection pattern in the fleur-de-lis abdominoplasty. Limited undermining outside of the area of resection preserves the perforating vessels adjacent to the vertical excision and improves the viability of the triple-point skin flaps.

Subcutaneous tissue can be debulked at the most cephalad extent of the incision to prevent contour irregularities and dog-ear formation. The T-junction is then tailor tacked in both the vertical and horizontal directions and can be adjusted to ensure the optimal amount of soft tissue is removed to obtain an ideal contour. Closure of the resection pattern is accomplished with reapproximation of the superficial fascial system at the level of the mons beginning with the transverse incision. If there is tissue thickness discrepancy, or the mons is in an inferiorly displaced position, the mons area can be debulked with direct fat excision and suspended to the abdominal wall fascia. Drainage tubes are placed in the abdominal dead space and the vertical limb is then closed with a deep layer approximating the superficial fascial system. To prevent excess widening of the

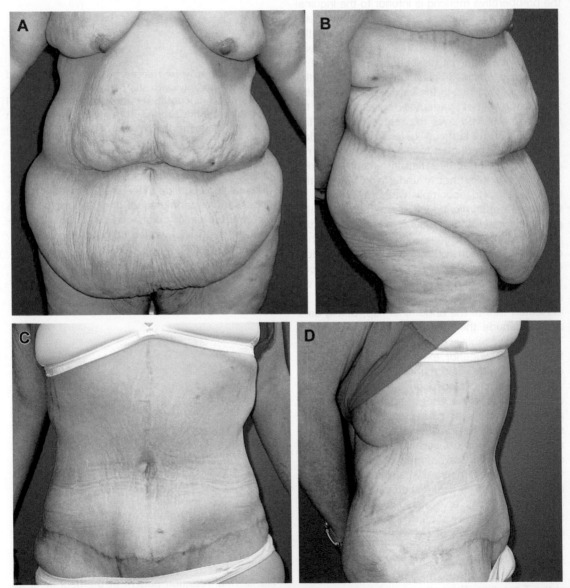

Fig. 4. Case 1: 33-year-old woman with Roux-En-Y bypass. BMI reduction from 70.7 to 37.4 was associated with resolution of sleep apnea, hypertension, diabetes, and gastroesophageal reflux disease. (*A*) Preoperative anteroposterior (AP) view. (*B*) Preoperative lateral view. (*C*) Nine-month postoperative AP view. (*D*) Nine-month postoperative lateral view.

umbilicus, the umbilicus is inset directly into the vertical closure without additional skin excision. Final skin closure is obtained with a running intradermal barbed suture.

POSTOPERATIVE MANAGEMENT

On completion of the procedure, the patient is maintained in a flexed position and transferred from the operative table to the stretcher. The stretcher is adjusted to maintain flexion at the hips. An abdominal binder is placed. Drain output is monitored and the drains are removed when the output is less than 30 mL over a 24-hour period. When the drains are removed, the patient can

transition into a compression garment for a total period of 4 to 6 weeks. Aggressive physical activity is also minimized during the recovery period of 4 to 6 weeks.

OUTCOMES AND COMPLICATIONS

Previous reports have suggested the superiority of a vertical abdominoplasty in obtaining an ideal cosmetic result In the population with massive weight loss and epigastric skin excess.[3,9,14,16] As stated, the main concern with this operative procedure is a theoretic increase in wound-related complications, particularly at the T-junction. The overall complication rate for this procedure is not

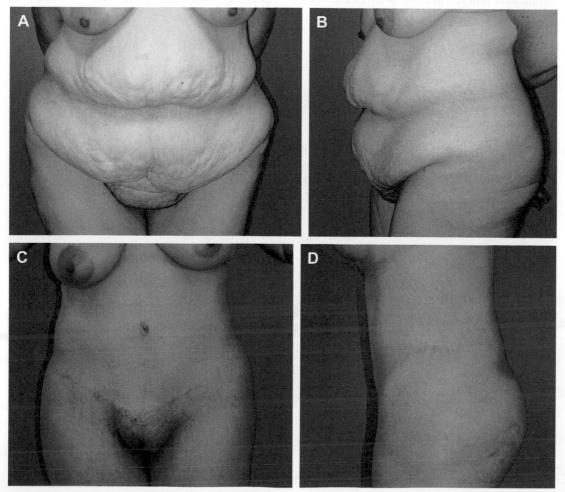

Fig. 5. Case 2: 42-year-old woman with gastric bypass who underwent Fleur-De-Lis abdominoplasty with circumferential lower body lift. (*A*) Preoperative AP view. (*B*) Preoperative lateral view. (*C*) 5 year postoperative AP view. (*D*) 5 year postoperative lateral view.

well described in the literature because of small patient populations relative to studies focused on the standard abdominoplasty. However, with the rise in bariatric surgery, and the subsequent rise in individuals with massive weight loss who are seeking contour correction, the patient demographic is expanding. In the limited literature, the most common complications encountered with this procedure are wound dehiscence, infection, hematoma, seroma, and skin necrosis.[2,3,9,14,17,18] It is difficult to compare the complication rates between the vertical abdominoplasty and the traditional abdominoplasty, as the patient demographics between the 2 populations vary widely. Most of the data regarding vertical abdominoplasties is from the population with massive weight loss, with complication rates ranging from 3.0% to 35.5%,[3,4,6,9,16,17] and is heavily influenced by preoperative BMI, absolute change in BMI, smoking status, and coexisting medical conditions. A comparative analysis in 2010[3] showed that within

a population with massive weight loss, the transverse and vertical abdominoplasty had similar rates of complications (30.5% for vertical abdominoplasty vs 24.6% for traditional abdominoplasty) with no statistical difference regarding major complications (5% overall). In multivariate analysis, the vertical abdominoplasty procedure was associated with a statistically significant increase in wound infection. However, wound dehiscence, hematoma, seroma, and skin necrosis rates were similar between the 2 groups.

SUMMARY

Vertical abdominoplasty is a safe and effective procedure to correct abdominal contour abnormalities in individuals with excessive soft tissue in both the vertical and transverse orientation (**Figs. 4–6**). The literature, although limited, supports the effectiveness of this procedure in addressing this clinical scenario. Further, the

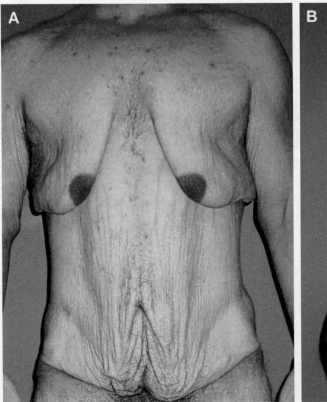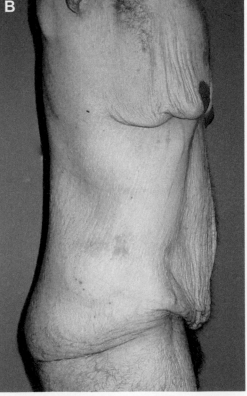

Fig. 6. Case 3: 26-year-old male with weight loss through diet and exercise. Fleur-De-Lis abdominoplasty was performed as part of staged plan along with gynecomastia correction, brachioplasty, and lower body lift. (*A*) Preoperative AP view. (*B*) Preoperative lateral view.

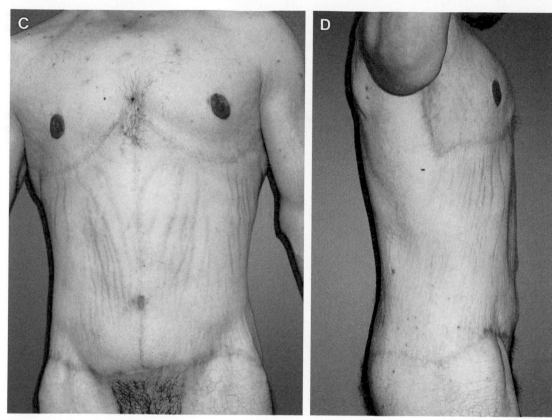

Fig. 6. (*continued*). 26-year-old male with weight loss through diet and exercise. Fleur-De-Lis abdominoplasty was performed as part of staged plan along with gynecomastia correction, brachioplasty, and lower body lift. (*C*) Ten-month postoperative AP view. (*D*) Ten-month postoperative lateral view.

complication rates are comparable to a standard transverse abdominoplasty.

REFERENCES

1. Strauch B, Herman C, Rohde C, et al. Mid-body contouring in the post-bariatric surgery patient. Plast Reconstr Surg 2006;117(7):2200–11.
2. Wallach SG. Abdominal contour surgery for the massive weight loss patient: the Fleur-de-Lis approach. Aesthet Surg J 2005;25(5):454–65.
3. Friedman T, O'Brien Coon D, Michaels J, et al. Fleur-de-Lis abdominoplasty: a safe alternative to traditional abdominoplasty for the massive weight loss patient. Plast Reconstr Surg 2010;125(5):1525–35.
4. Borud LJ, Warren AG. Modified vertical abdominoplasty in the massive weight loss patient. Plast Reconstr Surg 2007;119(6):1911–21.
5. Greco JA, Castaldo ET, Nanney LB, et al. The effect of weight loss surgery and body mass index on wound complications after abdominal contouring operations. Ann Plast Surg 2008;61(3): 235–42.
6. Moya AP, Sharma D. A modified technique combining vertical and high lateral incisions for abdominal-to-hip contouring following massive weight loss in persistently obese patients. J Plast Reconstr Aesthet Surg 2009;62(1):56–64.
7. Fraccalvieri M, Datta G, Bogetti P, et al. Abdominoplasty after weight loss in morbidly obese patients: a 4 year clinical experience. Obes Surg 2007;17: 1319–24.
8. Ramsey-Stewart G. Radical "Fleur-de-Lis" abdominoplasty after bariatric surgery. Obes Surg 1993;3: 410–4.
9. Costa LF, Landecker A, Manta AM. Optimizing body contour in massive weight loss patients: the modified vertical abdominoplasty. Plast Reconstr Surg 2004;114(7):1917–23.
10. Young S, Freiberg A. A critical look at abdominal lipectomy following morbid obesity surgery. Aesthetic Plast Surg 1991;15:81–4.
11. Castanares S, Goethel JA. Abdominal lipectomy: a modification in technique. Plast Reconstr Surg 1967;40:378–83.
12. Dellon AL. Fleur-de-lis abdominoplasty. Aesthetic Plast Surg 1985;9:27–32.

13. Sugarbaker PH. Vertical abdominoplasty. J Surg Oncol 2001;78(3):217–9.

14. Rieger UM, Erba P, Kalbermatten DF, et al. An individualized approach to abdominoplasty in the presence of bilateral subcostal scars after open gastric bypass. Obes Surg 2008;18(7):863–9.

15. de Castro CC, Salema R, Aboudib JH. T abdominoplasty to remove multiple scars from the abdomen. Ann Plast Surg 1984;12:269–73.

16. Duff CG, Aslam S, Griffiths RW. Fleur-de-Lys abdominoplasty—a consecutive case series. Br J Plast Surg 2003;56(6):557–66.

17. Chaouat M, Levan P, Lalanne B, et al. Abdominal dermolipectomies: early postoperative complications and long-term unfavorable results. Plast Reconstr Surg 2000;106(7):1614–8.

18. Beraka GJ. Modified vertical abdominoplasty in the massive weight loss patient. Plast Reconstr Surg 2008;121(2):686.

Two Position Comprehensive Approach to Abdominoplasty

Renato Saltz, MD, FACS

KEYWORDS

- Abdominoplasty • Body contouring • Preoperative planning • Positive outcomes

KEY POINTS

- The two position comprehensive abdominoplasty is a powerful and safe body sculpturing tool.
- In combination with other body contouring procedures, abdominoplasty can lead to a comprehensive body transformation; anatomic, physiologic, and psychological.
- Ultimately, a combined procedure should be attempted with a clean preoperative workup and by a surgical team who can complete multiple procedures in an efficient and timely fashion.
- Postoperative care should include instructions for early ambulation and adequate analgesia.
- Consistent application of safe practices is paramount in maximizing positive outcomes and minimizing negative events.

 Six abdominoplasty videos accompany this article, showing the Author's approach to:
1) Liposuction; 2) Patient turning; 3) Tunnel Undermining; 4) Sharp knife dissection;
5) Sharp lipectomy; and 6) Umbilical location.

INTRODUCTION

Globalization and the Internet, with easy exchange of news, technology, and ideas, have had a significant impact on medicine, especially on esthetic plastic surgery.

The impact on esthetic plastic surgery is mostly observed by the decrease and sometimes elimination of "the esthetic cultural divide," which for so long separated facial and body contouring standards in different societies kept apart by traditions, geography, customs, and old habits.

The concept of beauty no longer follows traditional cultural/geographic patterns but is now mostly determined by modern universal trends often dictated by the fashion and entertainment industry and distributed worldwide through highly sought magazines, Web sites, and the multitude of social media venues now available.

The free international exchange of new ideas and innovative techniques has allowed patients to identify themselves with many international models and celebrities and seek improvements in facial and body contouring beyond their traditional cultural and geographic differences.

The ideal modern "global woman" has a very similar shape and size of breasts, contouring of the abdomen, shape and definition of the extremities, and projection of the buttocks. From the original soft and delicate abdomens of Botticelli and other renaissance artists, patients now seek a much more defined etched, toned, flat abdomen. The two-position body contouring surgeon must be aware of the concept of the "global woman" and remain in tune with the modern concepts of abdominoplasty and body contouring surgery. Names of famous top models and actresses like Gisele Bundchen, Jennifer Lopez, Kim Kardashian, and others are often mentioned during the body contouring consultation. As long as patient expectations are reasonable and results are achievable, the esthetic body contouring surgeon's failure to recognize this "new normal" of the ideal torso will compromise his/her ability to offer the patient's desired result and lose the patient to another colleague.

Saltz Plastic Surgery & Spa Vitória, Salt Lake City and Park City, Utah, USA
E-mail address: rsaltz@saltzplasticsurgery.com

Clin Plastic Surg 41 (2014) 681–704
http://dx.doi.org/10.1016/j.cps.2014.07.008

This article illustrates details of the two position comprehensive abdominoplasty and provides safety tips for the young and also for the experienced body contouring surgeon. Preoperative tips on patient clinical and anatomic evaluation combined with a full medical clearance will help the surgeon provide a safe and excellent result. Detailed and well-illustrated intraoperative pearls will allow well-trained esthetic surgeons to easily duplicate the technique and obtain excellent results.

Postoperative care and safety issues related to abdominoplasty and combined body contouring procedures are also included to help the reader make the right selection for each individual patient and to obtain better and safer results.

The ultimate goal of this article is to provide the body contouring surgeon with the necessary tools for an optimal surgical result, fulfilling patient expectations by using state-of the-art modern and safe techniques in abdominoplasty.

HISTORY OF ABDOMINOPLASTY

Abdominoplasty was first described by Callia, and since then, many refinements have been published in the literature. Most recently, important contributions from Illouz with his "mesh undermining" by performing liposuction of the abdomen and then "end-block" removal of all infraumbilical tissue in selected patients started a new era in abdominoplasty. Matarasso described the treatment of different abdominal regions with major and minor risk of liposuction at the same time of the abdominoplasty. Avelar demonstrated a new technique for abdominoplasty by combining liposuction with a subdermal flap folded over itself. Suldanha combined many of these innovative and provocative techniques with his stellar contribution, lipoabdominoplasty, where liposuction of the abdomen was combined to rectus muscle plication through selective and safe undermining of the abdominal flap in the supraumbilical area by preserving the lateral rectus muscle perforators, thus increasing blood supply to the abdominal flap and its survival, decreasing the incidence of seroma and other complications of traditional abdominoplasty.

GOALS OF THE TWO POSITION COMPREHENSIVE ABDOMINOPLASTY

The goals of two position abdominoplasty include a total remodeling of the torso in a 360-degree view, the creation of a well-defined upper and lateral abdomen, a neo-supraumbilical sulcus, a small vertical "mysterious," attractive new umbilicus, a well-defined, symmetric and perfectly located low inconspicuous abdominal scar, and

a prepubic area that matches the anterior abdominal contouring with the prepubic (vulvar) tissue slightly rotated in a more cephalic position (Fig. 1). This technique can improve urinary and sexual functions in addition to a better cosmetic result. With the patient in a sitting position, one should see a much narrower waistline combined with a central depression at the level of the umbilicus, no "dog ears" at the end of the abdominal incision, and a continuous smooth transition from lower abdomen to prepubic area (Fig. 2). The rectus diastasis should be completely repaired, enhancing or eliminating the abdominal bulge on the lateral view and narrowing the transition of the lateral rectus to the external oblique aponeurosis in the frontal view (Fig. 3). Finally, the entire back should have a completely new definition with elimination of the lipodystrophies of the flanks as well as improving the hourglass figure and feminine appearance of the female torso (Fig. 4).

PRE-OPERATIVE PREPARATION

The safety issues related to the two position abdominoplasty start during the consultation. Patients are fully analyzed as to physical, intellectual, psychological, and financial aspects. All these aspects play an important role in the outcome of their surgery. Reasonable expectations are of paramount importance because much of the ultimate goal and results of the procedure will depend on patient health, understanding the limitations of the procedure, and intense cooperation before and after their surgery. Their daily habits regarding work, family, diet, and exercises are fully recognized by the surgeon and can impact the short-term and long-term outcome. A complete physical and full medical evaluation by their own internist is carefully reviewed by the surgical team. If necessary, anesthesia clearance is requested before surgery. More detailed workups are necessary in cases of a higher-risk patient, such as family history of deep venous thrombosis and pulmonary embolism (DVT/PE), hypertension, diabetes, in combined body contouring procedures. Patients are instructed regarding the postoperative care and the necessary help at home during the first few days after surgery. Ideal body mass index (BMI) is critical for the overall safety of abdominoplasty. If necessary, patients are referred to a nutritionist and a personal trainer in an attempt to bring their weight down to a safer BMI.

PATIENT MARKINGS

Preoperative pictures are taken during the preoperative visit. On the day of surgery, the patient is

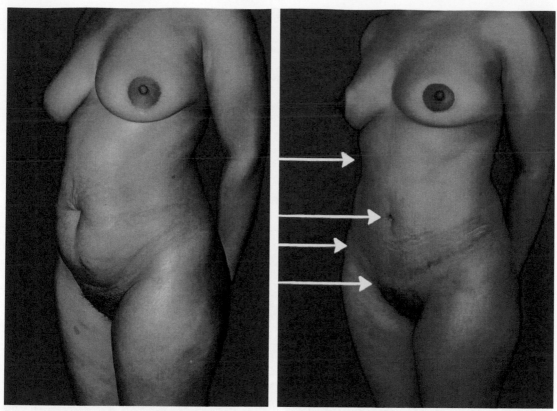

Fig. 1. Before and after combined procedure: abdominoplasty, liposuction of the back and flanks, and masto-pexy. Arrows from top to bottom outline the improved contoured flanks, small "mysterious" umbilicus, lower abdominal inconspicuous scar with excellent symmetry, and simultaneous lifting of prepubic area, restoring pre-pregnancy "natural anatomy."

marked in a standing position starting with the up-per back, lower back, and flank lipodystrophic areas. The upper and lower abdomen are also marked in a standing position, by defining the mar-gins of the lateral rectus diastasis, external oblique aponeurosis, the abdominal midline with a straight line from xiphoid to the pubis, and the excess of skin and fat in the lower abdomen. With the patient in a semi-sitting position at the edge of the oper-ating room table, the lowest abdominal crease, anterior superior iliac spine, and the most lateral aspect of the abdominal incision is marked, which should match the most lateral skin fold of the abdomen. This minor detail will avoid "dog ears" often seen in the postoperative period and requiring late revisions. After general anesthesia, airway control, and the patient in a supine position, the markings are finalized by placing the lowest portion of the abdominal incision at approximately 6 to 7 cm from the labia major vertex.

ANATOMIC PEARLS

Anatomic details of importance in the two position comprehensive abdominoplasty as emphasized

by Saldanha include preservation of the scarpa's fascia in the abdominal flap for increased blood supply to the dermis and skin. Also, by performing a selective tunnel undermining (instead of total undermining) over the rectus diastasis, only pre-serving the lateral rectus muscle perforators, 80% of the blood supply to the abdominal wall is protected (**Figs. 5** and **6**), thus reducing complica-tions when compared with traditional abdomino-plasty and also combined bariatric surgery (Video 3).

ANESTHESIA

General anesthesia should always be used in body contouring procedures. Excellent control of the airway is critical because the patient is moved and turned a great deal during the procedure: initially from supine to prone when transferred from stretcher to the surgical table for the back liposuction portion of the procedure and later back to a supine position for the abdominoplasty portion of the procedure. Compression boots (sequential compression devices) are in place before induction, continued in the recovery room,

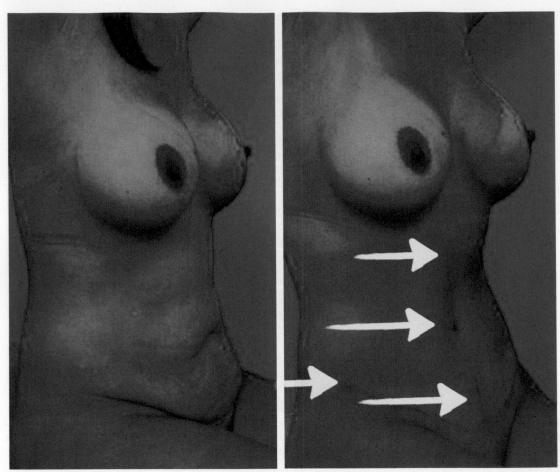

Fig. 2. Before and after "sit-down position" after combined procedure: abdominoplasty, liposuction back and flanks, implant exchange, and capsulotomies. Arrows from top to bottom outline the supraumbilical midline sulcus, a small, "mysterious" umbilicus. The length of the lower abdominal scar is determined by the location and length of the most lateral skin fold, and the infraumbilical short vertical scar from previous umbilical location is strategically placed below the top of the bikini line.

and during the overnight stay. All patients are kept warm with the use of a warm blanket and warm fluids. Hypothermia, a common problem in prolonged body contouring procedures with significant body exposure, can be completely avoided or prevented if appropriate preventative measures are taken at all times.

PATIENT POSITIONING

Once the patient is intubated and the endotracheal tube is secured, the patient is carefully placed in a prone position with padding under the arms, breasts, and hips. The table is flexed and the reverse Trendelenburg position is applied to avoid the head being down for prolonged periods and to avoid significant facial swelling (**Fig. 7**). At this point, warm tumescent solution is injected through 1 or 2 small incisions on the back. The superior midline incision is placed at the level of the

brassiere and the inferior midline incision at the top portion of the intragluteal fold. This process is followed by preparing and draping of the surgical area. After adequate time to allow the tumescent solution to work, the liposuction is completed in all of the premarked areas using the power-assisted liposuction system. If fat injection is anticipated, fat collection is done during this part of the procedure (Video 1).

PATIENT TURNING

Patient turning is a critical part of two position comprehensive abdominoplasty surgery. It is done by a well-trained team in a safe and quick manner by protecting the airway, intravenous sites, and all patient extremities. The author uses a draw sheet and 4 team members to perform this part of the procedure. An effective and safe turning should be done in less than 15 seconds by protecting the

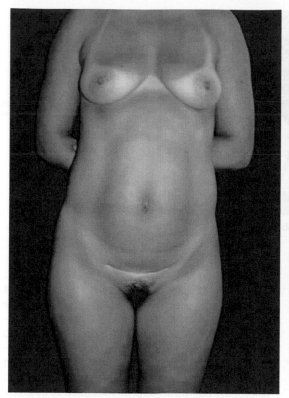
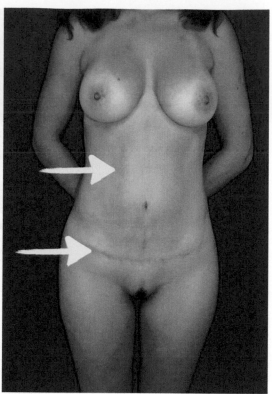

Fig. 3. Before and after combined procedure: abdominoplasty with repair of large rectus diastasis, liposuction of back and flanks, breast augmentation. Arrows from top to bottom outline improvement of the rectus lateral margin after diastasis repair, with well-healed scar with excellent placement below the bikini line.

patient, the airway, intravenous lines, and all other important accessories of the operation (Video 2).

Once turning is completed, the abdominal markings are double-checked and only then injected with vasoconstriction solution. The patient is re-prepared and redraped. Team members scrub again and change gowns and gloves. Before

making the first cut, incision marking symmetry is verified by the *"triangulation technique."* The triangulation technique consists of 2-0 silk sutures placed above the xyphoid and above the pubic bone that are then "triangulated" using a hemostat. Moving the hemostat from corner to corner helps to verify the markings' symmetry as well as

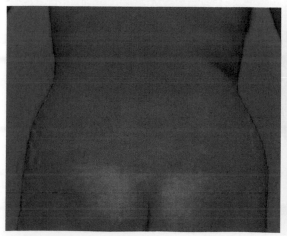
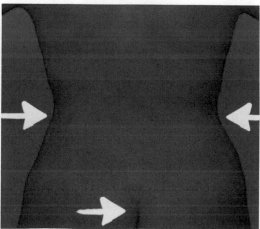

Fig. 4. Improved waist contouring and waistline after liposuction of the upper and lower back, with placement of incision at intragluteal fold.

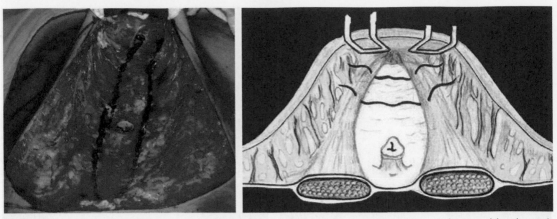

Fig. 5. Selective and safe undermining of the superior abdomen for preservation of the perforating blood vessels. (*Courtesy* of Dr. Saldanha.)

the perfect midline for future umbilical repositioning (**Fig. 8**).

The first incision is around the umbilicus. By using 2 single hooks at 12 and 6 o'clock, the umbilicus is incised with a number 11 blade. Dissection is carried down to the anterior fascia in a perpendicular fashion by using a Metzenbaum scissors and preserving a small amount of periumbilical tissue to improve umbilical blood supply. Complete undermining and defatting of the umbilicus can compromise its blood supply and create unnecessary postoperative complications, such as partial tissue necrosis, persistent drainage, and hypertrophic scarring with later umbilical scar contracture. At this point, the surgeon must judge the ability to resect the entire abdominal flap (en bloc), or if a partial resection will be preferable. In this case, a midline infraumbilical scar from the original umbilical excision site will result. If in doubt, it is

recommended to incise the upper abdomen first. During the dissection, a narrow undermining of the midline by preserving the lateral rectus muscle perforators is critical (see **Fig. 5**). The supraumbilical tunnel is undermined all the way above the xiphoid process, preserving the lateral neurovascular bundles that support the abdominal flap (see **Fig. 6**). Once the entire supraumbilical flap is free, the pull-down approach is used to estimate where the inferior flap or the lower resection can be made en bloc and without much tension. This maneuver is critical to determine whether the defect can be closed without stretching or putting tension on the lower abdominal scar. The risk of elevating the prepubic hair to the lower abdomen must be avoided at all times. The author tests the pull-down approach without flexing the table. The entire lower abdominal flap is then elevated off the anterior abdominal aponeurosis and

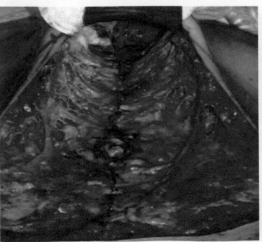
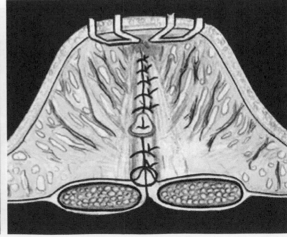

Fig. 6. Plication of rectus diastasis should not go beyond the lateral border of the abdominal rectus muscle to preserve perforators. (*Courtesy* of Dr. Saldanha.)

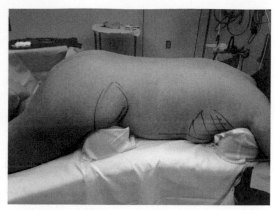

Fig. 7. Initial patient prone position ready for tumescent infiltration: surgical table flexed with padded hips, breasts, knees, and arms. Heating blanket is used below the knees and above the upper back immediately after patient is prepared.

discarded. In case the pull-down test fails, the patient will require an infraumbilical midline scar and a partial excision of the lower abdominal flap.

TREATMENT OF THE RECTUS DIASTASIS

The rectus muscle diastasis is identified and 2 lines are drawn from the xiphoid appendix to the suprapubic area. Any supraumbilical, infraumbilical, or umbilical hernias must be identified and treated appropriately. An interrupted layer following by a running layer of 0- Prolene® sutures are used to repair the diastasis. The knots are buried to avoid any postoperative complaints. At this point, the plication is evaluated as well as the position and laxity of external oblique aponeurosis at the junction of the lateral abdominal rectus muscle. If there is persistent laxity at this level, advancement of external oblique aponeurosis is indicated as demonstrated by Psillakis and de la Plaza in their color atlas of esthetic surgery of the abdomen. Plication of the rectus diastasis should not go beyond the lateral border of the abdominal rectus muscle perforators (**Figs. 9–13**).

ABDOMINAL FLAP THINNING

Shaping and contouring of the flank areas is best and safely achieved by sharp lipectomy. The scarpa's layer is identified by a perpendicular retraction of the superior abdominal flap and by pulling the lower abdominal flap until the scarpa's layer is identified laterally (**Fig. 14**). Sharp knife dissection under tension is then carried out below the scarpa's layer, removing a uniform thick layer of fat (Video 4). The intact scarpa's fascia is

Fig. 8. Triangulation technique with silk sutures at xyphoid and pubic bone. It is helpful to check markings for symmetry, final scar symmetry, and midline position for proper new umbilical scar placement.

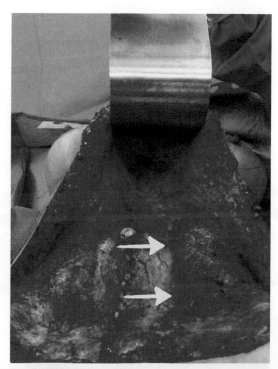

Fig. 9. Midline plication had been completed, and lateral rectus muscle perforators are preserved, with identification of lateral abdomen laxity at defining the external oblique muscle aponeurosis.

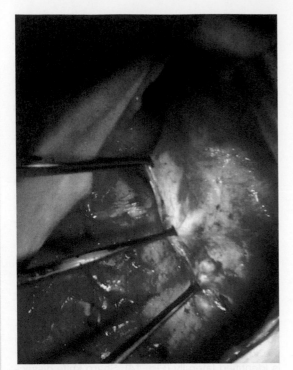

Fig. 10. Incision of the external oblique muscle aponeurosis.

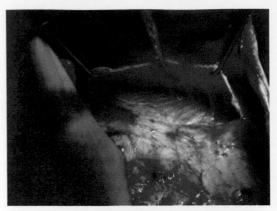

Fig. 12. External oblique muscle aponeurosis free for advancement.

protected and maintained with the abdominal flap (**Figs. 15** and **16**). This maneuver, known as "sharp lipectomy," helps to thin the flap and better define and contour the lateral abdomen (Video 5).

UMBILICAL PLACEMENT AND FIXATION

Ribeiro and Saltz recommend very specific shape, size, and location for the umbilicus in most patients while performing an abdominoplasty. They have defined the exact location, the width, length, and depth of the new umbilicus based on

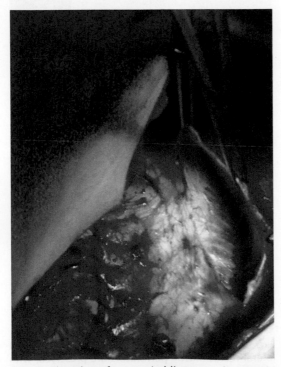

Fig. 11. Elevation of external oblique muscle aponeurosis preserving neurovascular supply to the muscle.

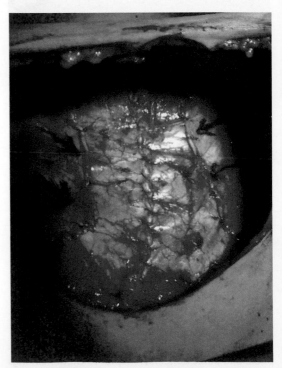

Fig. 13. External oblique muscle aponeurosis advanced bilaterally.

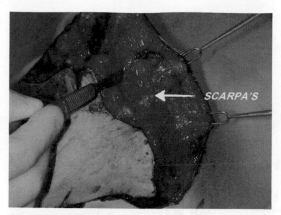

Fig. 14. Identifying scarpa's fascia.

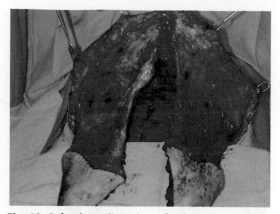

Fig. 16. Safe plane dissection of subcutaneous tissue below scarpa's fascia (*anterior view*).

measurements and ratios between xiphoid process, symphysis pubis, and anterior superior iliac spine to the umbilicus, all recorded in a large South and North American population. The umbilicus is first secured to the abdominal fascia at 12, 6, 3, and 9 o'clock after completion of the rectus diastasis plication. In case one cannot remove the entire lower abdominal flap, it is better to turn the old umbilical scar into a vertical scar at the infraumbilical lower abdominal midline area. A short infraumbilical midline scar is always better tolerated by the patient than a tight suprapubic closure with possible pubic hair migrating cephalic, resulting in hair growing in the lower abdomen. The author recommendations are to avoid flexing the table, avoid pulling the supraumbilical flap too hard, and avoid "forcing" the supraumbilical flap. The umbilical scar should be placed where it wants to go (**Figs. 17–20**).

PAIN CONTROL, DRAINS, AND THE UMBILICAL LOCATOR

Before closing the lower abdominal wound, drains, pain pumps, or fascia injections of Exparel®

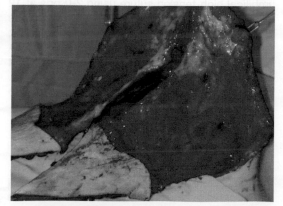

Fig. 15. Safe plane dissection of subcutaneous tissue below scarpa's fascia (*lateral view*).

(bupivacaine liposome injectable suspension) and the umbilical locator are placed. The drains are extended to the lower back and brought out through the suprapubic area. They drain the liposuctioned areas and lower abdomen, therefore decreasing the amount of swelling and bruising in the lower back. During the early postoperative period, the author recommends the drains be on low suction during the recovery room stay and overnight admission.

The pain pump catheters are placed at the junction of the lateral rectus aponeurosis and the medial external oblique aponeurosis. Catheters are then brought out at the corners of the incision. If one elects to use Exparel®, the injections should follow the manufacturer's recommendations and cover the rectus aponeurosis, external oblique aponeurosis (if the extended technique was used), and around the incision sites.

The midline supraumbilical sulcus is developed by a very narrow tunnel made with a 4-mm liposuction cannula. This maneuver is followed by advancement and plication of the midline soft tissues to the fascia underneath the xiphoid to the umbilicus using interrupted sutures. It defines the upper abdomen and closes the dead space, avoiding future seroma formation in that area.

The umbilical locator is then secured to the umbilicus with nylon sutures at 12 and 6 o'clock (see **Fig. 22**). The abdominal flap is pulled down and approximated at the lower abdominal incision with temporary staples.

ABDOMINAL CLOSURE

With the patient in a semi-sitting position, the patient is observed for extra skin or fat in the lower aspects of the incision. Treatment of future "dog ears" is done at this point by liposuction and/or skin incision with extension of the final lateral

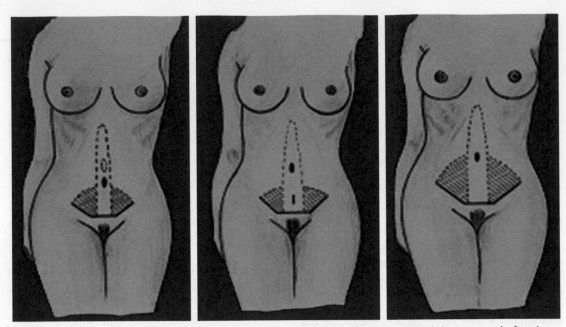

Fig. 17. Different placement of umbilical scar based on the amount of supraumbilical skin present before lower abdominal skin resection. Do not flex the table; do not pull the flap too hard, and do not force it. Place the old umbilical scar where it wants to go. A short midline infraumbilical vertical scar is always better than pubic hair growing in the lower abdomen.

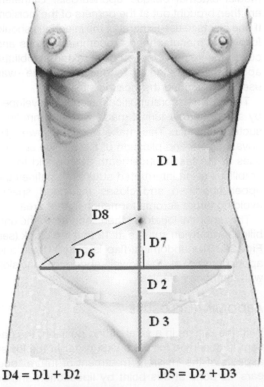

D 1

D 8

D 7

D 6

D 2

D 3

D4 = D1 + D2   D5 = D2 + D3

Fig. 18. Umbilicus study.

scar. Finally, the length and symmetry of the lower abdominal scar are checked by the "triangulation technique." The midline is determined and marked using the same technique. The second component of the umbilical locator is then applied and the future location of the umbilicus is determined (**Fig. 21**; **Figs. 22** and **23**, Video 6). That position should be verified also by measurements and positioning in relation to the iliac crest (see **Figs. 18** and **19**). The excess skin is removed through an elliptical excision. The umbilical locator is removed and the umbilicus is set through a supra-umbilical high-tension suture using 2-0 pds at 12 and 6 o'clock. The remaining umbilical closure is secured with dermal sutures of 4-0 Monocryl®; the skin margins are sealed with Dermabond®. A lateral view of the new abdomen with its elegant new contouring should be observed at this point. Dressings include topifoam® and girdle for 4 to 6 weeks.

Figs. 24–30 display various clinical cases.

OPTIMIZING OUTCOMES

Promoting safe surgical practice and prevention of catastrophic events is the surest way to optimize outcomes. Before the operating room, there should be a vigilant investigation of both personal

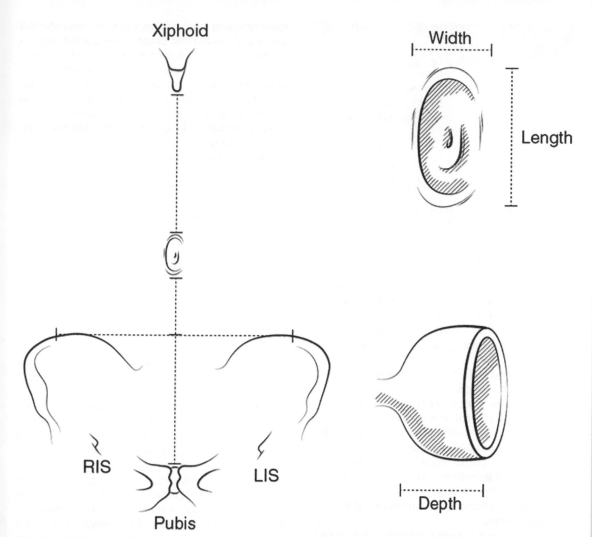

Fig. 19. Umbilicus study.

Width 1-2cm (1.65cm)
Length 1-2.5cm (1.38cm)
Depth 1-2cm (1.42cm)

Fig. 20. Umbilicus study.

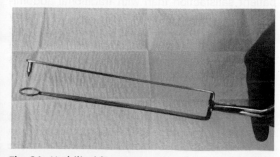

Fig. 21. Umbilical locator.

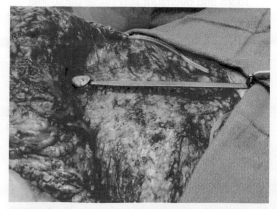

Fig. 22. First component of umbilical locator secured to umbilical stalk with 4-0 nylon sutures at 12 and 6 o'clock.

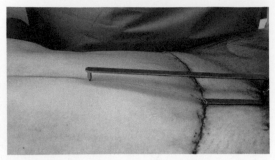

Fig. 23. Second component of umbilical locator in place after abdominal closure. The midline has been defined by the triangulation technique with silk sutures at xyphoid and pubic bone locations.

and family history of thrombotic events. Guidelines in clinical practice are as follows:

- Hematologic and/or appropriate specialist consultation for patient or family history of coagulopathy, including miscarriages, early myocardial infarction, prior thromboembolic events.
- Cancellation of immediate preoperative trips via airplane or car
- A baseline preoperative duplex scan with even a minor clinical suspicion
- Oral contraceptives and hormones stopped at least a month before surgery
- Sequential compression devices before induction of anesthesia, in recovery room, and during overnight stay
- Adequate temperature management to avoid hypothermia
- Low-molecular-weight heparins (Lovenox®) starting at 8 to 10 hours after completion of surgical procedure and to continue 3 to 5 days until fully ambulatory
- Aggressive early ambulation by recovery room and overnight stay nurse personnel
- Patient and family to be educated about the importance of ambulation in the immediate postoperative period so it continues at home after discharge from the surgical facility.

An outstanding postoperative appearance does not guarantee that an outcome is satisfactory to the parties involved. A postoperative period that is free of major clinical complications, delayed healing, and catastrophic events can significantly enhance both patient and surgeon satisfaction.

POSTOPERATIVE CARE

All patients should be placed in a semi-compressive dressing after abdominoplasty and other ancillary procedures. Initial dressing with foam dressing, such as Reston, over liposuctioned areas and abdominal binders are appropriate. In the author's practice, patients are instructed to purchase compressive garments that encompass the abdomen and hips and wear the garments continuously for 6 weeks after surgery. Both medical grade and commercially available compressive garments are appropriate as long as they are worn with consistency. Surgical edema often persists for several months and inconsistent use of garments can exacerbate the unflattering appearance.

Scar massage, lymphatic massage, and topical therapies such as silicone sheets are frequently used among patients, with the understanding that the therapeutic outcomes are highly variable. Frequent wound checks, frequent wound hygiene, and frequent and regular postoperative visits are essential in impeding wound problems before they flare out of proportion.

After surgery weight control is regularly discussed with patients, so that the surgical results are maintained. Postsurgery weight control is especially crucial in the postoperative period, when the patient may be more sedentary than usual, and activity restrictions prevent them from strenuous exercise.

Patients are kept in the surgery center overnight for safe postoperative management (pain control, fluid management, and DVT/PE prevention) when abdominoplasty is combined with other body contouring procedures or patient's health conditions warrant closer observation and care. The compression girdle is recommended for the first 4 to 6 weeks. Patients are then allowed to resume regular exercises. Their weight is checked and documented in the chart during all office visits.

Abdominoplasty in Combined Body Contouring Procedures

The two position comprehensive abdominoplasty has reliably demonstrated equal or superior esthetic results compared with traditional abdominoplasty while minimizing complications. Significant decrease in revision surgery signifies greater patient satisfaction than with traditional abdominoplasty. When the two position abdominoplasty is performed in conjunction with other esthetic procedures, there should not be an increase in abdominoplasty-related complications, such as seroma, hematoma, wound dehiscence, and tissue necrosis.

In the past, abdominoplasty has been implicated in a higher incidence of complications when performed in a combined procedure. In the 2001 American Society for Aesthetic Plastic Surgery (ASAPS) Lipoplasty Survey performed

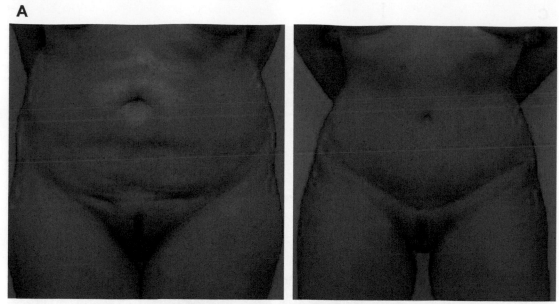

40y - Revision abdominoplasty & SAL back
after Laser Liposuction by local Dermatologist

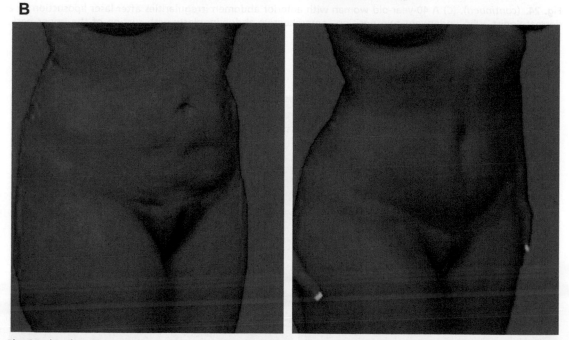

Fig. 24. (*A–C*) A 40-year-old woman with anterior abdomen irregularities after laser liposuction by a dermatologist, who underwent two position comprehensive abdominoplasty with suction of the upper back, lower back, and flanks.

between 1998 and 2000, data from 159 procedures were collected: 66% were suction-assisted lipectomy (SAL) alone, and 14% of the SALs were combined with abdominoplasty. The addition of abdominoplasty to SAL increased the likelihood of postoperative complications by a factor of 14 (1). Although this demonstrates that abdominoplasty is the more frequent culprit in postoperative complications compared with SAL, addition of ancillary procedures should not increase this risk further.

C

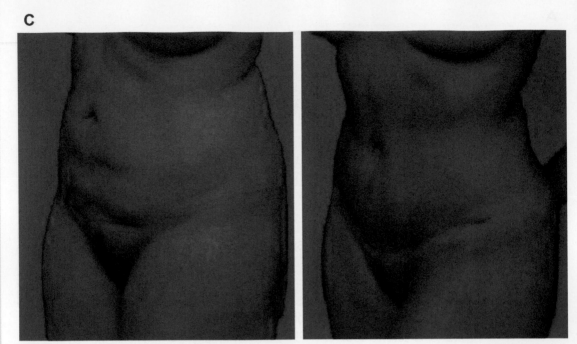

Fig. 24. (*continued*). (*C*) A 40-year-old woman with anterior abdomen irregularities after laser liposuction by a dermatologist, who underwent two position comprehensive abdominoplasty with suction of the upper back, lower back, and flanks.

A

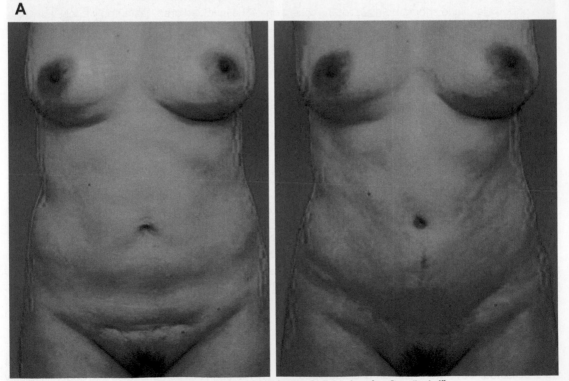

32y - Revision abdominoplasty & SAL back after "mini"

Fig. 25. (*A, B*) A 32-year-old woman underwent two position comprehensive abdominoplasty with rectus muscle plication and suction of the upper back, lower back, and flanks.

B

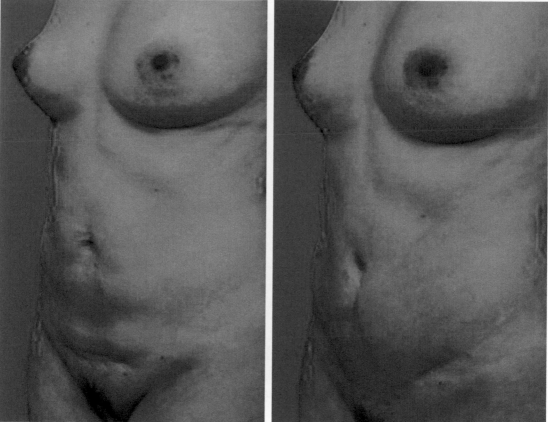

Fig. 25. (*continued*). (*B*) A 32-year-old woman underwent two position comprehensive abdominoplasty with rectus muscle plication and suction of the upper back, lower back, and flanks.

At the University of Utah, Voss and colleagues reported a very high incidence of PE (6.6%, 5 of 76 patients) that had combined abdominoplasty with a gynecologic procedure. They also noted the combined procedures had an increased operative time, increased blood loss, and increased hospital stay (2). However, this clinical study was reviewed and repeated at the same institution by the author 14 years later. There were no thromboembolic events after the same number of patients and similar cases.

Institutional changes implemented for combined gynecologic and plastic surgery procedures during the time interval included a more detailed preoperative screening, sequential compression devices in all cases, postoperative low-molecular-weight heparins in selective cases, early ambulation and discharge, and a significant increase in outpatient surgery. The recent addition of local

anesthestic pain pumps in all abdominoplasty cases has allowed patients to ambulate earlier and with greater ease. Decreased narcotic intake was also observed, hastening patient mobility and physical recovery.

By better preserving the nerves and vasculature to the anterior abdominal wall, the two position comprehensive abdominoplasty likely reduces much of the most common and aggravating complications of traditional abdominoplasty, including seromas and lower skin flap necrosis. This procedure should potentially be safely combined with other esthetic procedures to produce a more dramatic transformation.

PREOPERATIVE PREPARATION

Although liposuction of adjacent areas and breast contouring surgeries are the most often requested

A

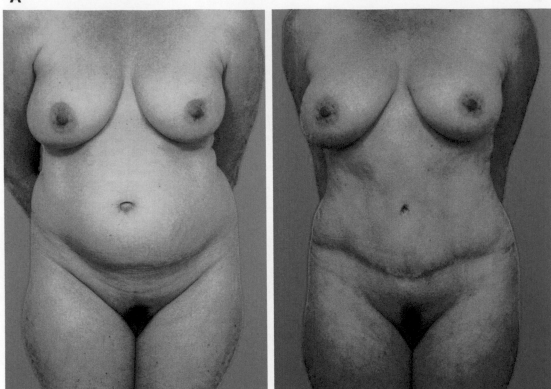

30y - Abdominoplasty, hernia repair & SAL back, flanks

B

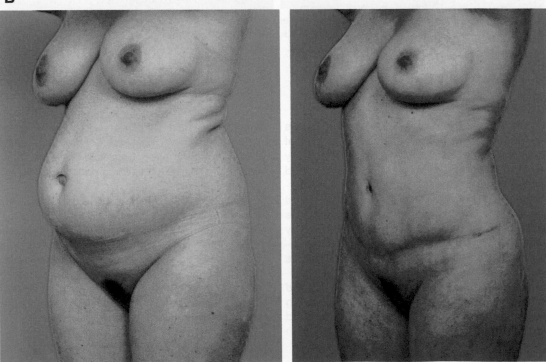

Fig. 26. (*A–C*) A 30-year-old woman with large rectus diastasis, umbilical hernia after twin pregnancy, who underwent two position comprehensive abdominoplasty, umbilical hernia repair, and liposuction of the upper back, lower back, and flanks.

C

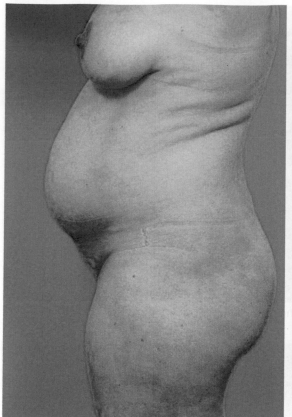

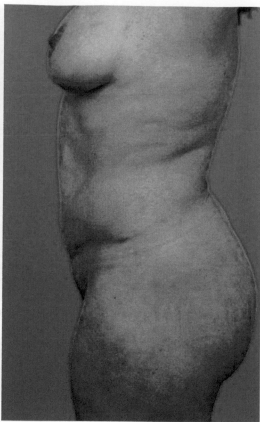

Fig. 26. (*continued*). (*C*) A 30-year-old woman with large rectus diastasis, umbilical hernia after twin pregnancy, who underwent two position comprehensive abdominoplasty, umbilical hernia repair, and liposuction of the upper back, lower back, and flanks.

procedures along with abdominoplasty, patients may also request distant ancillary procedures, including facial rejuvenation. Tackling several areas during a single trip to the operating room is a tempting prospect, and in the right patient, appropriate. With optimal patient selection and preoperative planning, two position comprehensive abdominoplasty can be safely combined with other esthetic procedures.

In the decision to perform a combined procedure with abdominoplasty, patient selection is of significant consequence. Before any elective surgery, the surgeon should confirm that no preexisting heath conditions preclude lengthy general anesthesia. Preoperative laboratory work would be prudent before a multiregion combined procedure. In cases of prior cardiac or pulmonary conditions, appropriate specialists should be consulted in addition to an anesthesiologist. The surgeon should also provide an honest estimate of the total

length of the combined procedure, depending on prior surgical experience and availability of appropriate assistants. The concept of a "surgical team" familiar with combined body contouring procedures and the importance of "time efficiency" cannot be overemphasized in these types of cases.

Patients should be weight stable for several months and nutritionally stable before surgery. Although a normal BMI is not always a realistic goal, an obese patient should be counseled on further weight loss before surgery, as they are not likely to derive optimal results from surgery.

Preoperative evaluation should focus on both personal and family history of coagulopathy, including a history of multiple miscarriages. Smokers should not undergo abdominoploasty or combined procedures, because of the high likelihood of wound complication and pulmonary compromise. Oral contraceptives and hormone

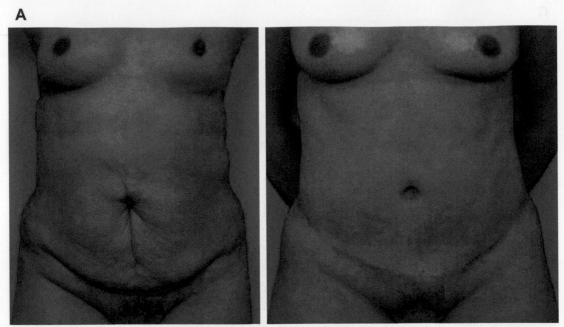

58y - Revision abdominoplasty & SAL back, flanks

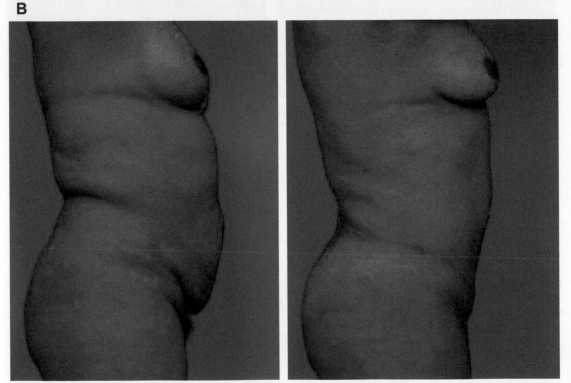

Fig. 27. (*A, B*) A 58-year-old patient underwent two position comprehensive abdominoplasty with combined liposuction of the upper back, lower back, and flanks.

replacement therapies can increase thrombotic risk and should be stopped weeks before surgery.

In the combined procedure population, the patient's dedication to total body transformation is extremely high, and the expectation no less so. The outcome of the surgery is expected to be transformative and staggering, given the monetary and time commitment of the patient. It is

A

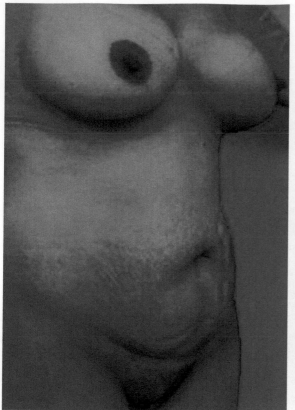 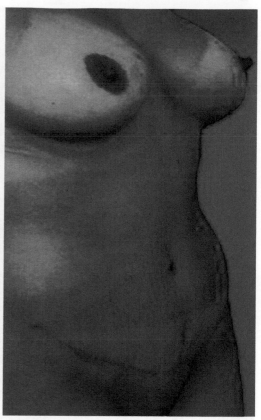

Fig. 28. (*A*, *B*) Patient after combined procedures: implant exchange, two position comprehensive abdomino-plasty, and liposuction of the upper, lower, and flank areas.

imperative that extensive preoperative discussions occur using the patient's own photographs outlining the realistic goals of surgery. When sharing photographs from prior surgeries, the representative photographs should be close in age and body habitus to the patient. The limits of the patient's own anatomy due to natural body shape, age, skin quality, and prior surgical scars should be carefully outlined. The patient should also be informed that in any esthetic surgery, there is always room for improvement and revision further down the line.

SURGICAL TECHNIQUE

Many patients present to the plastic surgeon desiring esthetic improvement of multiple regions. Among the author's abdominoplasty patients, the most frequent requests are for breast esthetic surgery and for SAL of adjacent areas, including flanks, back, hips, and thighs.

In the author's practice, they routinely adjoin liposuction of back and flank areas to their abdominoplasties. Starting in the prone position, the back and flank adiposities are addressed first before undertaking the anterior trunk. Circumferential reduction of excess adiposity produces a total torso transformation and improves the visual esthetic from every angle (see **Figs. 1**, **3**, and **4**). Liposuction of back and flanks further assists in creating a defined waist, where traditional abdominoplasty can blunt the waistline. Residual adiposity in the flanks and back can distract from an overall harmonious result from an abdominoplasty; when one area becomes smaller and tighter, it can call attention to other problem areas that were previously less noticeable.

Among the weight-loss and multiparous patients, the ptotic, involuted breasts can similarly detract from achieving a harmonious result. The huge popularity of the so-called mommy makeovers stems from the high incidence of simultaneous

B

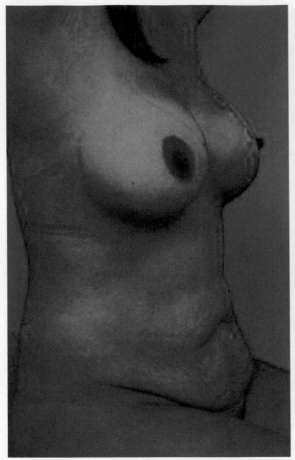
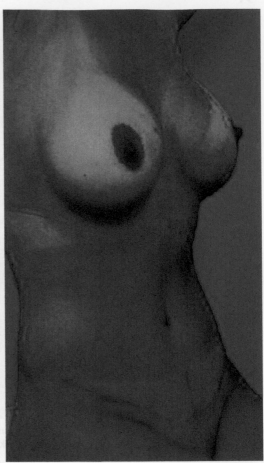

Fig. 28. (*continued*). (*B*) Patient after combined procedures: implant exchange, two position comprehensive abdominoplasty, and liposuction of the upper, lower, and flank areas.

deformities of the breasts and the abdomen. Augmentation, mastopexy, and augmentation-mastopexy are the most common procedures performed to rejuvenate and restore felicitous dimensions to the breasts. When combined with lipoabdominoplasty and SAL of the lower torso, breast esthetic surgery can facilitate a more complete transformation.

Facial esthetic surgery can be combined with two position comprehensive abdominoplasty, but with caution as to the length of the procedure. Patients often desire a combination procedure of the face (a rhytidectomy and a brow lift, for example) that would necessitate significant operative time and would result in excessive operative time if combined with body contouring procedures. If the patient also desires breast surgery and or

extensive SAL, other esthetic surgeries may be best performed on a separate date.

COMPLICATIONS AND THEIR MANAGEMENT IN COMBINED BODY CONTOURING PROCEDURES

Performing abdominoplasty in a combined body contouring procedure has the potential for increased postoperative pain limiting early ambulation, as well as the theoretic potential for increased incidence of thrombophilia, owing to the length of the procedure and prolonged immobilization. With cautious preoperative workup and limiting the number of hours under general anesthesia, combined procedures parlay the potential benefits of single anesthesia, decreased total

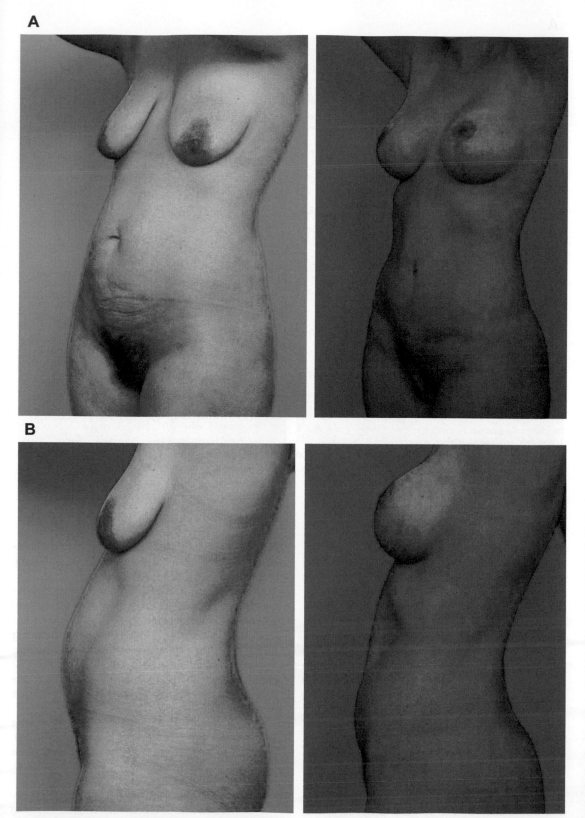

Fig. 29. (*A, B*) Massive weight-loss patient after combined procedures: two position comprehensive abdomino-plasty combined to breast augmentation, mastopexy, liposuction of the upper back, lower back, and flanks.

A

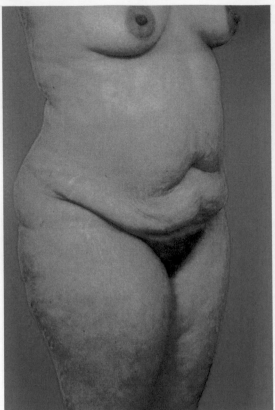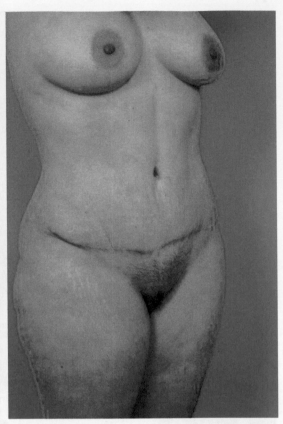

Fig. 30. (*A, B*) Massive weight-loss patient after combined procedures: breast augmentation, two position comprehensive abdominoplasty, breast augmentation, liposuction of the upper back, lower back, and flanks.

recovery time, and decreased expense to the patient. The author aims to establish that combining abdominoplasty with other esthetic procedures can be safe to the patient and result in the similar low rates of complications as with lipoabdominoplasty alone.

The risk of DVT/PT in this situation is likely multifactorial: prolonged operative time, increased pelvic vein compression due to rectus muscle diastasis repair, which increases intra-abdominal pressure, and a prolonged recovery period with relative immobility.

With implementation of safe clinical practices, such as preoperative screening, early ambulation, and multiple methods of anticoagulation, thromboembolic events do not appear closely correlated with abdominoplasty in combined procedures. Hester noted that it was obesity, rather than length and complexity of the surgical procedure, that increased the likelihood of thromboembolism. Another study of 103 abdominoplasties combined

with intra-abdominal surgeries reported no thromboembolic complications with ted hose and early ambulation as the sole interventions.

More recently, a retrospective review of 268 patients who underwent combined abdominoplasty and cosmetic breast surgery over a 10-year period found a 34% overall complication rate including minor seromas and wound dehiscence, but no thromboembolic events or death. Combining 2 procedures did not lead to an increase in complications when compared with individually staged procedures.

Over a 2-year period, 175 patients underwent lipoabdominoplasties in the author's practice. One hundred forty-one patients (80%) underwent combination procedures:

- Only lipoabdominoplasty: 34 (20%)
- Combined with SAL back/extremities: 79 (46%)
- Combined with breast surgery: 31 (17%)
- Combined with other surgeries: 31 (17%)

B

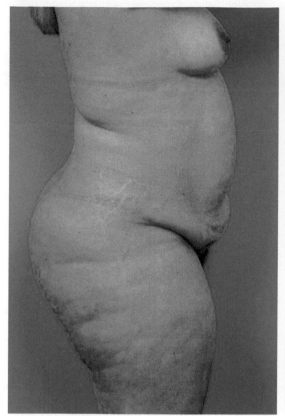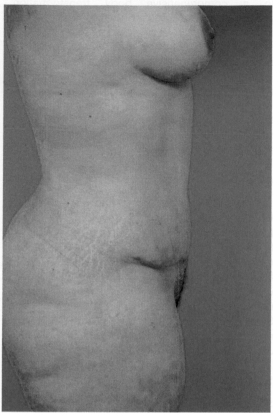

Fig. 30. (*continued*). (*B*) Massive weight-loss patient after combined procedures: breast augmentation, two position comprehensive abdominoplasty, breast augmentation, liposuction of the upper back, lower back, and flanks.

The complications of combined procedures were comparable to rates after lipoabdominoplasty alone, and superior to rates associated with traditional abdominoplasty in the author's practice. Three patients required hospitalization after a combined procedure: 2 admissions were for postsurgical complications and 1 patient for inadvertent narcotic overdose while at home. There was a single incidence of PE that recovered well with intravenous heparin therapy and hospitalization. This particular patient received both mechanical and chemical prophylaxis. It was discovered afterward that the patient had driven 10 hours the day before surgery (**Box 1**).

Box 1
Complications among 175 patients

- Seroma = 5 (2.85%)
- Pulmonary embolism = 1 (0.5%)
- Dehiscence = 1 (0.5%)
- Narcotic overdose = 1 (0.5%)

SUMMARY

Ultimately, a combined procedure should be attempted with a clean preoperative workup and by a surgical team who can complete multiple procedures in an efficient and timely fashion. Postoperative care should include instructions for early ambulation and adequate analgesia. Overnight stay is mandatory in the author's practice for all patients who undergo combined procedures in addition to lipoabdominoplasty or traditional abdominoplasty. Also, overnight stays are recommended for patients with any prior medical conditions or for significant blood loss, difficult pain control, or difficult recovery from anesthesia. The American Society of Plastic Surgeons (ASPS) Patient Safety Committee guidelines detail guidelines for appropriate preoperative workup, patient selection, and perioperative management of risk factors. Consistent application of safe practices is paramount in maximizing positive outcomes and minimizing negative events.

The two position comprehensive is a powerful and safe body sculpturing tool. In combination with other body contouring procedures, it can lead to a comprehensive body transformation: anatomic, physiologic, and psychological. A significant series from a single surgeon's office was obtained demonstrating that other procedures can be safely combined with abdominoplasty without multiplying the number of complications. With vigilant patient screening, preoperative planning, and aggressive postoperative management, two position comprehensive abdominoplasty in combination with other procedures can be safely and effectively performed.

ACKNOWLEDGMENTS

The Author would like to acknowledge and thank Dr. Ricardo Ribeiro and Dr. Osvaldo R. Saldanha for their contributions to this article. The Author acknowledges that portions of the text in the section COMPLICATIONS AND THEIR MANAGEMENT IN COMBINED BODY CONTOURING PROCEDURES were derived from Lipoabdominoplasty in Combined Body Contouring Procedures by Renato Saltz and Angela S. Landfair in Body Contouring and Liposuction, edited by Peter J. Rubin, Mark L Jewell, Dirk Richter, and Carlos O Uebel.

SUPPLEMENTARY DATA

Supplementary data related to this article can be found online at http://dx.doi.org/10.1016/j.cps.2014.07.008.

SUGGESTED READINGS

Callia WE. Dermolipectomia abdominal. Sao Paulo (Brazil): Carlo Erb; 1963.

Castro CC, Salema R, Atias P, et al. The abdominoplasty to remove multiple scars from the abdomen. Ann Plast Surg 1984;12:369.

Dillerud E. Abdominoplasty combined with suction lipoplasty: a study of complication, revisions, and risk factors in 487 cases. Ann Plast Surg 1990;25(5): 333–8.

El-Mrakby HH, Milner RH. The vascular anatomy of the lower anterior abdominal wall: a microdissection study on the deep inferior epigastric vessels and the perforators branches. Plast Reconstr Surg 2002;109(1):539–47.

Gemperli R, Neves RI, Tuma P Jr, et al. Abdominoplasty combined with other intraabdominal procedures. Ann Plast Surg 1992;29(1):18–22.

Haeck PC, Swanson JA, Iverson RE, et al, The ASPS Patient Safety Committee. Evidence-based patient safety advisory: patient assessment and prevention of pulmonary side effects in surgery. Part 2—patient and procedural risk factors. Plast Reconstr Surg 2009;124(4S):57S–67S.

Haeck PC, Swanson JA, Iverson RE, et al. The ASPS Patient Safety Committee evidence-based patient safety advisory: patient selection and procedures in ambulatory surgery. Plast Reconstr Surg 2009; 124(4S):6S–27S.

Hakme F. Technical details in the lipoaspiration associate with liposuction. Rev Bras Cir 1985;75(5): 331–7.

Hester TR, Baird W, Bostwick J 3rd, et al. Abdominoplasty combined with other major surgical procedures: safe or sorry? Plast Reconstr Surg 1989; 83(6):997–1004.

Huger WE Jr. The anatomic rationale for abdominal lipectomy. Am Surg 1979;45:612.

Hughes CE 3rd. Reduction of lipoplasty risks and mortality: an ASAPS survey. Aesthet Surg J 2001;21(2):120–7.

Illouz YG. A new safe and aesthetic approach to suction abdominoplasty. Aesthetic Plast Surg 1992; 16:237–45.

Lockwood T. Fegli-lateral-tension abdominoplasty with superficial fascial system suspension. Plast Reconstr Surg 1995;9:603–8.

Matarasso A. Liposuction as an adjunct to full abdominoplasty. Plast Reconstr Surg 1995;95:829–36.

Most D, Kozlow J, Heller J, et al. Thromboembolism in plastic surgery. Plast Reconstr Surg 2005;115(2): 20e–30e.

Pitanguy I. Abdominoplasty: classification and surgical techniques. Rev Bras Cir 1995;85:23–44.

Psillakis JM, de la Plaza R, Appiani E, et al. Color atlas of aesthetic surgery of the abdomen. Thieme Publishing Group; 1991.

Ribeiro R, Saltz R, et al. The ideal umbilicus – anthropometric measurements of a North and South American population. In preparation for publication.

Shestak KC. Marriage abdominoplasty expands the miniabdominoplasty concept. Plast Reconstr Surg 1999;103:1020–31.

Simons S, Thaller SR, Nathan N. Abdominoplasty combined with additional surgery: a safety issue. Aesthet Surg J 2006;26(4):413–6.

Stevens WG, Repta R, Pacella SJ, et al. Safe and consistent outcomes of successfully combining breast surgery and abdominoplasty: an update. Aesthet Surg J 2009;29(2):129–34.

Stokes RB, William S. Does concomitant breast surgery add morbidity to abdominoplasty? Aesthet Surg J 2007;27(6):612–5.

Taylor GI, Watterson PA, Zest RG. The vascular anatomy of the anterior abdominal wall: the basis for flap design. Perspect Plast Surg 1991;5:1–28.

Vernon S. Umbilical transplantation upward and abdominal contouring in lipectomy. Am J Surg 1957;94: 490–2.

Voss SC, Sharp HC, Scott JR. Abdominoplasty combined with gynecological surgical procedures. Obstet Gynecol 1986;67(2):181–5.

The Extended Abdominoplasty

Kenneth C. Shestak, MD[a,b,*]

KEYWORDS

- Abdominoplasty • Extended high lateral tension abdominoplasty
- Direct excision of hip soft tissue excess

KEY POINTS

- This article illustrates the author's approach of directly excising adipose tissue excess in the lateral and posterior hip region by extending the lateral extent of the horizontal incision in a full abdominoplasty toward the posterior axillary line to produce a superior contour in this region in a select group of patients.
- It is most applicable in patients with a significant adipose tissue excess in the lateral hip area that produces an outward convexity (a parenthesis deformity) seen in the frontal, posterior, or oblique view.
- Such an excess represents a soft tissue "dog ear" composed of skin, and adipose tissue both deep and superficial to the superficial fascial system or SFS.
- Direct excision of a various amount of skin and adipose tissue above and deep to the SFS with subsequent closure of the SFS optimizes the cosmetic appearance of the lateral hip and flank, thus creating an excellent transition between the lateral thigh and flank region while producing a modest upper thigh lift without discontinuous undermining.
- In the author's experience, the contour improvements produced in this area are superior to those that result from liposuction alone in this subset of patients presenting for full abdominoplasty.

INTRODUCTION

Full abdominoplasty is the cornerstone of body contouring of the trunk and most often it includes liposuction of the lateral hips and flanks to achieve 3-dimensional contour improvement. Modern abdominoplasty techniques were developed in the 1960s,[1–3] and many elements of the procedure remained largely unchanged for 3 decades. The features common to this technique have included a transverse lower abdominal incision, undermining of the abdominal skin flap often to the costal margins, tightening of the abdominal musculofascial layer by means of suture placation, and resection of the excess lower abdominal skin with inferior advancement of the abdominal flap and closure, with maximal tension at the line of skin closure occurring in the midline of the abdominal flap.[4] Although contour improvements are realized initially in many patients, often the long-term results were suboptimal because of overtightening of the central aspect of the abdomen with accompanying superior displacement of the pubic tissues and depressed or spread scar appearance. In addition, there was often laxity of the lateral lower abdominal tissues. These shortcomings were cited by several authors, who assessed their results noted in the 1980s from a long-term perspective.[5,6]

An important paradigm shift in the thinking about abdominoplasty was introduced by Lockwood,[7,8] when he introduced and refined the concept of high lateral tension abdominoplasty.[1]

[a] Department of Plastic Surgery, University of Pittsburgh School of Medicine, 3380 Boulevard of Allies, Islay's Building Suite 180, Pittsburgh, PA 15213, USA; [b] Plastic Surgery Service, Magee Womens Hospital, Pittsburgh, PA, USA
* Department of Plastic Surgery, University of Pittsburgh School of Medicine, Pittsburgh, PA.
E-mail address: Shestakkc@upmc.edu

Clin Plastic Surg 41 (2014) 705–713
http://dx.doi.org/10.1016/j.cps.2014.07.001

His insight was that the main deformity in the aging abdomen results from truncal laxity that occurred laterally in most patients and that this was not addressed by existing standard abdominoplasty approaches. To address this, he devised a procedure that entailed selective undermining of the central abdominal flap with a lesser excision of central skin and adipose excess but with a more aggressive excision of tissue in the lateral lower abdomen accompanied by a wound closure that incorporated the superficial fascial system (SFS)[8] that achieved improved lateral contours and a more natural appearance of the central abdomen. Importantly, the selective undermining done to allow musculofascial plication preserved perforating vessels from the rectus abdominis muscles and this in turn allowed the safe application of liposuction to the upper central abdominoplasty flap. In addition, he recognized the need for circumferential contouring of the trunk to achieve true 3-dimensional esthetic contour improvement. The incorporation of liposuction of the abdominal flap and posterior trunk was the essential element of the procedure. By the late 1990s, these concepts were quickly recognized as valid by plastic surgeons around the world and have been widely adopted.[9,10] In addition, they gave rise to even more aggressive approaches to body contouring in the form of body lift procedures.[11,12]

The author has employed this approach for almost 2 decades but has noted that even with the high lateral tension (HLT) design the lateral wound closure frequently resulted in some element of lateral tissue excess or a "lateral soft

tissue dog ear." Very frequently this dog ear must be excised at the end of the procedure by extending the incision posteriorly. Depending on the preoperative deformity and the selected incision plan, this additional incision extension can be somewhat lengthy and has frequently required a position adjustment from the supine to a modified oblique position at the latter stages of the procedure, which makes it especially onerous for the surgeon and the surgical team. It is precisely in this area where the transition of the posterior lateral thigh to lateral flank occurs, which is an esthetically important region. The author's experience quickly taught him that this "dog ear" consisted more of excess subcutaneous adipose tissue than a skin component in virtually all patients and is especially true for patients with thick adipose layers in the lateral and posterior hip (**Fig. 1**). Eventually the author came to recognize that this "soft tissue dog ear" was not as completely addressed by the liposuction of the posterior hip and flank regions (which is routinely performed in >95% of his full abdominoplasty patients) as it is by the combination of liposuction followed by direct excision.

Concurrently, the author began to see and treat more patients (see **Fig. 1**) who had significant tissue excess of adipose and skin tissue in the posterior hip and flank areas that did not extend to the midline posteriorly who therefore did not require a lower body lift but rather a more aggressive approach to contour of the hip and flank regions. Because it is the author's routine to begin almost every full abdominoplasty with liposuction

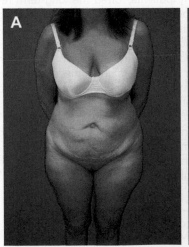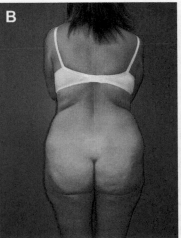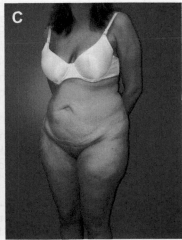

Fig. 1. (*A–C*) Preoperative anteroposterior (AP), lateral, oblique, and posterior view of a patient who will undergo an extended high lateral abdominoplasty with a posterior extension of the incision. Note the significant excess of adipose tissue in the lateral hips on AP and lateral view and blunted transition from lateral thigh to flank on the oblique view.

of the posterior trunk with the patient in the prone position to optimize the liposuction of the back, flanks, and posterior hips, the author decided to begin the abdominoplasty in the prone position using the preoperatively placed markings (**Fig. 2**), which were made to address the "lateral soft tissue dog ear" (see **Fig. 1**A, B; **Fig. 3**A), following the preliminary posterior trunk liposuction. This excision of skin and subcutaneous adipose tissue is performed down to and through the SFS. The wound closure begins medially on the posterior aspect of the trunk with apposition of the incised edges of the SFS on the posterior trunk and proceeds in a lateral direction. This SFS closure produces a modest lateral thigh lift without discontinuous undermining in the thigh area, and the contour of this area is optimized.

PREOPERATIVE EVALUATION

The consultation entails a detailed history focusing on the patient's chief complaint so the surgeon can be clear about the patient's goals and expectations relative to which areas of his or her abdominal and trunk contour are most objectionable. This history also includes recording data about the patient's body mass index, weight stability or fluctuations, dietary, bowel, and exercise habits, waist

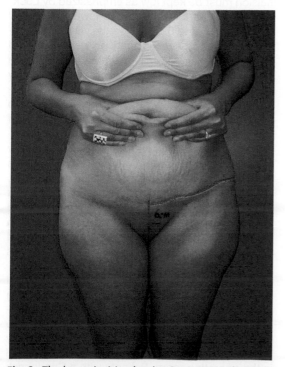

Fig. 2. The lower incision begins 6 cm above the superior aspect of the vulvar commissure and is kept low as it continues laterally.

measurement, dress size, and any history of previous abdominal surgery, types of incisions, and complications. Favorable candidates are patients who are nonsmokers, in good health, with stable weight over at least a 6-month period. A comprehensive medical history is done focusing on any history of previous venous thrombosis or other known coagulopathies, difficulty with previous anesthesia, or other significant medical problems.

Next, a careful examination of the abdomen from an esthetic standpoint is performed. The examination is carried out in both the supine and the standing positions, which enable an accurate assessment of the location and extent of skin and adipose excess and the degree of musculofascial laxity, permitting the surgeon to classify the patient's abdominal deformity preoperatively[13,14] and to select the most appropriate procedure to satisfy the patient's goals.

Full abdominoplasty is selected in patients with significant excess of upper and lower abdominal skin and adipose tissue along with musculofascial laxity of the abdominal wall (Matarasso type IV).[13,14] A detailed plan for surgery is then proposed and discussed with the patient, outlining the position and extent of incisions. As stated, it is the author's experience that the very large majority (>95%) of patients requesting abdominoplasty will have a significant excess of adipose tissue in the posterior hip, flank, and back regions. These areas of adipose excess are most often treated with liposuction. The method of liposuction is purely the surgeon's preference. The author strongly believes that not addressing these areas results in a significant missed opportunity to produce a balanced and harmonious 3-dimensional contour improvement in the trunk region.

Some patients present with a significant amount of adipose excess that results in a marked lateral convexity in the lateral and posterior hip region, which is immediately obvious when viewed from the anterior, posterior, or oblique vantage points (see **Fig. 1**). The author has come to think that in this subset of patients seeking 3-dimensional contour improvement liposuction alone is often not optimal. However, direct excision of this "soft tissue dog ear" performed by extending the incision posteriorly in a line similar to that used for a body lift, but not traversing the midline, addresses the problem in a more optimal way. The next section describes the technique the author uses.

TECHNIQUE

Marking occurs in the standing position (see **Figs. 2** and **3**; **Fig. 4**). To optimize esthetics, the anterior

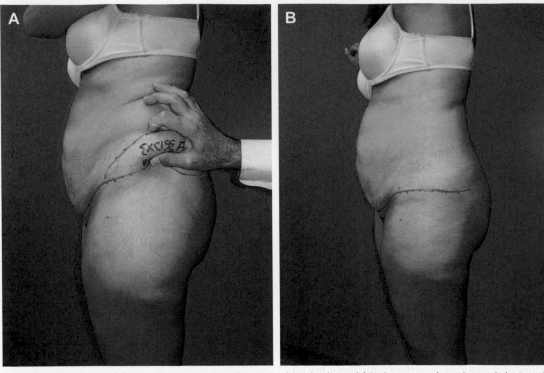

Fig. 3. (*A*, *B*) Excess skin and adipose tissue to be excised in the lateral hip is accurately estimated during the marking by gentle digital manipulation and is outlined.

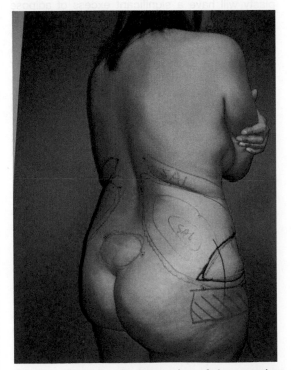

Fig. 4. Markings for the liposuction of the posterior trunk and the upper and lower limbs of the skin excision, which will be started posteriorly with the patient in the prone position.

incision must be kept low as emphasized by Lockwood,[10,11] and the plan for the lower abdominal incision is outlined 6 cm above the vulvar commissure with the tissues placed on gentle upward stretch (see **Fig. 2**). It extends laterally (see **Fig. 3**B) to a low position and continues posteriorly to excise the excess lateral tissue (see **Fig. 3**), carrying the incision as far posteriorly as necessary to excise the skin excess. An accurate estimate of skin resection in both the abdomen and the hip region is possible in virtually every patient by digitally manipulating the tissue (see **Fig. 3**A) in a gentle manner with the patient in the standing position, allowing an upper incision to be inscribed that laterally and posteriorly encompasses the planned "dog ear excision." Markings for the liposuction on the posterior trunk including the hips, flanks, and back region are made on the respective areas (see **Fig. 4**).

Sequential compression devices are used in all patients, are placed in the preoperative holding area, and are activated preoperatively by attaching them to the inflation pump before transport to the operating room. They are immediately attached to a similar inflation machine on arrival in the operating room. Patients with a Caprini risk assessment[15–18] equal to or greater than 6 are given chemoprophylaxis with 5000 units of

Heparin subcutaneously 1 hour before surgery. Heparin is followed by Lovenox, given in a single dose of 40 mg for 10 days postoperatively. General anesthesia is induced on the patient's transport gurney, which is positioned next to the operating table with the patient in the supine position. Inducing the anesthesia in this position allows the patient to be gently rolled onto the previously draped operating table for prone positioning with the padding of all bony prominences and with a pillow under the drape and placed transversely between the anterior superior iliac spines and the umbilicus. This pillow is critical for "presenting "the adipose tissue of the posterior hips and flanks to the surgeon for liposuction with the patient in the prone position. Positioning is conjointly supervised by the surgeon, anesthesiologist, and the operating room team. Intravenous antibiotics of choice are administered within 1 hour of the start of surgery. The author's antibiotic of choice is 2 g of Ancef, which is repeated every 4 hours. In

patients allergic to penicillin, 900 mg of Clindamycin or Vancomycin 1 g is administered. A Foley catheter is placed after the patient is induced. Careful padding of the face region and all bony prominences in the prone position is critical. Although the patient is in the prone position, the face is checked every 20 minutes by the anesthesia team. A warming blanket is placed on the operating table under the drapes on the table and a Bair Hugger is applied to the lower extremities.

The procedure begins with the subcutaneous infiltration of a wetting solution made with the addition of 12.5 mL of 1% Xylocaine and 1 ampule of epinephrine added to each liter of warmed lactated Ringer solution producing a 12.5 mg solution of xylocaine with epinephrine in a concentration of 1:1,000,000. A superwet infiltration technique is used. Liposuction (**Fig. 5**C) of the posterior trunk is performed first in the outlined areas with the surgeon's technique of choice (Suction assisted

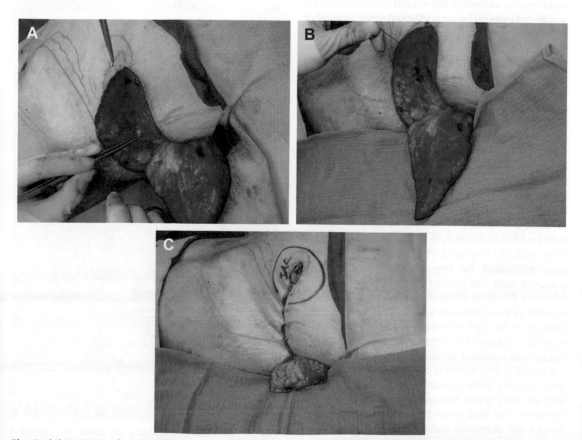

Fig. 5. (A) Excision of excess skin and subcutaneous adipose tissue is performed beginning posteriorly and extending laterally, including adipose tissue above and below the SFS with much less fat being excised deep to the SFS. (B) Closure of the SFS is performed in the posterior extent of the incision. (C) Liposuction is used to correct the prominence of subcutaneous tissue at the medial end of incision after SFS and skin closure.

Lipoplasty (liposuction) [SAL], Power assisted Lipoplasty (liposuction) [PAL], or Ultrasonic Assisted Lipoplasty (liposuction) [UAL]).

As noted previously, the abdominoplasty portion of the procedure (see **Fig. 5**A, B) then begins in the prone position, using the markings placed before surgery. The upper and lower incisions are made at the posterior aspect of the planned skin resection through the skin and subcutaneous tissue down to and through the superficial fascial system (SFS; see **Fig. 5**A) and are continued laterally toward the anterior surface of the abdomen. At the level of the midaxillary line, this skin segment excision can vary in width between 5 cm and 10 cm. More adipose tissue is excised above the SFS than below the SFS layer. The SFS layer is closed (see **Fig. 5**B) with interrupted 2-0 Polyglycolic acid suture (Vicryl; Ethicon (Ethicon a, Johnson and Johnson Company, Guaynabo, Puerto Rico), Somerville, NJ, USA) and the deep dermis and skin are closed with 3-0 and 4-0 running buried Vicryl absorbable suture. The closure of this wound may produce a prominence of adipose tissue at the most medial aspect of the wound closure, which is readily addressed by an additional small amount of liposuction of this prominence if it exists (see **Fig. 5**C) before turning the patient into the supine position to complete the abdominoplasty portion of the surgical procedure.

The patient is then repositioned by turning him or her into the supine position (**Fig. 6**), again with careful padding of bony prominences. The abdominoplasty is performed as described by Lockwood.[10] Undermining is limited to the area needed for musculofascial plication (**Fig. 7**) in a vertical midline orientation in the upper abdomen with additional lateral undermining if horizontal plication is necessary in the supra-umbilical or lower abdominal region. Plication is done with permanent braided Nylon suture (0-Surgilon; US Surgical Corporation). The abdominal tissue excess that was estimated by the preoperative marks is checked with the patient in the upright position with hips flexed to 60 degrees. The umbilicus is relocated in the midline at the level of the iliac crest. Closure of the SFS with the same 2-0 Polyglycolic acid suture placed using interrupted suture technique with maximal tension significantly lateral to the lateral pubic region is done, creating more tension laterally than medially. Skin closure is performed with more tension placed laterally than medially. The final maneuver is selective liposuction of the abdominoplasty flap as described by Lockwood[10] (which is well vascularized because of the selective undermining and preservation of the lateral row of rectus abdominis perforators on both sides[18–20]) with aspiration of fat mainly in

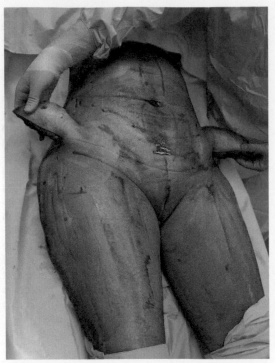

Fig. 6. Following closure of the incisions in the prone position, the patient is turned to the supine position.

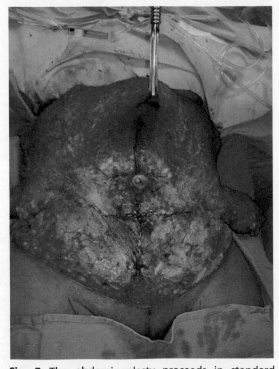

Fig. 7. The abdominoplasty proceeds in standard fashion. Selective undermining is illustrated in this case to permit vertically oriented midline musculofascial plication and transverse plication above and below the umbilicus.

the deep adipose layer as needed, through the "umbilical cutout" before reinsetting the umbilicus. Caution must be taken in preserving adequate circulation[21–23] to the flap during elevation, and selective central undermining will ensure this by preserving the vascular contributions in Zone 1.[18]

Three 10-mm suction drains are placed with small incisions in the pubic hair region, one vertically oriented in the midline toward and above the umbilicus, and the additional drains directed laterally toward the lateral dissection space, which is in continuity with the excision sites in the posterior hip regions. The skin wound is closed with absorbable sutures in the deep dermis and subcuticular portion of the skin.

Nonstick topical foam is placed over the areas on the posterior trunk, which have undergone liposuction, and an abdominal binder is placed to hold the gauze dressings. The drains are maintained until the output drops to less than 30 cc per 24 hours and are usually required for 7 to 10 days.

The postoperative recovery is exactly similar to that observed in patients undergoing an abdominoplasty. Most patients are hospitalized overnight following the procedure. Mobilization begins the night of surgery with the patient encouraged to get out of bed. Discontinuing the Foley catheter immediately after surgery provides an impetus for early mobilization. Sequential compression devices are maintained while the patient is in bed during his or her time in the hospital. Patient-controlled anesthesia (PCA pump) is administered until 6:00 AM the day after surgery. Early ambulation is encouraged. Chemoprophylaxis is administered as described. Patients are uniformly discharged on postoperative day 1 when they and their families are instructed in management and care of the Jackson-Pratt drains. Drains are discontinued when they drain less than 30 cc per 24 hours.

DISCUSSION

Virtually all body contouring operations involve the "tradeoff" of scars for shape. This tradeoff is certainly true of full abdominoplasty procedures wherein a lengthy lower abdominal scar is standard. This incision across the lower anterior allows direct excision of excess skin and redundant adipose tissue of the abdominal wall. Liposuction is applied to optimize contours of the posterior trunk in most patients.

The author has increasingly encountered patients who do not require total circumferential excision of tissue but who have significant excess tissue between the anterior and mid to posterior axillary lines. This will occasionally extend more medially than the posterior axillary line but often there is no excess skin or redundancy of skin in the midline. Such patients therefore do not require a body lift (see **Figs. 1**B and **4**). When such patients have abdominoplasty coupled with liposuction of the posterior hip and flank regions, frequently there remains a slight redundancy of both skin and adipose tissue with a lack of smooth contour transition in this area; this may even be evident when the abdominoplasty portion of the procedure is completed. It is disappointing to the patient when it is noted postoperatively.

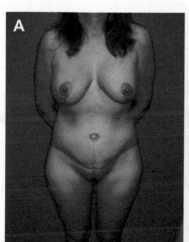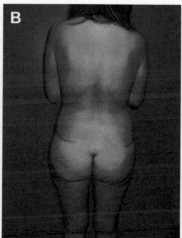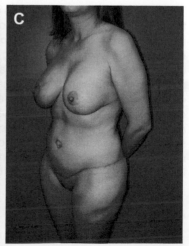

Fig. 8. (*A–C*) Postoperative AP, lateral, oblique, and posterior view of the patient shown in **Fig. 1**. Note the contour improvement on the posterior view and the esthetically enhanced transition between the lateral hip and flank seen on the oblique view, along with extension of the incision posteriorly.

In patients with thick adipose layers in the lateral and posterior hip, there is an excess in the subcutaneous adipose tissue in both its superficial and deep layers (see **Fig. 5**A) and skin laxity that will not optimally "redrape" in this area with liposuction alone, even when the liposuction is aggressively performed. The larger the amount of preoperative tissue excess in the lateral and posterior hip region, as noted by a distinct lateral convexity in multiple views, the more limited liposuction alone becomes.

To address this, the author suggests performing the liposuction of the posterior trunk in the prone procedure, treating the lateral and posterior hip, flank, and back regions in customary fashion and then beginning the abdominoplasty in the prone position as described, excising the posterior and lateral hip adipose rolls that have undergone preliminary liposuction. Excising the premarked skin excess along with adipose tissue superficial and deep to the SFS and reapproximating the SFS layer consistently produce an excellent contour in this area, along with a modest upper thigh lift (**Fig. 8**) and an esthetically pleasing transition between the lateral thigh and flank region. The subset of patients identified in this report is consistently benefited by this approach, and the author recommends it for consideration. In the author's experience over the past 10 years, this modification of the high lateral tension abdominoplasty operation has consistently delivered the best contours of the lateral and posterior lateral aspects of the trunk that the author has produced in the absence of performing a total body lift.

SUMMARY

The procedure described herein is an extension of the extended high lateral abdominoplasty concept introduced and refined by Lockwood. It grew out of the author's experience of excising the lateral "dog ear" at the completion of several abdominoplasty procedures in patients with the anatomic features described. Direct excision of skin and subcutaneous adipose tissue in the lateral and posterior hip region following preliminary liposuction in this subset of patients produces optimal contour improvement in patients whose presenting deformity includes a significant convexity in this area.

ACKNOWLEDGMENTS

The author would like to acknowledge the help in preparing this article from Edward H. Davidson, MD, Resident, Department of Plastic Surgery, University of Pittsburgh.

REFERENCES

1. Pitanguy I. Abdominal lipectomy: an approach to it through an analysis of 300 consecutive cases. Plast Reconstr Surg 1967;40:384.
2. Calia W. Dermolipectomia abdominal. Sao Paulo (Brazil): Centro de cinematografia Carlo Reba; 1965.
3. Baroudi R, Keppke EM, Netto FT. Abdominoplasty. Plast Reconstr Surg 1974;54(2):161–8.
4. Grazer FM. Abdominoplasty. Plast Reconstr Surg 1973;51:617–23.
5. Guerrerosantis J, Spaillat L, Morales F. Some problems and solutions in abdominoplasty. Aesthet Plast Surg 1980;4:227–37.
6. Baroudi R, Moraes M. Philosophy, technical principles, selection, and indication in body contouring surgery. Aesthet Plast Surg 1991;15(1):1–18.
7. Lockwood T. High lateral tension abdominoplasty with superficial fascial system suspension. Plast Reconstr Surg 1995;96:603–15.
8. Lockwood T. Superficial fascial system (SFS) of the trunk and extremities: a new concept. Plast Reconstr Surg 1991;87:1009–18.
9. Hughes CE, Baroudi R, Lockwood TE, et al. Abdominoplasty. Aesthet Surg J 2002;22:465–73.
10. Lockwood TE. Maximizing aesthetics in lateral-tension abdominoplasty and body lifts. Clin Plast Surg 2004;31:523–37.
11. Lockwood T. Lower body lift with superficial fascial system suspension. Plast Reconstr Surg 1993;92: 1112–22.
12. Lockwood T. Lower body lift. Aesthet Surg J 2001; 21:355–70.
13. Matarasso A. Abdominolipoplasty: a system of classification and treatment for combined abdominoplasty and suction-assisted lipectomy. Aesthet Plast Surg 1991;15:111–21.
14. Bozola AR, Psillakis JM. Abdominoplasty: a new concept and classification for treatment. Plast Reconstr Surg 1988;82:983.
15. Young VL, Watson ME. The need for venous thromboembolism(VTE) prophylaxis in plastic surgery. Aesthet Surg J 2006;26(2):157–75.
16. Venturi ML, Davison SP, Caprini JA. Prevention of venous thromboembolism in the plastic surgery patient: current guidelines and recommendations. Aesthet Surg J 2009;29(5):421–8.
17. Pannucci CJ, Bailey SH, Dreszer G, et al. Validation of the Caprini risk assessment model in plastic and reconstructive surgery patients. J Am Coll Surg 2011;212(1):105–12.
18. Huger WE Jr. The anatomic rationale for abdominal lipectomy. Am Surg 1979;45:612.
19. Boyd JB, Taylor GI, Corlett R. The vascular anatomy of the superior epigastric and the deep inferior epigastric systems. Plast Reconstr Surg 1984;73: 1–16.

20. Taylor GI, Watterson PA, Zelt RG. The vascular anatomy of the abdominal wall. The basis for flap design. Plast Reconstr Surg 1991;5:1–10.

21. Matarasso A. Liposuction as an adjunct to a full abdominoplasty. Plast Reconstr Surg 1995;95(5):829–36.

22. Matarasso A. Liposuction as an adjunct to a full abdominoplasty revisited. Plast Reconstr Surg 2000; 106(5):1197–202.

23. Saldanha OR, Federico R, Daher PF, et al. Lipoabdominoplasty. Plast Reconstr Surg 2009;124(3):934–42.

The Bra-Line Back Lift
A Simple Approach to Correcting Severe Back Rolls

Joseph P. Hunstad, MD[a,b,c],*, Phillip D. Khan, MD[c]

KEYWORDS

- Bra line back lift • Back contouring • Upper body lift • Back rolls

KEY POINTS

- Laxity in the upper back is not corrected by the traditional lower body lift. The midline zone of adherence prevents transmission of contouring tension to the upper back, creating and sometimes accentuating prior contour deformities.
- The comprehensive upper back deformity, which includes laxity of the skin, excess adiposity, and redundant lateral breast tissue, can be corrected using the bra line back lift.
- This versatile technique can be used in massive-weight-loss patients or in individuals showing signs of redundant skin and adiposity as a result of age.
- Candidates for the procedure have graspable soft tissue laxity in the mid and lateral upper back.
- The surgical scar is well tolerated by patients and easily concealed beneath a bra or bathing suit top of the patients' choice.
- The resection pattern extends to the anterior axillary line at the level of the inframammary fold.
- Preservation of the loose areolar tissue over the underlying muscle fascia will help minimize pain and swelling.
- A 3-layer space-obliterating suture closure method prevents seroma.
- Laxity from the neck to the lower back is addressed.
- The procedural learning curve is gentle for surgeons with experience in excisional body contouring, yielding consistent and predictable results.
- Patient acceptance of the procedure and its results has been universal.

INTRODUCTION/OVERVIEW

Several methods have been described to address the natural tissue effects that occur as a result of normal aging or fluctuations in weight.[1–23] Distribution of subcutaneous fat and change/differences in skin elasticity can create effects on the skin that are cosmetically and functionally unappealing to patients. These effects are accentuated by natural zones of adherence for soft tissue in the body contour.

Anatomic sequelae in the upper back in particular have been somewhat underserved. Natural upper torso adherence zones in the posterior midline create tether points that lead to both horizontal and vertical laxity.[1,4] A lampshade effect is created on the skin and soft tissue of the upper torso.[3] These tether points hinder contouring of the upper back from procedures such as lower body lifts by preventing transmission of forces to this area (**Fig. 1**). Contouring procedures of the

[a] Plastic Surgery Carolinas Medical Center, University Hospital, Charlotte, North Carolina, USA; [b] Division of Plastic Surgery, University of North Carolina, Chapel Hill, North Carolina, USA; [c] Hunstad-Kortesis Center for Cosmetic Plastic Surgery and Medical Spa, 11208 Statesville Road, Suite Number 300, Huntersville, North Carolina 28078, USA
* Corresponding author.
E-mail address: Jph1@hunstadcenter.com

Clin Plastic Surg 41 (2014) 715–726
http://dx.doi.org/10.1016/j.cps.2014.06.007
0094-1298/14/$ – see front matter © 2014 Elsevier Inc. All rights reserved

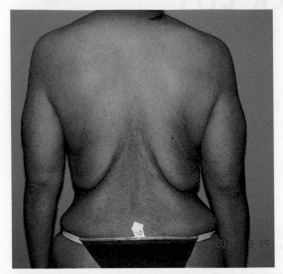

Fig. 1. Patients are evaluated for skin quality, stretch marks, subcutaneous adiposity, and excess or hanging skin. Note the tethering points at the midline creating both horizontal and vertical folding into skin and subcutaneous tissues. This tissue redundancy compromises a smooth transition while wearing clothing for most patients.

lower and midtrunk, in fact, may even accentuate these deformities in some instances.[4–10]

Treatment of this area must be tailored to the particular patient. Some may be candidates for standard tumescent liposuction or adjunctive liposuction procedures using laser or ultrasound.[1,4] Skin in the upper back is robust, with thicker epidermis and dermis to aid in retraction following liposuction. With this, however, fat in the upper back, being thicker and fibrous, can make it relatively more resistant to traditional methods of liposuction.[4] Because of this, many may be candidates for direct excision of this tissue.[1,4,24]

Excisional methods of excess tissue in the past have been described with skin resection in a dermatomal pattern. This, however, tends to leave an oblique scar that is impossible to conceal in normal clothing.[1] These scars are often disfiguring.

The authors present the bra line back lift, a consistent and reliable method of addressing these issues by completely eliminating both excess skin and subcutaneous fat from the region while correcting excess skin laxity in both normal-weight and massive-weight-loss populations.

TREATMENT GOALS AND PLANNED OUTCOMES

The goals of the bra line back lift are to consistently and safely eliminate the skin and subcutaneous fat from the posterior upper torso while correcting

excess skin laxity. The well-accepted position of the scar beneath the bra line without the need for a drain enhances patient satisfaction and minimizes postoperative complications. Patients are able to achieve an ideal contour with relatively minimal morbidity and downtime. The procedure may be combined safely with other body contouring procedures, such as reverse abdominoplasty, mastopexy, and breast reduction, in order to maximize patient outcomes.

PREOPERATIVE PLANNING AND PREPARATION

The patients are given a comprehensive understanding of body contouring procedures and how they relate to their particular situation and deformity. Diagrams and photographs are reviewed and tailored to the patients' particular goals and desires. The authors discuss a comprehensive approach to the area of treatment and how it will affect their long-term goals.

Routine complete blood counts, comprehensive metabolic panels, and coagulation profiles are drawn and reviewed. Patients are instructed to discontinue and nonsteroidal antiinflammatory drugs and herbal medications 2 weeks before surgery. Smoking is a relative contraindication.

PATIENT EVALUATION

Patients with concerns of upper back tissue excess are evaluated for skin quality, stretch marks, subcutaneous adiposity, and excess or hanging skin (see **Fig. 1**).

Most patients will grasp the redundant skin and excess adiposity of the upper back to demonstrate areas they would like to see improvement. In the full-length mirror, the surgeon shows the patients how much will be removed and the contour improvement that they will expect from the neck to the back. Redundant tissue is firmly grasped with bimanual palpation to demonstrate the final outcome in terms of tissue resection (**Figs. 2 and 3**). The day of surgery, patients are encouraged to bring their most revealing bra or bathing suit top in order to plan the area of scar placement and ensure that their expectations will be met (**Fig. 4**).

Patients are counseled on the importance of keeping the arms adducted until full tissue relaxation. Full range of motion will be permitted in 6 weeks or less.

PREOPERATIVE MARKINGS

Patients are marked in a standing position with arms at the sides. This position allows for the maximum amount of tissue to be to be safely

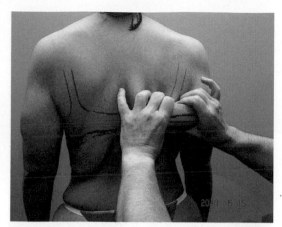

Fig. 2. Strong bimanual palpation helps to demonstrate the final outcome in terms of tissue resection. It shows the surgeon and patients the expected contour after resection.

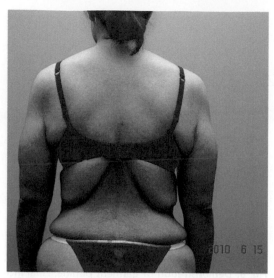

Fig. 4. Patients are encouraged to bring their most revealing bra or bathing suit top in order to plan the incision-line placement and ensure that their expectations will be met.

removed. A standard photographic technique is used to record the entire lateral and upper back condition. These photographs consist of left and right lateral and oblique images as well as a posterior image with the patients' arms down at the sides.

The boundary of the patients' ideal scar position is marked to fall within the outlined margins of the bra or bathing suit top of choice (**Figs. 5** and **6**). If there is not a preferred undergarment, then the ideal final incision line is determined by first identifying the level of the inframammary fold bilaterally. This mark is transcribed across the back in a horizontal fashion (**Figs. 7** and **8**).

Bimanual palpation is then used to strongly gather the redundant skin and excess adiposity such that it centers on the final incision line (**Figs. 9–11**). This technique is performed at multiple points across the ideal incision, and the line is marked superiorly and inferiorly. The markings are subsequently connected identifying the final area of resection (**Figs. 12–14**). Because of the strong zone of adherence in the midline, the resection will be least at this position. The resection pattern is strongly tapered into the inframammary fold at the level of the anterior axillary line in order to avoid a dog-ear (**Fig. 15**). Realignment markings are

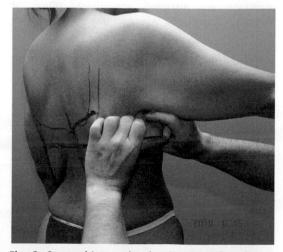

Fig. 3. Strong bimanual palpation identifies the redundancy throughout the entire back. It is important to aggressively gather the tissues in the midaxillary line with the arms relaxed. This allows complete redundant tissue resection achieving maximum improvement in shape and contour.

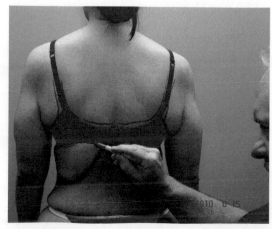

Fig. 5. The boundary of the patients' ideal incision position is marked to fall within the outlined margins of the bra or bathing suit top of choice.

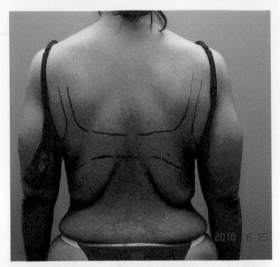

Fig. 6. Demonstration of garment outline. Final incision lines will be planned within these markings.

made to aid in intraoperative assessment of resection patterns.

The marks are reviewed with patients with the aid of a mirror. A full set of postmarking photographs is also taken.

PATIENT POSITIONING

Following the induction of general anesthesia, patients are carefully turned to the prone position. Chest rolls are used along with padding at the knees and ankles. Sequential compression devices are used on the lower extremities.

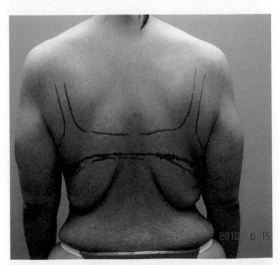

Fig. 7. The final incision line is marked in black, within the garment outline preferred by patients. If there is not an ideal garment, this line is marked at the level of the inframammary fold and transcribed in horizontal fashion across the back.

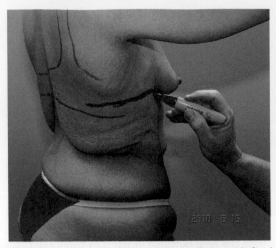

Fig. 8. Oblique view of the patient in **Fig. 7**, with final incision line (marked in *black*) corresponding to the level of the inframammary fold.

Arms are placed on the adjustable arm boards with the elbows flexed and upper arms only moderately abducted. This position aids in reducing tension on closure in the midaxillary line. Adjustable arm boards allow further arm adduction, if needed, in order to decrease tissue tension during closure.

PROCEDURAL APPROACH

A penetrating towel clip is used to the confirm preoperative markings and assess tension at multiple points (**Figs. 16–19**). Difficulty in closing the clamp signifies excessive tension and more conservative markings are adjusted accordingly (**Figs. 20 and 21**). Admittedly a subjective measurement,

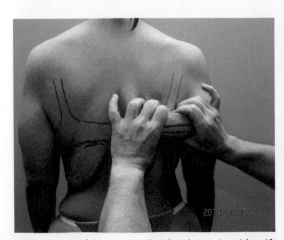

Fig. 9. Strong bimanual palpation is used to identify the resection pattern and center the superior and inferior resection markings on the final proposed incision line, marked in black.

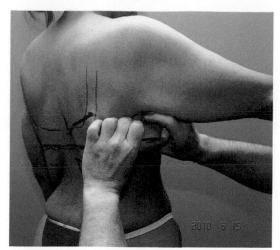

Fig. 10. This palpation is continued at multiple points in order to keep resection patterns within the areas of concealed tissue. Final closure line is marked in black.

the experienced surgeon can accurately assess appropriate tension with this maneuver. These markings are then subsequently tattooed with methylene blue at the realignment points (**Fig. 22**), which aids in reapproximation of tissues, as marked lines will invariably be wiped off during the procedure. It is important to note that these marks should be made outside of the pattern of resection so that they may be seen at the time of closure.

Dilute lidocaine with epinephrine may used to infiltrate the incision lines. In addition, the authors infuse the loose areolar tissue and incision lines above the muscular fascia with a dilute tumescent infiltration. Full prepping and draping is performed.

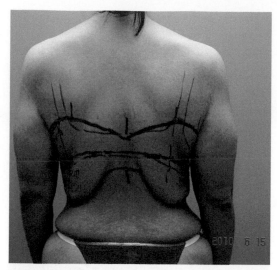

Fig. 12. Markings are connected in order to outline the superior and inferior resection patterns for the procedure. These lines are strongly marked in black, superior and inferior to the final incision line pattern.

Incisions are made into the dermis (**Fig. 23**). Electrocautery is then used to continue the incision through the dermis, sealing the subdermal plexus in order to minimize bleeding (**Fig. 24**). Dissection proceeds, without beveling or undermining, straight down to the loose areolar plane above the muscle fascia. Leaving this layer of tissue will facilitate closure. It allows room for space obliterating sutures.

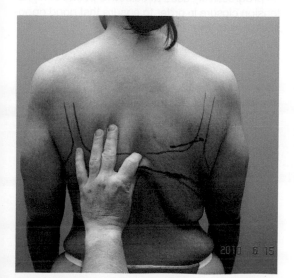

Fig. 11. Because of the strong points of adherence, the narrowest area of resection will be in the midline.

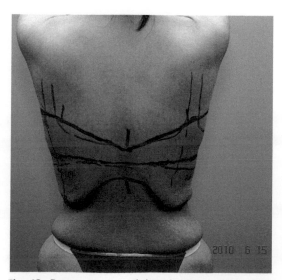

Fig. 13. Demonstration of the resection margins falling outside of the margins of the proposed garment (which is marked in *blue*). Hatch markings are made in order to facilitate in realignment following resection.

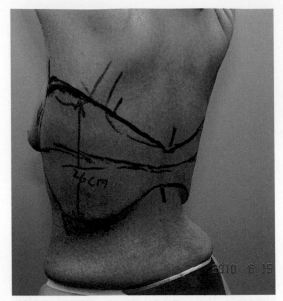

Fig. 14. As seen in this photograph, the widest margins of resection will fall within the area of the posterior axillary line, the most distant from the midline zone of adherence. The resection width demonstrated is 26 cm in this patient.

The resection is completed and tissue passed off for weighing. Meticulous hemostasis is ensured. Skin edges are temporarily closed with penetrating towel clamps, using previously placed realignment marks as reference points. A 3-layered closure is then performed to create space obliteration. This closure is done by taking bites of

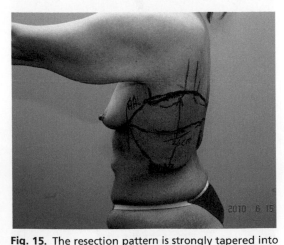

Fig. 15. The resection pattern is strongly tapered into the inframammary fold at the level of the anterior axillary line in order to avoid a dog-ear. Note the superior and inferior resection margins marked in black with a maximum width of 26 cm. *AA* signifies the anterior axillary line, where the resection pattern is tapered to avoid a dog-ear with closure.

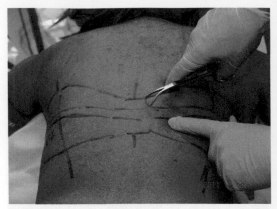

Fig. 16. Penetrating towel clamps are used to assess tension on incision lines at multiple points.

the superficial fascial system, then underlying muscular fascia, and then the opposite side of the superficial fascia (SFS) (**Figs. 25–27**).

Taking care to take accurate bites of the SFS layers is of vital importance to the closure. It is important to recognize that the SFS may seem to retract in relation to the overlying dermis when the towel clamps are placed. Understanding this and insuring strong and accurate bites of this layer will optimize closure and decrease the chance of scar widening. Conveniently for the patients and surgeon, if this is performed meticulously, it eliminates the need for drains.

Based on tension, either a 0 or number 1 polyglactin (Vicryl, Ethicon Inc, Somerville, NJ) suture is used. The closure begins laterally and progresses toward the spine, selectively removing towel clamps along the way. Towel clamps can be progressively used at selective points of higher tension closure in order to ensure that good opposition is secured.

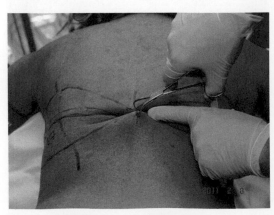

Fig. 17. Penetrating towel clamps are used to assess tension on incision lines at multiple points.

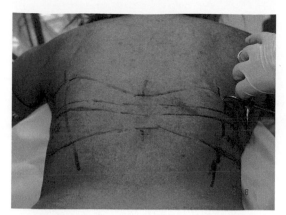

Fig. 18. Penetrating towel clamps are used to assess tension on incision lines at multiple points.

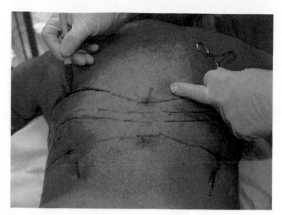

Fig. 21. Incisions lines are reinforced or readjusted according to clamp tension.

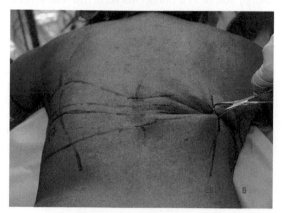

Fig. 19. Penetrating towel clamps are used to assess tension on incision lines at multiple points.

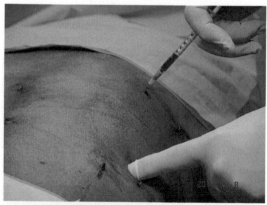

Fig. 22. Realignment markings are tattooed with methylene blue, as they will invariably be lost during the procedure. Note how the tattooing is performed outside of the resection pattern so that they may be seen at the time of closure.

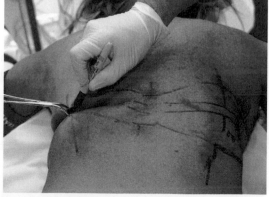

Fig. 20. Markings are made again on the inferior and superior portions of the tissue brought together by the clamps. Difficulty in closure signifies excess tension and the resection lines should be remarked inward removing less tissue and lessening tension.

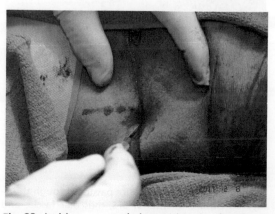

Fig. 23. Incisions are made just within the dermis.

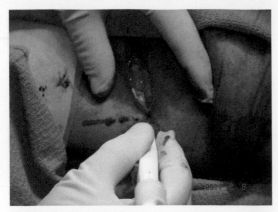

Fig. 24. Electrocautery is used to continue the incision through the dermis, thus, sealing the subdermal plexus and minimizing bleeding.

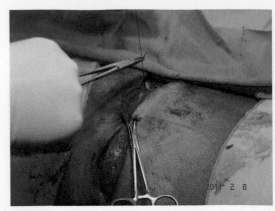

Fig. 27. The 3-layered closure obliterates dead space and eliminates the need for drains postoperatively.

The deep dermis is closed with a 2-0 polyglactin (Vicryl) suture in a buried fashion. The final layer is finished with an intracuticular running 4-0 poliglecaprone suture (Monocryl, Ethicon Inc, Somerville, NJ). Alternatively, a 3-0 Quill SRS Monoderm™ (Surgical Specialties Corporation, Vancouver, B.C. Canada) suture may also be used. Should this procedure be combined with a mastopexy, breast reduction, or reverse abdominoplasty, a temporary V-Y closure can be performed laterally as far as the table permits. Closure on the back can proceed and then the V-Y closure released when patients are subsequently turned supine.

The suture line is then treated with either tissue adhesive or taping. In taping, it is important to split the tapes periodically to allow for swelling and to avoid shearing forces. This splitting avoids blistering and subsequent hyperpigmentation of the incision line.

POTENTIAL COMPLICATIONS AND MANAGEMENT

The most common complication after a bra line back lift is scar widening. The primary author's experience reveals that all patients have been unconcerned with the minor widening that may occur with the incision

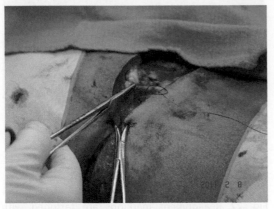

Fig. 25. Towel clamps are used to facilitate a temporary closure of the wound. A 3-point closure is performed by taking a bite of the SFS, then underlying muscular fascia, then the opposite side superficial fascia. Closure begins laterally and progresses medially.

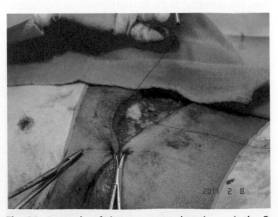

Fig. 26. Example of the suture passing through the 3-layered closure of inferior SFS, muscular fascia, and then superior SFS.

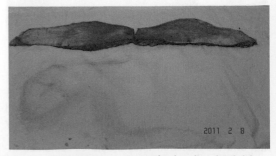

Fig. 28. Resected tissue from the bra line back lift.

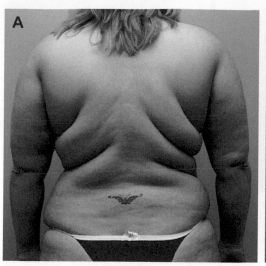
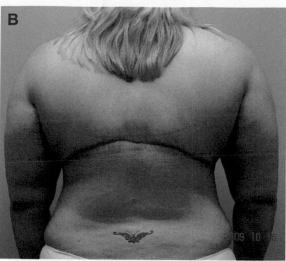

Fig. 29. (*A*) A 32-year-old 100-kg (221-lb) woman concerned with multiple skin folds of the upper back and flanks. (*B*) After bra line back lift, a smooth contour is achieved.

over time. Early experience with this method revealed widening concerning to patients to be the case in less than 5% of cases.[10] If this occurs, a scar revision is offered no sooner than 3 months after healing to allow for full relaxation of the tissues. These revisions subsequently do not widen.

Rarely, a patient may be concerned of a possible undercorrection. In these cases, additional resection can usually be performed under local anesthesia. Lateral dog-ears will generally settle out over several months. Revision under local anesthesia is occasionally required.

Local wound healing complications are managed with debridement and secondary intention healing or delayed primary closure. Seroma, hematoma, and infection have not been experienced in the authors' series; however, they are still discussed as a part of the informed-consent process. Should they occur, standard surgical techniques, including drainage, debridement, and wound care, are recommended.

POSTPROCEDURAL CARE

Patients are allowed to shower on postoperative day one. It is important to remind them to leave their arms adducted when shampooing their hair. Range of motion and arm abduction is increased

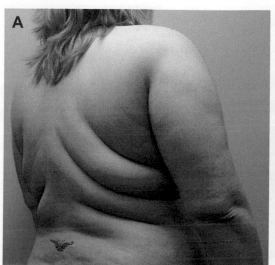
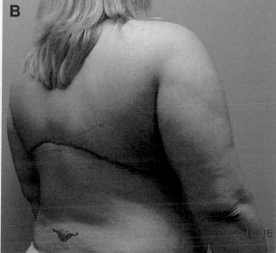

Fig. 30. (*A*, *B*) Oblique photographs of the patient in **Fig. 29**. Overall, a 22-cm resection width of tissue was performed.

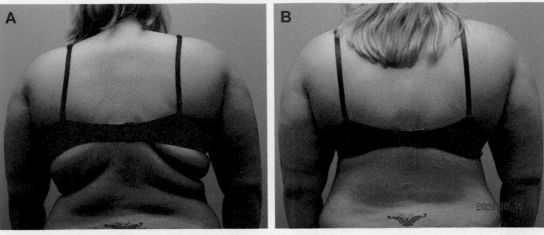

Fig. 31. (*A, B*) The final scar in this patient seen in **Figs. 29** and **30** is concealed easily within the bra line.

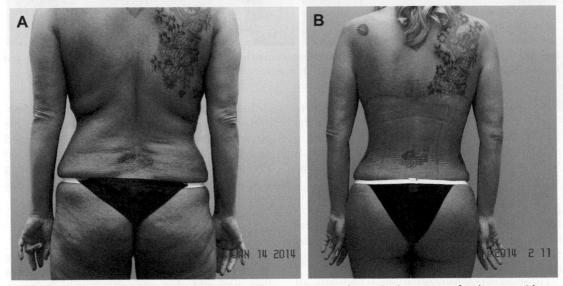

Fig. 32. (*A*) A 44-year-old woman who desired contouring to correct skin and subcutaneous fat changes with age. (*B*) An ideal contour can be seen along the flanks at this 2-month postoperative photograph.

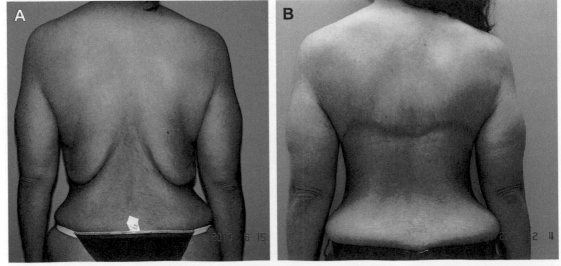

Fig. 33. (*A, B*) A 30-year-old 70-kg (155-lb) woman following massive weight loss. The bra line back lift achieved a complete correction of dramatic excess of skin and subcutaneous tissue in the flank and back. Her marking photographs can be seen in **Figs. 1–15**.

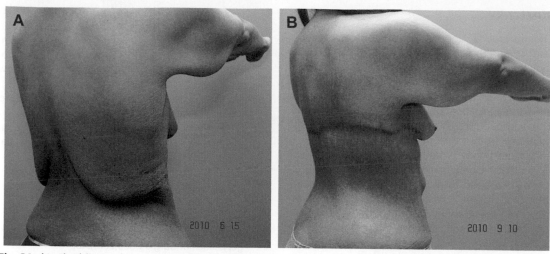

Fig. 34. (*A, B*) Oblique photographs of the patient in **Fig. 33**.

gradually based on patient comfort. If abducting the arms is painful or creates undo tension, they are advised to scale back their activity. Common sense in matters of activity is stressed with patients as well as their family. Skin tapes are removed between the third and fifth postoperative days. Scar therapy is begun at that time, consisting of applying a topical hydrocortisone, vitamin E, and silicone cream 3 times daily.

OUTCOMES AND EVIDENCE

Over a 13-year period, more than 46 procedures have been performed in the authors' practice either as isolated cases or in combination with others. The overall complication rate of scar widening requiring minor revision has been less than 5%. Even with minor widening, patients have been overwhelmingly pleased with the outcome and contour. There are no documented cases of infection, seroma, or hematoma over this period, which can be attributed to the 3-point space-obliterating closure that is used.

In postoperative photographs and patient records, this case series reveals increased patient satisfaction with minimal postoperative morbidity. The results were predictable and consistent throughout. See **Figs. 28–35** for some postoperative examples of resected tissue as well as patient examples.

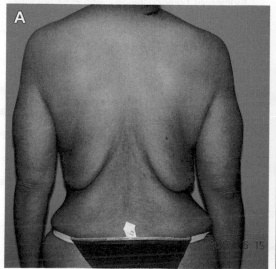
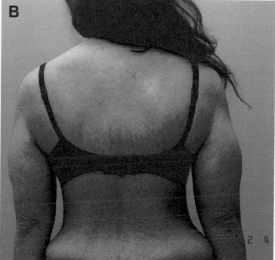

Fig. 35. (*A, B*) The incision line is well hidden within the bra coverage, an ideal position for the patient.

SUMMARY

The transverse upper body lift that the authors refer to as the *bra line back lift*[1,2,10] is a powerful tool that delivers consistent and safe results. It has proven useful for both normal-weight and massive-weight-loss patients who have experienced weight fluctuations and subsequent laxity. The procedure eliminates skin excess and adiposity from the upper back. The final scar is concealed beneath the bra line and tolerated well by patients. Complications are rare and can usually be managed by minor wound care or revision under local anesthetic. The overall patient satisfaction in the authors' practice has been universally high. Mastering this technique has a gentle learning curve and serves as a useful tool in the armamentarium of excisional body contouring.

REFERENCES

1. Hunstad JP, Knotts CD. Transverse upper body lift. In: Rubin JP, editor. Body contouring and liposuction. Elsevier; 2013. p. 159–65.

2. Hunstad JP, Repta R. Bra-line back lift. Plast Reconstr Surg 2008;122(4):1225–8.

3. Solimen S, Aly A. Upper body lift. Clin Plast Surg 2008;35:107–14.

4. Shermak M. Management of back rolls. Aesthet Surg J 2008;28:348–56.

5. Strauch B, Rohde C, Patel MK, et al. Back contouring in massive weight loss patients. Plast Reconstr Surg 2007;120:1692.

6. Aly AS, Cram AE, Chao M, et al. Belt lipectomy for circumferential truncal excess: the University of Iowa experience. Plast Reconstr Surg 2003;111:398.

7. Van Geertruyden JP, Vandeweyer E, De Fontaine S, et al. Circumferential torsoplasty. Br J Plast Surg 1999;52:623.

8. Carwell GR, Horton CE. Circumferential torsoplasty. Ann Plast Surg 1997;38:213.

9. Hurwitz DJ. Optimizing body contour in massive weight loss patients: the modified vertical abdomi-

noplasty. Plast Reconstr Surg 2004;114:1917–23 [discussion: 1924–6].

10. Hunstad JP, Urbaniak RM. Bra-line back lift. In: Strauch B, Herman CK, editors. Encyclopedia of body sculpting after massive weight loss. New York: Thieme; 2011. p. 230–9.

11. Shermak M. Body contouring. Plast Reconstr Surg 2012;129:963e.

12. Huemer GM. Upper body reshaping for the woman with massive weight loss: an algorithmic approach. Aesthetic Plast Surg 2010;34(5):561–9.

13. Strauch B, Herman C, Rohde C, et al. Mid-body contouring in the post bariatric surgery patient. Plast Reconstr Surg 2006;117(7):2200–11.

14. Gusenoff JA, Rubin JP. Plastic surgery after weight loss: current concepts in massive weight loss surgery. Aesthet Surg J 2008;28(4):452–5.

15. Aly AS. Upper body lift. In: Als AS, editor. Body contouring after massive weight loss. St Louis (MO): Quality Medical Publishing Inc; 2006. p. 235–60.

16. Rubin JP, Aly AS, Eaves FF III. Approaches to upper body rolls. In: Rubin JP, Matarasso A, editors. Aesthetic surgery after massive weight loss. Philadelphia: Elsevier; 2007. p. 101–12.

17. Cannistra C, Rodrigo V, Marmuse JP. Torsoplasty after important weight loss. Aesthetic Plast Surg 2006; 30:667.

18. Gonzalez-Ulloa M. Belt lipectomy. Br J Plast Surg 1961;13:179.

19. Hamra ST. Circumferential body lift. Aesthet Surg J 1999;19:244.

20. Hunstad JP. Addressing difficult areas in body contouring with emphasis on combined tumescent and syringe techniques. Clin Plast Surg 1996;23:57.

21. Hunstad JP. Body contouring in the obese patient. Clin Plast Surg 1996;23:647.

22. Baroudi R. Flankplasty: a specific treatment to improve body contouring. Ann Plast Surg 1991; 27:404.

23. Hurwitz DJ. Single stage total body lift after massive weight loss. Ann Plast Surg 2004;52:435.

24. Chamosa M. Lipectomy of fat rolls. Aesthetic Plast Surg 2006;30:417–21.

The Vertical Medial Thigh Lift

Joseph F. Capella, MD[a,b,*]

KEYWORDS

- Excess skin • Body contouring • Medial thigh lift • Inner thigh lift • Surgical technique
- Plastic surgery • Cosmetic surgery

KEY POINTS

- Careful patient screening and education are critical to optimizing the outcome of medial lift procedures.
- Major variables contributing to the thigh deformity include descent of the soft tissues of the hips, lower abdomen and mons pubis; inferomedial migration of thigh soft tissues; descent of the buttocks; and circumferential thigh soft tissue excess secondary to weight changes and aging. Prior liposuction may also contribute to thigh contour deformities.
- An effective medial thigh lift requires prior correction of soft tissue excess along the lower body.
- Thigh lift procedures with an excisional component limited to the thigh perineal crease usually provide little if any additional benefit to individuals who have undergone an effective circumferential lower body lift procedure.
- Liposuction in vertical medial thigh lift procedures serves to create a readily identifiable and safe plane of dissection and to improve outcome by optimizing the amount of soft tissue that can be removed.
- A lower body lifting procedure and subsequent medial thigh lift with a vertical component help minimize the likelihood of the well-described complications associated with medial thigh lifts with an approach limited to the thigh perineal crease: labial spreading and scar migration.

INTRODUCTION

Thigh contour deformities, and in particular those of the medial thighs, are a frequent concern for individuals seeking body contouring. The deformity is usually secondary to weight loss and is often associated with prior pregnancy and, in many instances, liposuction of the thighs. Despite the frequency of this concern, plastic surgeons have often been reluctant to use the medial thigh lift procedure because of the risk for significant complications and poor results, and the potential for readily visible scars.[1–4] Until recently, nearly all medial thigh lift techniques described in the literature attempted to address the medial thigh deformity by removing soft tissue excess in a vertical vector alone. An exception was the first description of a medial thigh lift in 1957 by Lewis.[5–15] He advocated both a horizontal and vertical component to the procedure. Lockwood[3], a proponent of vertical vector excision alone, described minimizing complications such as labial spreading and scar migration and improving outcome by securing the medial thigh flap to Colles fascia. Although the concept seemed to be a logical approach to address problems associated with medial thigh lifts, it added little to existing procedures. In recent years, primarily in response to the increase in numbers of individuals with postbariatric body

Disclosures: The author has received royalties from Addicus Books.
a Capella Plastic Surgery, 545 Island Road, Suite 2A, Ramsey, NJ 07446, USA; b Division of Plastic Surgery, Hackensack University Medical Center, 30 Prospect Avenue, Hackensack, NJ 07601, USA
* Capella Plastic Surgery, 545 Island Road, Suite 2A, Ramsey, NJ 07446.
E-mail address: jfcapella@aol.com

Clin Plastic Surg 41 (2014) 727–743
http://dx.doi.org/10.1016/j.cps.2014.06.005
0094-1298/14/$ – see front matter © 2014 Elsevier Inc. All rights reserved.

contour concerns, plastic surgeons have again advocated the excision of soft excess in both a vertical and horizontal vector to address medial thigh deformities.[4,16–20] In addition, the significance of addressing the vertical soft tissue excess of the lower abdomen, hips, thighs, and buttocks before performing an effective medial thigh lift has become more generally accepted.

Our approach to medial thigh contouring is to address the variables outside the medial thighs affecting the medial thighs before performing a medial thigh lift procedure. In most instances, a body lift or simultaneous abdominoplasty, thigh lift, and buttock lift is performed first.[21] For a small number of individuals, only an abdominoplasty is

performed initially. For some patients, the need for a medial thigh lift may be eliminated by these techniques (**Fig. 1**). For patients with a remaining deformity, a medial thigh lift with a vertical component is performed (**Fig. 2**).[4,22–24] For data and discussion purposes, this article classifies our various forms of medial thigh lift (**Box 1**).

PATIENT SELECTION AND SCREENING

As with all surgical candidates, individuals seeking surgical correction of their medial thigh deformities should undergo a thorough history and physical examination. Information particularly relevant to medial thigh lift surgery includes a history of weight

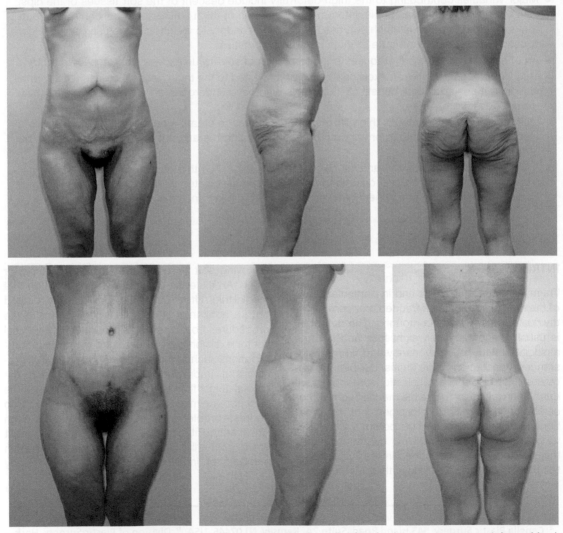

Fig. 1. (*Top*) A 27-year-old woman who lost 74 kg (163 lb) through lifestyle changes. Current weight and body mass index (BMI): 53 kg (117 lb) and 19.5 respectively. Highest weight and BMI ever achieved: 127 kg (280 lb) and 47. The medial thigh deformity was one of her primary concerns. (*Bottom*) Eighteen months following body lift. The body lift provided sufficient improvement of her medial thighs for her to forgo any further surgery to her medial thighs.

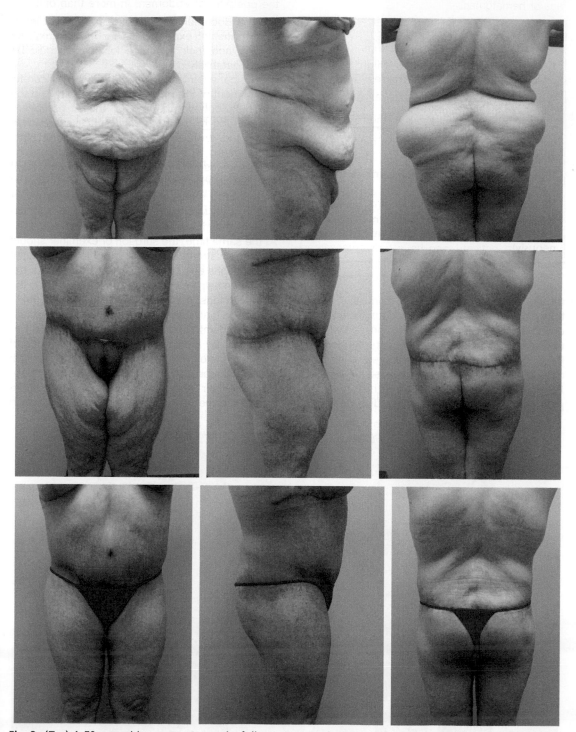

Fig. 2. (*Top*) A 50-year-old woman 42 months following gastric bypass surgery and weight loss of 36 kg (80 lb). Current weight and BMI: 77 kg (170 lb) and 31 respectively. Highest weight and BMI ever achieved: 114 kg (250 lb) and 46. (*Middle*) Three months following body lift. (*Bottom*) Three months following medial thigh lift with vertical component extending to junction of knee with leg; type III medial thigh lift.

change, and whether secondary to bariatric surgery, lifestyle changes, or pregnancy. The patient's height, current weight, and maximum weight should be noted, as should the time interval between their maximum and current weights. If weight loss was achieved through bariatric surgery, the technique and when it was performed should be noted. For patients who have lost weight

Box 1
Classification system for medial thigh lifts

Type I: approach limited to thigh perineal crease and proximal gluteal crease

Type II: type I approach plus vertical component limited to medial thigh

Type III: type I approach plus vertical component extending to junction of medial knee with leg.

Type IV: type I approach plus vertical component extending to medial leg

Type V: type IV technique plus transverse component over distal anterior thigh (type IV and type V not usually performed simultaneously)

also be documented. As part of the initial interview, patients' expectations for medial thigh lift surgery and their tolerance for scars should be clearly established.

Physical examination should focus on a careful assessment of the medial thigh deformity and the variables outside the medial thighs potentially contributing to the deformity: soft tissue excess along the lower abdomen, mons pubis, hips, lateral thighs, and buttocks. In an effort to assess the variables contributing to the medial thigh deformity during the examination, patients should be asked to stand in front of a full-length mirror and to apply strong upward traction to the soft tissues of their lower abdomens with their 2 hands. At the same time, the surgeon or examiner should then apply strong upward traction to the patient's lateral thighs and buttocks. This technique for examination helps eliminate the variables outside the medial thighs contributing to the medial thigh deformity. It also serves to show patients the function of circumferential body lifting procedures. Patients usually are not aware of the significance of these variables (**Fig. 3**). A second maneuver that should also be considered is to have patients abduct one their thighs (**Fig. 4**). Grasping the soft tissue of the medial thigh with the patient standing

through lifestyle changes, some discussion should take place as to how this was accomplished (ie exercise, diet and exercise, medication, and whether they are being supervised by a professional).[25] Prior body contouring procedures should be noted, including liposuction because it may affect the surgical plan and outcome. A history of lymphedema or peripheral vascular disease should

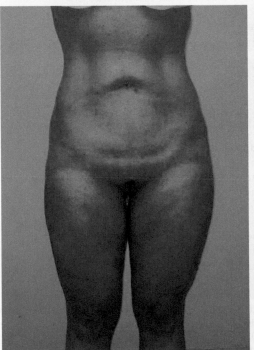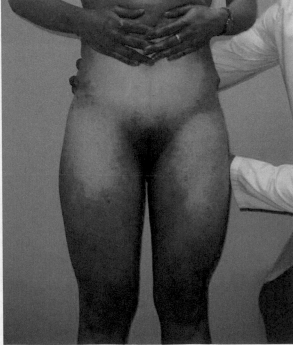

Fig. 3. This maneuver is the application of upward traction to the lower abdomen by the patient and the lateral thighs by the examiner, which helps eliminate the variables outside of the medial thighs contributing to the medial thigh deformity. It also serves to show patients the function of circumferential body lifting procedures. (*From* Capella JF, Woehrle, S. Vertical medial thigh lift with liposuction. In: Rubin PJ, Richter DF, Jewell ML, et al, editors. Body contouring and liposuction. London: Elsevier; 2013; with permission.)

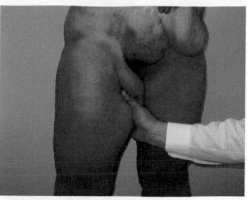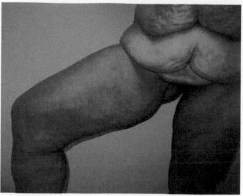

Fig. 4. Traction on the soft tissues of the medial thigh with the patient standing and abducting a lower extremity highlights soft tissue excess in the horizontal vector and shows the function of the vertical medial thigh lift. (*From* Capella JF, Woehrle, S. Vertical medial thigh lift with liposuction. In: Rubin PJ, Richter DF, Jewell ML, et al, editors. Body contouring and liposuction. London: Elsevier; 2013; with permission.)

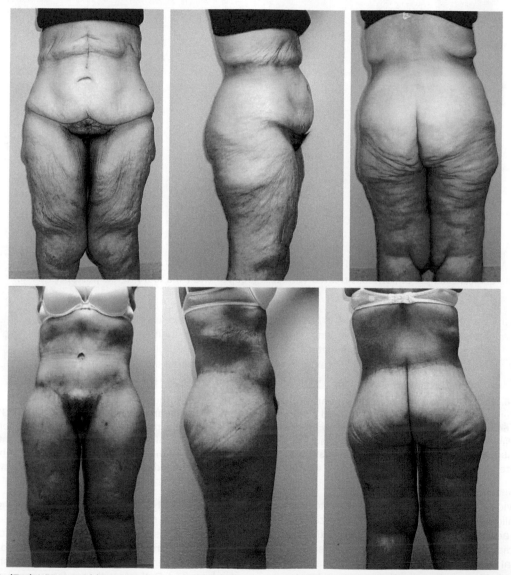

Fig. 5. (*Top*) A 55-year-old woman 13 months following gastric bypass surgery and weight loss of 52 kg (115 lb). Current weight and BMI: 71 kg (156 lb) and 30 respectively. Highest weight and BMI ever achieved: 123 kg (271 lb) and 53. (*Bottom*) The same patient 22 months following body lift and 10 months following medial thigh lift with a vertical component extending onto leg; type IV thigh lift. (*From* Capella JF, Woehrle, S. Vertical medial thigh lift with liposuction. In: Rubin PJ, Richter DF, Jewell ML, et al, editors. Body contouring and liposuction. London: Elsevier; 2013; with permission.)

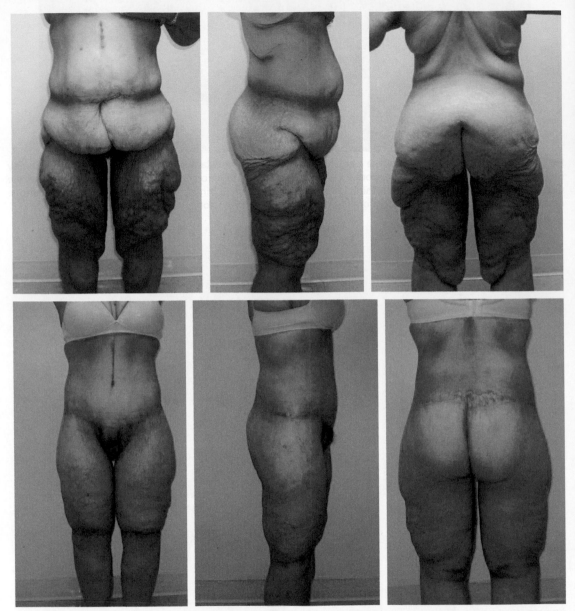

Fig. 6. (*Top*) A 59-year-old woman 18 months following gastric bypass surgery and weight loss of 89 kg (196 lb). Current weight and BMI: 55 kg (122 lb) and 25 respectively. Highest weight and BMI ever achieved: 145 kg (319 lb) and 64. (*Bottom*) One year following body lift, 6 months following medial thigh lift with vertical component extending to leg, medial thigh lift type IV, and 3 months following addition of transverse component over anterior distal thigh; type V thigh lift. (*From* Capella JF, Woehrle, S. Vertical medial thigh lift with liposuction. In: Rubin PJ, Richter DF, Jewell ML, et al, editors. Body contouring and liposuction. London: Elsevier; 2013; with permission.)

provides similar information. These techniques highlight soft tissue excess in the horizontal vector, accurately showing the function of the vertical medial thigh lift with liposuction procedure. The distal extent of the thigh deformity should be noted. Many women and some men have concerns about the excess soft tissue along the medial aspect of the knee and, in some instances, the leg as well (**Fig. 5**). Some women following

extreme weight loss have soft tissue draping the anterior aspect of the knee (**Fig. 6**). Tissue elasticity can be assessed by evaluating the skin for the presence of striae and cellulite. The fat content of the thighs and surrounding structures should also be noted. Patients with less fat excess usually have a more deflated appearance (see **Fig. 1**). Any intertriginous dermatitis, potentially along the proximal medial thigh, is noted. Lymphedema and/or stigmata of lymphedema should be documented, as should the presence of arterial or vascular insufficiency. Scars from previous surgery along the lower body and extremities should be documented, as should contour irregularities secondary to liposuction. The quality of existing scars is important to note. Medial thigh lifting surgery may result in scars that are more perceptible than with other more traditional procedures.

TREATMENT GOALS AND PLANNED OUTCOMES

A clear understanding of the variables contributing to a patient's medial thigh deformity is critical to optimizing outcomes following medial thigh lift surgery. An analysis of the medial thighs is complicated by its dependent position. Unlike many other areas of the body commonly treated by plastic surgeons, the medial thigh contour is strongly affected by the status of the soft tissues immediately cephalad to it, particularly in patients after weight loss. A failure to address deformities along the mons pubis, hips, thighs and buttocks, or lower body produces suboptimal results. Circumferential lower body lift procedures effectively address these concerns (see **Fig. 1**). Efforts to approach the medial thighs before addressing the lower body deformities usually lead to undesirable outcomes (**Fig. 7**). Equally important is the recognition of soft tissue excess in the horizontal vector.

Almost all patients after weight loss and many individuals who have undergone significant liposuction have soft tissue excess in the horizontal vector.

The lack of enthusiasm of many plastic surgeons for medial thigh lift procedures has much to do with the well-described complications associated with these techniques: labial spreading and scar migration and the potential for lymphedema.[1–3] Some of these complications relate to excessive tension along the thigh perineal closure. The combination of a prior lower body lifting procedure to address the vertical vector soft tissue excess and a subsequent vertical medial thigh lift with liposuction to address the horizontal vector of excess diminishes the need for tension along the thigh perineal closure, decreasing the likelihood of these classic complications (**Fig. 8**). When a medial thigh lift is performed from a thigh perineal approach alone, the surgeon often resects a substantial amount of soft tissue along the proximal medial thigh in an effort to effect change to the midthigh and distal thigh. Securing the thigh flap to an immobile structure such as Colles fascia is a logical strategy for preventing complications. However, the combination of a wide range of motion at the thigh perineal interface and the diminished elastic qualities of the soft tissues of most patients seeking contouring invariably leads to a change in the anticipated location of the scar at the thigh perineal junction and some transference of tension to the labia.

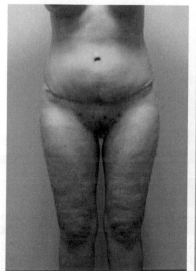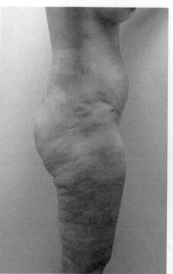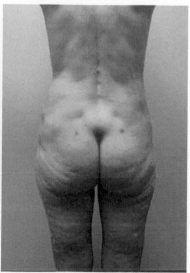

Fig. 7. This 53-year-old woman had lost 34 kg (74 lb) through lifestyle changes before undergoing concomitant liposuction of the thighs, a thigh lift limited to the thigh perineal crease, and abdominoplasty. Her surgeries were performed by another surgeon. She presented to us with concerns about thigh cellulite, thigh contour irregularities, and excess skin along her abdomen, thighs, and buttocks. Our plan for her is a body lift and possibly second-stage medial thigh lift type III, which are the procedures she most likely would have benefited from the most initially.

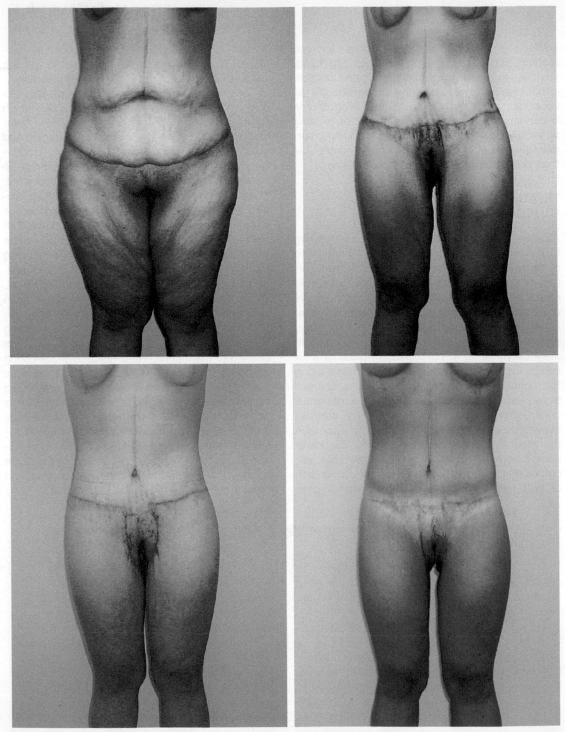

Fig. 8. (*Top left*) This 33-year-old woman with a presenting weight of 81 kg (179 lb), BMI of 31, lost 78 kg (172 lb) following gastric bypass performed 11 years previously. (*Top right*) She is now 3 months following the body lift and has concerns about remaining excess skin along her medial thighs. (*Bottom left*) Three months following bilateral medial thigh lift with approach limited to thigh perineal and gluteal crease; type I medial thigh lift. The patient was now primarily concerned about the lack of improvement of her medial thighs and was concerned about the distortion of her labia and the migration of the scar. (*Bottom right*) Two years following body lift and 18 months following revision medial thigh lift. A vertical component was added, extending to the junction of the knee with the leg; type III medial thigh lift. In addition to the improvement in the contour of her thighs, note correction of the thigh perineal scar migration. (*From* Capella JF, Woehrle, S. Vertical medial thigh lift with liposuction. In: Rubin PJ, Richter DF, Jewell ML, et al, editors. Body contouring and liposuction. London: Elsevier; 2013; with permission.)

In our plastic surgery practice, we rarely use liposuction as a sole procedure on postpartum or postbariatric individuals. The risk for contour irregularities is significant and the aesthetic benefits marginal.[26,27] However, we have embraced liposuction as an adjunct to soft tissue excisional procedures such as brachioplasty and vertical medial thigh lifts. Liposuction serves several functions in these procedures.[4,28] The first is to create a readily identifiable and safe plane of dissection. The evacuation of fat from the soft tissues deep to the superficial fascial system (SFS) facilitates dissection and the identification and preservation of nerves and veins (**Fig. 9**). The second is to reduce the volume of the extremity being treated. A smaller volume allows more skin and soft to be removed, improving the aesthetic outcome of a broad range of patients, particularly individuals with high body mass index (BMI) (see **Fig. 2**). On several occasions we have performed liposuction as a separate procedure before the medial thigh lift. We soon abandoned this approach in favor of concomitant liposuction. The scar tissue resulting from prior liposuction made dissection more difficult and less precise. In addition, the aesthetics of the patient's medial thighs are worsened by the liposuction, creating an unpleasant situation

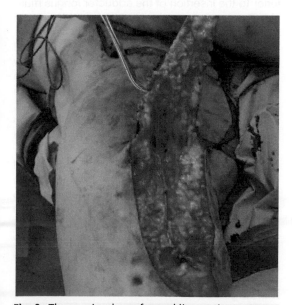

Fig. 9. The previously performed liposuction creates a readily identifiable plane of dissection with a characteristic honeycomb appearance. An effort is made to preserve the greater saphenous vein and its tributaries, although this is not always possible. (*From* Capella JF, Woehrle, S. Vertical medial thigh lift with liposuction. In: Rubin PJ, Richter DF, Jewell ML, et al, editors. Body contouring and liposuction. London: Elsevier; 2013; with permission.)

if the patient cannot undergo a medial thigh lift in the near future.

PREOPERATIVE PLANNING AND PREPARATION

The goal of the technique is to have the scars lie along the thigh perineal crease, proximal gluteal crease, and the medial aspect of the thigh. The patient is evaluated for marking while standing and facing the surgeon. The lower extremities should be parallel and several centimeters apart from each. A vertical line is drawn along the medial thighs from the thigh perineal crease to the medial aspect of the knees. The line should terminate at a point just distal to the deformity to be treated; typically the junction of the knee with the leg. The scar terminates in this region in approximately 90% of our cases and is classified as a medial thigh lift type III in our practice (see **Box 1**). The line should not be visible when evaluating the standing patient from either an anterior or posterior perspective. The remaining marks are made with the patient supine and following anesthesia.

PATIENT POSITIONING

Standing in a warm operating room, the patient is prepped with Betadine from the shoulders to the ankles. The patient then steps backward and sits on an operating table draped with sterile sheets. The patient is then rotated into the supine position on the operating table with the assistance of one individual holding the upper extremities and another holding the lower extremities. Before placing the lower extremities on the operating table, sterile stockings are applied. Immediately afterward and before induction, sterile sequential lower extremity compression devices are placed. A first-generation cephalosporin is given intravenously.

PROCEDURAL APPROACH
Patient Preparation

Following induction and with the patient under general anesthesia, a grounding pad is placed on one of the arms and the upper body is draped in the usual sterile fashion. A cotton swab soaked in methylene blue is used to delineate a line extending from just inferior to the preexisting scar from a circumferential body lift or abdominoplasty to the thigh perineal crease on either side of the mons pubis (**Fig. 10**). The marking should then transition from the thigh perineal crease to the proximal gluteal crease. The gluteal crease typically becomes visible along the proximal posterior medial thigh. The marking should stop several

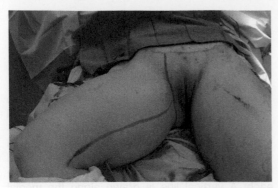

Fig. 10. A cotton swab soaked in methylene blue is used to delineate a line extending from just inferior to the preexisting scar from a circumferential body lift or abdominoplasty to the thigh perineal and gluteal crease on either side of the mons pubis. (*From* Capella JF, Woehrle, S. Vertical medial thigh lift with liposuction. In: Rubin PJ, Richter DF, Jewell ML, et al, editors. Body contouring and liposuction. London: Elsevier; 2013; with permission.)

centimeters before the gluteal crease makes contact with the operating table. This ensures that the proximal medial thigh scar will not be visible along the lower buttocks from a posterior perspective.

Tumescent Fluid

Tumescent fluid (50 mL of 1% lidocaine and 1 mL of 1:1000 epinephrine in 1 L of normal saline) is then injected into the soft tissues of the right medial thigh and knee. We typically begin with the right side. The volume of tumescent fluid injected is approximately equal to what is expected in effluent, or even less. Injecting excessive tumescent fluid makes an accurate assessment of the soft tissue to be removed difficult.

Dissection

While the tumescent fluid is taking effect, the skin along the marking at the right thigh perineal and gluteal crease is incised. Liposuction is usually not performed on individuals with a BMI of less than 21. Less benefit is seen in this patient population.

- Superior to the insertion of the adductor longus muscle, the dissection is limited to the superficial subcutaneous fat. The lymph nodes and other vital structures in this region are avoided.
- Posterior to the muscle insertion, the dissection is continued to the level of the muscle fascia.
- In the region of the gluteal crease, the dissection is limited to just deep to the superficial fascial system (SFS).

- Liposuction is then performed along the medial thigh and knee areas, deep to the superficial fascial system (SFS).

In many instances, more effluent can be removed than the tumescent volume injected. The pinch technique is then used by the surgeon to estimate the excess skin and soft tissue to be removed. The index finger of both hands is used to depress the previously made marking along the medial thigh and knee (**Fig. 11**). This technique maintains the final closure centered on the least perceptible location. The first pinch is usually over the area of greatest soft tissue excess, often the middle one-third of the medial thigh.

Clamping

The assistant then uses Adair or towel clamps to maintain the position of the estimated tissue to be removed. The process is continued distally to just beyond to the knee/leg junction and proximally to a point approximately 8 cm from the thigh perineal crease.

With the patient supine and flat, with the lower extremities slightly abducted, and the feet in the line with the shoulders, the most proximal medial thigh clamp is advanced cephalad until the pubic bone limits further advancement at a level just posterior to the insertion of the adductor longus muscle. The tension required to advance the clamp should be minimal. If moderate or significant tension is required, an additional more proximal clamp should be placed. This clamp should only maintain the same estimated amount of soft tissue to be removed in the horizontal vector as the clamp immediately caudal to it.

This most proximal clamp should then be advanced toward the pelvis. If it can be advanced toward the bone with minimal tension, no further clamps are placed along the proximal medial thigh. With the most proximal medial thigh clamp in place and the assistant advancing that clamp to the pelvic bone, the surgeon approximates the skin edge of the midportion of the lateral mons pubis to the skin along the medial thigh flap directly across from it to estimate skin redundancy in this portion of the medial thigh flap (**Fig. 12**).

Marking

Methylene blue is used to mark that spot along the medial thigh flap. The assistant releases the clamp that has been advanced toward the pelvis.

- The methylene blue–soaked cotton swab is used to make a line from the superior extent of the skin edge along the right side of the mons pubis to the spot marked along the thigh

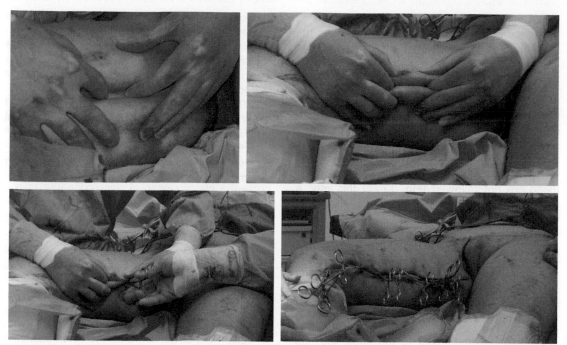

Fig. 11. The pinch technique is used by the surgeon to estimate the excess skin and soft tissue to be removed. The index fingers of both hands depress the previously made marking along the medial thigh and knee. This technique maintains the final closure centered on the least perceptible location. The first pinch is usually over the area of greatest soft tissue excess, often the middle one-third of the medial thigh. The assistant then uses Adair or towel clamps to maintain the position of the estimated tissue to be removed. (*From* Capella JF, Woehrle, S. Vertical medial thigh lift with liposuction. In: Rubin PJ, Richter DF, Jewell ML, et al, editors. Body contouring and liposuction. London: Elsevier; 2013; with permission.)

flap and extended to the most proximal medial thigh clamp.

- The mark is then extended to the most posterior extent of the gluteal crease incision in the form of a gentle arc.

- Hatch marks are made in the skin with a blade at the site of the most proximal clamp to help identify the intersection of the planned closure at the thigh perineal crease.

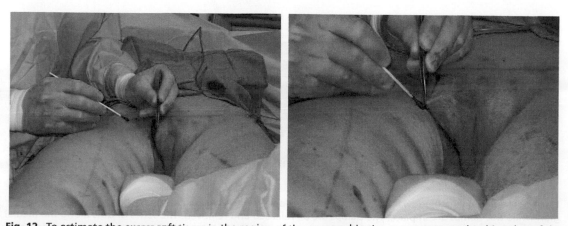

Fig. 12. To estimate the excess soft tissue in the region of the mons pubis, the surgeon grasps the skin edge of the midportion of the lateral mons pubis and the skin along the medial thigh flap directly across from it. Methylene blue is used to mark that spot along the medial thigh flap. (*From* Capella JF, Woehrle, S. Vertical medial thigh lift with liposuction. In: Rubin PJ, Richter DF, Jewell ML, et al, editors. Body contouring and liposuction. London: Elsevier; 2013; with permission.)

- The methylene blue swab is then used to place dots on either skin edge all along the medial thigh and knee region where the clamps are in place.
- The clamps are all released and removed.

The series of dots along the medial thigh and knee delineate the pattern of the skin and soft tissue to be removed.

The cotton swab is used to connect the dots. Some of the dots may not correspond exactly with the overall pattern being produced and those are not followed (**Fig. 13**). In this way, a smooth contour is maintained along the medial thighs.

Incision, Dissection, Closure

Having completely demarcated an area of skin and soft tissue to be removed both along the proximal and medial thighs and knee areas, the skin along the marking is incised completely.

- Beginning just distal to the knee, the flap is elevated under moderate tension. The previously performed liposuction creates a readily identifiable plane of dissection with a characteristic honeycomb appearance (see **Fig. 9**).
- An effort is made to preserve the greater saphenous vein and its tributaries, although this is not always possible.
- Along the proximal thigh the dissection is at the level previously described for the incision at the thigh perineal and gluteal creases.
- After gaining careful hemostasis, the skin edges are undermined for a distance of approximately 1 cm in the midthigh and knee areas, which facilitates wound closure and skin eversion.
- The skin and soft tissue edges along the medial thighs, the vertical component of the procedure, are approximated with Adair or towel clamps.
- The closure is performed with interrupted 2-0 Vicryl sutures placed through the superficial fascial system and deep dermis approximately 1 cm from the skin edge. The technique everts and diminishes tension along the skin edges.
- The vertical closure is completed with a continuous, intracuticular 3-0 Monocryl suture.
- Attention is directed toward the proximal medial thighs. The cephalad tissue edge along the most posterior extent of the gluteal crease wound is approximated to the caudal tissue edge in a manner that does not produce a standing cone or dog ear on the buttocks. Avoidance of this problem is facilitated by flexing the right hip and knees to 90° with slight hip abduction and having an assistant align the tissue edges.
- The tissue edges in the gluteal crease region are approximated initially with a #1 Vicryl suture placed through the FS and deep dermis approximately 1 cm from the tissue edge (**Fig. 14**).
- The closure continues into the thigh perineal area in a similar fashion.
- The hip is gradually extended from its flexed position as the closure proceeds.
- Anterior to the gluteal crease and posterior to the insertion of the adductor longus muscle, Colles fascia is readily identifiable. The sutures placed in the cephalad tissue edge

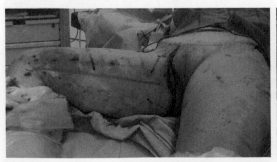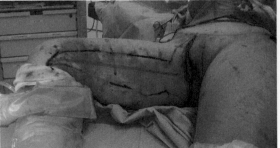

Fig. 13. The methylene blue swab is used to place dots on either skin edge along the medial thigh and knee region while the clamps are in place. The clamps are all released and removed. The series of dots along the medial thigh and knee delineate the pattern of the skin and soft tissue to be removed. The cotton swab is used to connect the dots. Some of the dots may not correspond exactly with the overall pattern being produced and those are not followed. In this way, a smooth contour is maintained along the medial thighs. (*From* Capella JF, Woehrle, S. Vertical medial thigh lift with liposuction. In: Rubin PJ, Richter DF, Jewell ML, et al, editors. Body contouring and liposuction. London: Elsevier; 2013; with permission.)

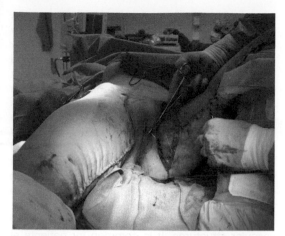

Fig. 14. The cephalad tissue edge along the most posterior extent of the gluteal crease wound is approximated to the caudal tissue edge in a manner that does not produce a standing cone or dog ear on the buttocks. Avoidance of this problem is facilitated by flexing the right hip and knees to 90° with slight hip abduction and having an assistant align the tissue edges. (*From* Capella JF, Woehrle, S. Vertical medial thigh lift with liposuction. In: Rubin PJ, Richter DF, Jewell ML, et al, editors. Body contouring and liposuction. London: Elsevier; 2013; with permission.)

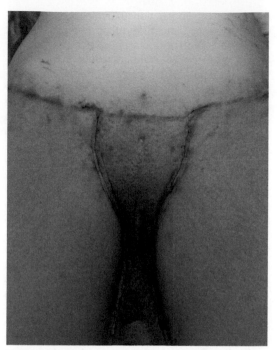

Fig. 15. The excess length of the thigh flap should be excised along the scar of the previously performed abdominoplasty or body lift. (*From* Capella JF, Woehrle, S. Vertical medial thigh lift with liposuction. In: Rubin PJ, Richter DF, Jewell ML, et al, editors. Body contouring and liposuction. London: Elsevier; 2013; with permission.)

may incorporate this structure along with the SFS and deep dermis; however, no sutures are placed specifically in this structure.

- The closure continues into the region of the mons pubis. The hip should now be fully extended.
- The greater length of the thigh flap tissue edge versus the cephalad edge of the wound in many instances leads to a closure mismatch in the region of the mons pubis. Rather than attempt to manipulate the thigh flap tissues edge to facilitate the closure, the excess length of the thigh flap should be excised along the scar of the previously performed abdominoplasty or body lift (**Fig. 15**).
- If a body lift or abdominoplasty is being performed at the same time as a medial thigh lift, the abdominoplasty closure on either side of the mons pubis is finalized after the excess thigh tissue has excised along this closure. A failure to excise the excess length of the thigh flap may lead to a distortion in the appearance of the mons pubis.
- Vicryl sutures (size 0) are placed along the wound at a deep dermal level to further reinforce the closure, and intracuticular 3-0 Monocryl completes the closure.
- Sterile dressings are applied, followed by elastic wraps.

POTENTIAL COMPLICATIONS AND MANAGEMENT

Complications following medial thigh lift procedures are usually minor but are more frequent than with other more traditional body contouring procedures (**Table 1**). The complications and their management are similar to those following brachioplasty.[27] In our review of 335 cases of vertical

Table 1
Complication rates associated with vertical medial thigh lift	

Vertical Medial Thigh Lift Complication Rates (%) N = 335 Cases (670 Thighs)	
Skin dehiscence	28.4
Seroma	19
Infection	1
Hematoma	0.3
Skin necrosis	0.3
Deep vein thrombosis	0.3
Pulmonary embolism	0.0

medial lift with liposuction (670 thighs), skin dehiscence was the most frequent complication at 28.4%. Only 1 of the dehiscences occurred acutely (ie within the first 24–48 hours following the operation). Most began to become evident approximately 2 weeks following the procedure. Nearly all (95%) occurred at the intersection of the closure at the thigh perineal crease. As in many instances in plastic surgery in which a skin flap narrows, the tip of the flap may have a compromised blood supply. In the days following the procedure the tip may become increasingly ischemic and take on a dusky appearance, and at 2 weeks skin separation may take place. Most skin dehiscences are less than 3 cm in size. Avoiding this complication is challenging. A technique that avoids a closure intersection at the thigh perineal crease is unlikely to produce optimal results. We advise patients to limit abduction of the thighs; however, this restriction is unlikely to prevent this problem. The dehiscences are treated with dressing changes. In some instances, hypergranulation tissue may arise in the area of skin dehiscence. Silver nitrate application is effective. Seromas are the second most common complication at 19%. Approximately 90% occur along the distal medial one-third of the thigh and are positioned immediately beneath the scar. Most become evident at about 3 weeks after surgery and range in diameter from 1 to 4 cm. At first we manage them by needle aspiration. However, this technique has a high recurrence rate, particularly with seromas larger than 1 cm in diameter. The technique of marsupialization (ie, incising the skin over the seroma, draining the seroma, and suturing the seroma cavity to the skin) is 100% effective but results in a scar that may be wider than the adjoining scar and often results in a prolonged healing process. Our preference at this time is to drain the seroma via the scar and place a secured Penrose-type drain into the seroma cavity. This technique has also proved to be effective. In several instances, a localized cellulitis has resulted from this approach. We now prescribe a first-generation cephalosporin while the drain is in place. Infections have been infrequent, as have bleeding and hematomas. Skin necrosis has also been infrequent despite liposuction being performed in virtually all cases. We have only 1 documented instance of deep vein thrombosis in a patient undergoing vertical medial thigh lift with liposuction. There have been no instances of pulmonary embolism.

Chronic lower extremity edema is often considered to be a significant risk for patients undergoing a medial thigh lift procedure.[2] However, this has not been the case in our series. We have had only 2 cases in which lower extremity edema has persisted beyond 3 months and in both instances the patients returned to their presurgical states by 6 months. A significant number of patients after massive weight loss, particularly those who had weighed more than 160 kg (350 lb) before weight loss, have some degree of chronic stable edema and skin changes consistent with the sequelae of lymphedema. It is important during the preoperative assessment to document these clinical findings because they are unlikely to be improved by a medial thigh lift. Preserving lymph nodes at the femoral triangle and perhaps the incorporation of liposuction in the areas of tissue removal have helped minimize this complication in our series. Liposuction may facilitate the preservation of vascular structures. It is common for patients at the 2-week postoperative period, a time when many are resuming their normal daily activities, to develop more lower extremity swelling than they had in the immediate postoperative period. If the swelling is limited to a single extremity, we advise them to undergo a lower extremity venous Doppler. If the swelling is symmetric and bilateral, supportive stockings are prescribed and the findings are followed closely with expectation that it should resolve gradually over the next several weeks.

Scar quality is often of great concern to patients following a vertical medial thigh lift procedure. As described earlier, we do not routinely make any particular recommendation regarding scars, aside from the avoidance of ultraviolet light during the period of scar maturation. If patients are not satisfied with the quality of their scars and if the potential for improvement exists, we perform a scar revision, often with local anesthesia or at the time when another procedure requiring general anesthesia is being performed. The revisions are usually not considered before 1 year. Revisions performed at this time nearly always produce a less perceptible scar, probably because of diminished tension along the closure.

POSTPROCEDURAL CARE

Patients are advised that they may ambulate immediately after surgery as tolerated. Dressings and elastic wraps are removed 48 hours after surgery, at which time showering is permissible. Thereafter, patients are not advised to wear any supportive garments unless swelling of the legs or feet become evident. In these cases supportive stockings are suggested. Any exercise or activity that may lead to significant perspiration is discouraged for 2 weeks. In addition, patients are advised to avoid abducting their thighs beyond 45° to avoid excessive tension along the thigh perineal closure during this time.

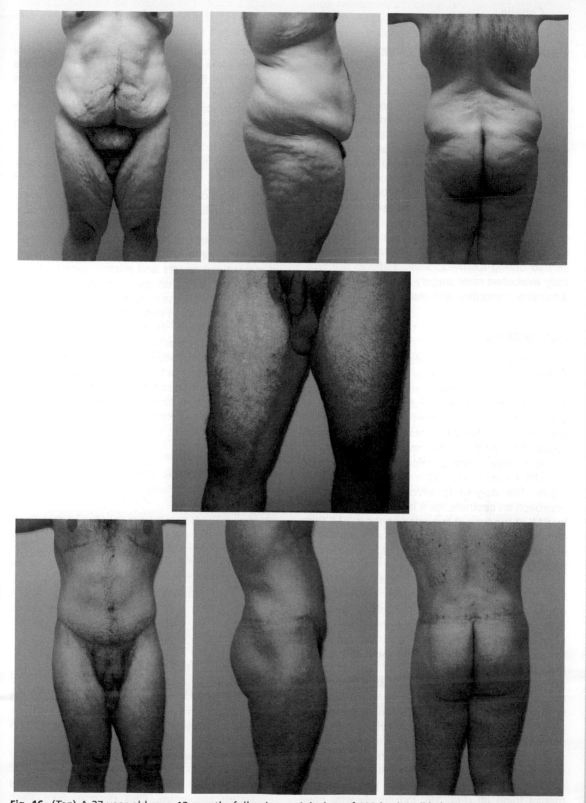

Fig. 16. (*Top*) A 27-year-old man 12 months following weight loss of 102 kg (225 lb) through lifestyle changes. Current weight and BMI: 80 kg (175 lb) and 27 respectively. Highest weight and BMI ever achieved: 182 kg (400 lb) and 61. (*Bottom*) Thirteen months following body lift and simultaneous vertical medial thigh lift: thigh with vertical component extending to junction of medial knee with leg; type III medial thigh lift. (*Middle*) Vertical component of medial thigh lift. (*From* Capella JF, Woehrle, S. Vertical medial thigh lift with liposuction. In: Rubin PJ, Richter DF, Jewell ML, et al, editors. Body contouring and liposuction. London: Elsevier; 2013; with permission.)

REHABILITATION AND RECOVERY

Vigorous upper body activities are permitted after 2 weeks and lower body activities after 6 weeks. Patients are not advised to apply or consume any products or perform any particular therapy for the purpose of improving scar quality. Patients who are determined to use a particular product are informed that silicon gel sheeting is the only product with scientific data to support its use in scar therapy. Silicon gel sheeting may be applied after 2 weeks. All patients are advised to minimize ultraviolet light exposure to the scar while it is hyperemic to avoid permanent hyperpigmentation. The normal process of scar maturation is often reviewed during follow-up visits. Patients are typically evaluated after surgery at 1 week, 6 weeks, 3 months, 6 months, and yearly.

OUTCOMES

Achieving optimal and consistent results with our technique for vertical medial thigh lifting requires careful patient education, screening, and selection, and effective prior treatment of the vertical vector soft tissue variables contributing to the thigh deformity. Most patients who have had satisfactory treatment of their lower body vertical vector soft tissue excess before a vertical medial thigh lift are pleased with the outcome of our technique. The degree to which our patients can approach an aesthetic ideal is influenced primarily by BMI at the time of surgery, change in BMI from highest weight, body type, and the extent of deformities created by prior liposuction. Patients who present for body contouring at or near ideal BMI are most likely to obtain near-ideal results (see **Fig. 8**). Individuals who present overweight or obese but who have had substantial changes in BMI from their highest weight have significant improvement in appearance but may not reach the same level of result as the prior group (see **Fig. 2**). Patients with a gynoid body habitus, almost exclusively women, present a greater challenge than individuals with a more android body type (see **Fig. 6**). Almost all men and a substantial percentage of women have an android or near-android body type. The thigh deformity in the near-android group is more proximal and usually limited to the medial thighs, and thus is effectively treated by the sequence of lower body lift and a medial thigh lift (**Fig. 16**). Individuals who have had prior liposuction of the midthighs and distal anterior and/or posterior thighs represent a great challenge. Liposuction may have taken place when these patients were younger and the deleterious consequences unnoticed until later, or the liposuction may have been done more recently as a mistaken approach to addressing soft tissue excess. The lack of deep fat compartments in these 2 zones of the thighs makes contour deformities secondary to liposuction particularly difficult to correct despite the use of excision techniques (see **Fig. 7**).

SUMMARY

Medial thigh deformities are a concern for many patients seeking body contouring. Despite this, many plastic surgeons are reluctant to approach this region with soft tissue excisional procedures. The lack of enthusiasm relates to the frequency of suboptimal results and related complications. Medial thigh lifts that are consistently effective are possible when the vertical and horizontal components of the thigh deformity and their relationship to the lower body are recognized. Our approach to the medial thighs, the correction of lower body deformities before a vertical medial thigh lift with liposuction, has been used in hundreds of cases with satisfying results. Medial thigh lift surgery is a routine and essential part of our plastic surgery practice.

REFERENCES

1. Leitner DW, Sherwood RC. Inguinal lymphocele as a complication of thighplasty. Plast Reconstr Surg 1983;72:878.
2. Moreno CH, Neto HJ, Junior AH, et al. Thighplasty after bariatric surgery: evaluation of lymphatic drainage in lower extremities. Obes Surg 2008;18:1160.
3. Lockwood T. Fascial anchoring technique in medial thigh lifts. Plast Reconstr Surg 1988;82(2):299–304.
4. Capella JF, Woehrle S. Vertical medial thigh lift with liposuction. In: Rubin PJ, Richter DF, Jewell ML, et al, editors. Body contouring and liposuction. London: Elsevier; 2013. p. 353–65.
5. Lewis JR. The thigh lift. J Int Coll Surg 1957;27:330.
6. Pitanguy I. Trochanteric lipodystrophy. Plast Reconstr Surg 1964;34:280.
7. Planas J. Crural meloplasty for lifting the thighs. Clin Plast Surg 1975;2:495.
8. Vilain R. Surgical correction of steatomeries. Clin Plast Surg 1975;2:467.
9. Schultz RC, Feinberg LA. Medial thigh lift. Ann Plast Surg 1979;2:404.
10. Lockwood T. Lower body lift with superficial fascial system suspension. Plast Reconstr Surg 1993;92(6):1112–22.
11. Spirito D. Medial thigh lift and DE.C.LI.VE. Aesthetic Plast Surg 1998;22:298.
12. Le Louarn C, Pascal JF. The concentric medial thigh lift. Aesthetic Plast Surg 2004;28:20.

13. Kirwan L. Anchor thighplasty. Aesthet Surg J 2004; 24:61.
14. Sozer SO, Agullo FJ, Palladino H. Spiral lift: medial and lateral thigh lift with buttock lift and augmentation. Aesthetic Plast Surg 2008;32:120.
15. Shermak MA, Mallalieu J, Chang D. Does thighplasty for upper thigh laxity after weight loss require a vertical scar? Aesthet Surg J 2009;29:513.
16. Baker. Medial Thigh Lift. Gordon Symposium on Cosmetic Surgery. Miami, Florida. February 4, 2005.
17. Hurwitz DJ. Medial thighplasty. Aesthet Surg J 2005; 25:180.
18. Kenkel JM, Aly AS, Capella JF, et al. Body contouring after massive weight loss. Plast Reconstr Surg 2006;117(1 Suppl):45S–73S.
19. Mathes DW, Kenkel JM. Current concepts in medial thighplasty. Clin Plast Surg 2008;35:151–63.
20. Cram A, Aly A. Thigh reduction in the massive weight loss patient. Clin Plast Surg 2008;35:165.
21. Aly AS, Capella JF. Staging, reoperation and treatment of complications after body contouring in the massive-weight-loss patient. In: Grotting J, editor. Reoperative aesthetic and reconstructive surgery. 2nd edition. St Louis (MO): Quality Medical Publishing; 2007. p. 1701–40.
22. Nemerofsky RB, Oliak DA, Capella JF. Body lift: an account of 200 consecutive cases in the massive weight loss patient. Plast Reconstr Surg 2006;117:414.
23. Capella JF. An approach to the lower body after weight loss. In: Matarasso A, Rubin P, editors. Aesthetic surgery in the massive weight loss patient. New York: Elsevier; 2007. p. 69–99.
24. Capella JF. Body lift. Clin Plast Surg 2008;35:27–51.
25. Capella JF, Travato M, Woehrle S. Screening and safety issues in the massive-weight loss patient. In: Nahai F, editor. Art of aesthetic surgery: principles and technique, 2E. St Louis (MO): Quality Medical Publishing; 2010. p. 2797–817.
26. Capella JF. Special problems in re-operative body contouring. In: Nahai F, editor. Art of aesthetic surgery: principles and technique, 2E. St Louis (MO): Quality Medical Publishing; 2010. p. 3169–80.
27. Capella JF. Role of suction assisted liposuction. In: Thaller S, Cohen M, editors. Cosmetic surgery after weight loss. London, UK: JP Medical Publishers; 2013. p. 165–78.
28. Capella JF, Travato M, Woehrle S. Brachioplasty. In: Nahai F, editor. Art of aesthetic surgery: principles and technique, 2E. St Louis (MO): Quality Medical Publishing; 2010. p. 2819–52.

Brachioplasty

Dennis Hurwitz, MD

KEYWORDS

- Brachioplasty • Arm • Aesthetics • Deformity

KEY POINTS

- The arm is shaped by muscular and adipose disposition and mass.
- Because the loose skin and fat predominantly sag along the laminar-related posterior border, the triceps-related contours can be obscured.
- The goal of plastic surgery of the arm is to approximate the ideal arm by removal and/or redistribution of tissues leaving the least conspicuous scars and as few complications and deformity as possible.
- In borderline cases of excess adipose and skin, liposuction is the preferred approach, particularly in young patients after massive weight loss.
- When skin laxity is excessive, even in young patients, an extensive arm-long operation that extends across the axilla and onto the lateral chest is indicated.

Although the demand for brachioplasty has increased greatly over the past 10 years, there has been little attention to the aesthetics of the arm and avoidance of brachioplasty deformity. There is no consensus on technique. There also remains uncertainty as to the role of liposuction as an adjunct or alternative.

This article contrasts the ideal appearance of the female upper arm, axilla, and upper midlateral chest with the sagging and/or oversized deformity. The constellation of postbrachioplasty aesthetic deformity is introduced. These aesthetic shortcomings are best avoided, because they are difficult, if not impossible, to correct. The L brachioplasty with liposuction[1,2] is briefly described in a recent case and applied to a variety of deformities to show the range of applicability and quality of results. The role of liposuction in arm reshaping is examined. The aesthetic advantages and low complication rate of the L brachioplasty, when precisely performed, are contrasted with other currently popular brachioplasties.[3–5]

Women's upper arms are tapering undulating cones extending from shoulders to elbows. A recent 1-year postoperative L brachioplasty result in a thin and muscular 67-year-old woman shows the salient aesthetics that apply across genders (**Fig. 1**). Her frontal, right anterior oblique, and posterior images are all taken in standardized positions of the upper arm abducted 90° from the body and flexed at right angles with the arm supine. These are also the positions that the patient is asked to take when assessing redundancy of skin and fat. The extended elbow is not used, because the skin laxity about the elbow slides to the distal arm and this should not be accounted for in the upper arm resection.

The arm is shaped by muscular and adipose disposition and mass. Description of the arm, which can be rotated into numerous positions, was standardized by Avelar[6] in assigning the 4 sides (1) anterior, (2) external, (3) posterior, and (4) internal (see **Fig. 1**). There are 2 layers of fat. The arm is surrounded by the subdermal areolar layer of vertically segmented adipose containing the superficial neurovasculature. Only posterior is there a lamellar layer (deep) composed of horizontally oriented adipose. This deep layer is more prone to storing fat.[7] Except for the thinnest women (as seen in **Fig. 1**), muscular definition is muted by less muscular bulk and a fuller alveolar layer. Regardless, the ideal aesthetic result in

Department of Plastic Surgery, Hurwitz Center for Plastic Surgery, University of Pittsburgh Medical Center, 6B Scaife Hall, 3550 Terrace Street, Pittsburgh, PA 15261, USA
E-mail address: drhurwitz@hurwitzcenter.com

Clin Plastic Surg 41 (2014) 745–751
http://dx.doi.org/10.1016/j.cps.2014.07.003
0094-1298/14/$ – see front matter © 2014 Elsevier Inc. All rights reserved.

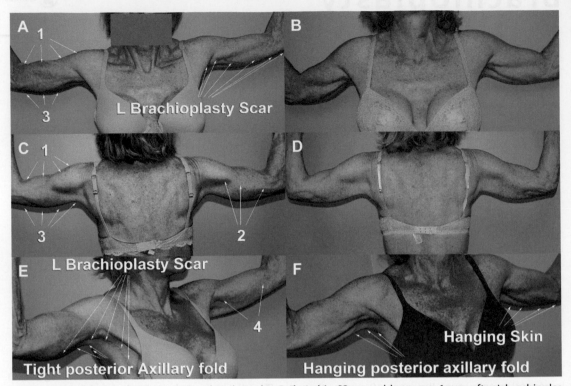

Fig. 1. Aesthetics after and before L brachioplasty. (*A, C, E*). A thin 68-year-old woman, 1 year after L brachioplasties, models aesthetic muscular arms. The 4 sides are (1) anterior, (2) external, (3) posterior, and (4) internal. Her skin is tightly wrapped about underlying muscles and intermuscular clefts. The posterior axillary folds hug the proximal triceps and latissimus dorsi muscles. The midarm has the greatest muscle-related convexities on the anterior and posterior surfaces. At 1 year, the L-shaped scar is difficult to see. In contrast with the preoperative views (*B, D, F*), there is no loose or hanging skin.

either gender is tight skin enveloping muscular curves. The deltoid and biceps muscles clearly define the bulging curves of the anterior and external arms. Separated from the biceps and brachioradialis by transverse grooves, the hanging triceps supplemented by a deposit of lamellar fat imparts a central convexity to the posterior arm. This muscle, with tightly adherent skin, acutely rises to attach to the chest to create the posterior axillary fold. The width of the most proximal arm from its attachment to the chest and the deltoid prominence is equal to the midarm from the deepest curvature of the triceps to the bulge of the biceps. The flat internal arm is accentuated by the bicipital groove, which leads to the axilla.

The axilla is a shallow dome created by the suspended clavipectoral fascia and bordered by the triceps, latissimus dorsi, and pectoralis muscles. There is a dynamic aesthetic relationship of the depth of the axilla to the position of the arm. As the arm rises from resting against the chest to full abduction and extension, the axillary recession increases to its greatest depth at 90° of abduction

and progressively flattens as the arm is further raised. The central axilla is recessed by its clavipectoral fascia roof and its adherent hair-bearing skin tethered by fascia extensions through the lymph nodal area to the upper chest. Massive weight loss increases axillary depth and size.

Excess skin and fat blunt the muscle-related contours. Because the loose skin and fat predominantly sag along the laminar-related posterior border, the triceps-related contours can be obscured. Along with even more descent of the posterior axillary fold, the posterior margin evolves from curved to flat. The axillary hollow may have rolls of excess skin or deepen and widen, which is called hyperaxilla.[2] The upper lateral chest is too full, often leading to a lateral bra roll. The definition between the lateral borders of the pectoralis major and latissimus dorsi muscles is lost.

The goal of plastic surgery of the arm is to approximate the ideal arm by removal and/or redistribution of tissues leaving the least conspicuous scars, as few complications, and as little deformity as possible. An assessment is made of the undesirable deposits of adipose and skin redundancy and laxity. Healthy youth have greater skin retraction than the aged.

In borderline cases of excess adipose and skin, liposuction is the preferred approach, particularly in young patients after massive weight loss. It is the experience of this author that preliminary focused energy results in better skin retraction to encompass the smaller volume. Radiofrequency-assisted lipoplasty of the arms has the added benefit of inducing collagen retraction through sublethal injury in borderline cases.[8] Prolonged induration and scattered residual pockets of scarring are drawbacks. The most advanced minimally invasive bipolar technology is the BodyTite (InVasix, Israel), which remains in prolonged trials and has not yet obtained US Food and Drug Administration approval. Meanwhile, improvements in design have advanced VASERlipo to the forefront. Through 3 incisions of 4 mm, 1 in the posterior fold and 2 across the elbow, the arm is evacuated of excess superficial and deep adipose (**Fig. 2**). Even following 54-kg (120 pound) weight loss, the resulting contours are improved with no increased laxity of skin.

When skin laxity is excessive, even in young patients, an extensive arm-long operation that extends across the axilla and onto the lateral chest is indicated. Full-length and more limited L brachioplasty has been the workhorse arm reduction operation for more than 120 cases. The goal is reduction of excess skin and fat along the internal and posterior arm, through the axilla, and then along the lateral chest. The technique for the L brachioplasty has not changed since it was last published in 2011. The long arm excision is a hemiellipse along the inferior aspect of the internal arm. The resulting scar along the internal arm dips toward the posterior margin and then ascends to the deltopectoral groove superior to the axilla. The short arm excision along the upper midlateral chest meets the arm pattern at right angles across the axilla. This angulation forms a broad-based triangular flap with the base along the posterior axillary fold. After the excess skin in the axilla is excised, this flap is advanced across the axilla, thereby making the hollow smaller.

A recent case of a 33-year-old woman after massive weight loss shows the preoperative markings, intraoperative critical events, and early

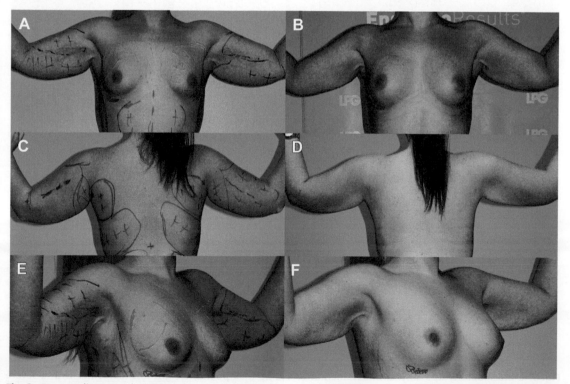

Fig. 2. Excess adipose and sagging skin in a 23-year-old patient after massive weight loss. (*A, C, E*) Despite losing more than 45 kg (100 pounds), she has excessive adipose throughout her upper torso and arms. Her small breasts are widely spaced. She has no definition of her upper arm musculature. The planned liposuction is marked in black with breast lipoaugmentation marked in green. (*B, D, F*) The 6-month result of VASERlipo of the arms and torso as previously marked, along with an abdominoplasty and 300-mL lipoaugmentation of each breast.

excellent postoperative results along with a minor delayed healing complication of the right axilla. She is 170 cm (5′ 7″) tall and weighs 91 kg (200 pounds; BMI 30), down from 204 kg (450 pounds) through diet and exercise. She desires removal of considerable excess skin followed by aesthetic reshaping of her arms (**Fig. 3**A, C, D). There is massive descending tissue along the posterior arm and posterior axillary fold with hyperaxilla. With sculptured reflections of her deltoid and biceps bulges, posterior/internal and axillary resections with a superior advancement are needed. Radical excision site and cosmetic posterior arm liposuction is planned. The result 3 months later shows aesthetically sculptured arms with a proportional axillary hollow and reduced upper lateral chest (see **Fig. 3**B, D, F). She had 2 cm of dehiscence along the apex of the right axillary closure, which healed with limited debridement over 2 months. The stepwise preoperative arm markings are precisely drawn and then measured to leave a cookie-cutter pattern for excision (**Fig. 4**). Three points are placed for the anterior incision from the

deltopectoral groove[1] and the medial condyle,[3] with the midarm number 2 along the bicipital groove. The maximal width of resection is made at the midarm at 2 and is determined by pinching the tissues together to point 4 (see **Fig. 4**B). The posterior incision sweeps upward to toward the axilla for point 5 and the completion of the posterior incision. The straight anterior incision, 1 to 3, is measured and equals the curving posterior incision, 3 to 5 (see **Fig. 4**C, D). The axillary and lateral chest excision is through equidistant lines 1 to 6 and 5 to 6 (see **Fig. 4**E, F). **Fig. 5** shows the 6 essential steps of her L brachioplasty. The prepped arm lies on an arm board extending 90° from the side of the operating room table. The area of arm excision is radically suctioned of fat (see **Fig. 4**A). Limited cosmetic removal of fat is performed in the posterior portion. The perimeter incision of the L brachioplasty is made perpendicular through the skin and subcutaneous tissue until a gap is present (see **Fig. 5**B). The skin of the arm is avulsed proximal to distal with the assistance of scalpel cuts (see **Fig. 5**C). The proximal posterior inverted V flap is

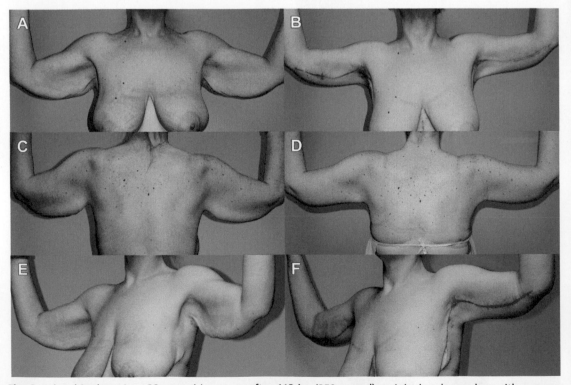

Fig. 3. L brachioplasty in a 38-year-old woman after 113-kg (250 pound) weight loss leaves her with a severe deformity. (*A, C, E*) There is hanging skin and adipose along the posterior and external aspects of her arm, and oversized and deep axillary hollows. The posterior arm is flat, has no muscular definition, and the axillary fold is descended. (*B, D, F*) Five months after L brachioplasty, the shape is aesthetic with ascend of the posterior axillary fold, definition of the triceps, and normal axillary hollow. The undulating scar is still reddened and has no contracture across the axilla.

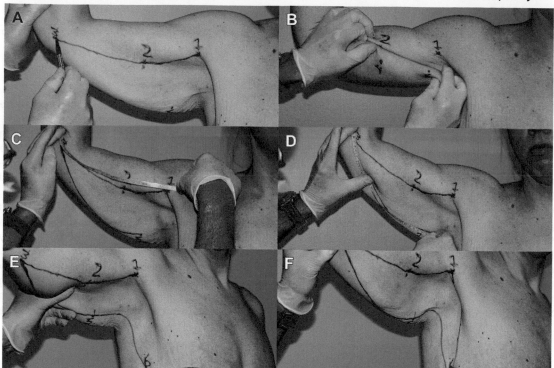

Fig. 4. Presurgical markings for right arm L brachioplasty of the patient in **Fig. 3**. (*A*) A straight line is drawn across points 1, 2, and 3. (*B*) The midarm width of excision at point 4 is determined by direct squeeze of the tissues. Point 5 is advanced across the axilla. (*C, D*) The linear distance from 1 to 3 is equal to the distance from 3 to 5. (*E, F*) The short limbs of the L brachioplasty are lines of equal length from 5 to 6 and 1 to 6 that include excision of excess skin in the axilla and upper lateral chest.

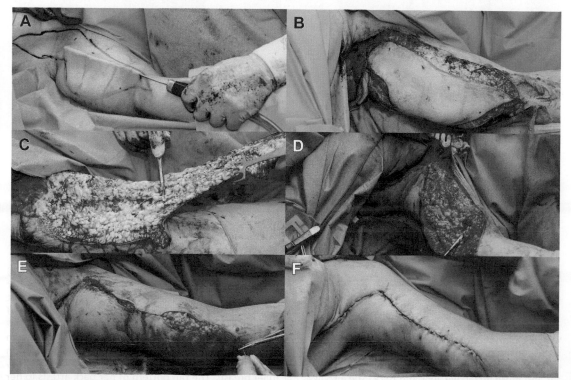

Fig. 5. The 6 critical stages of L brachioplasty of the patient in **Figs. 3** and **4** are (*A*) excision site liposuction, (*B*) perimeter incision, (*C*) skin avulsion/excision, (*D*) anchor suture of point 5 to point 1, (*E*) first layer Quill closure, and (*F*) second layer running dermal closure.

suture advanced across the central axilla to the del-topectoral fascia with 2-0 absorbable braided suture (see **Fig. 5**D). The first layer is closed with double-armed, bidirectional #0 barbed poly-dioxanone suture (see **Fig. 5**E). The second layer is a 3-0 Monoderm intradermal closure. The L-shaped line of tight closure leaves a curvilinear scar that descends to the posterior margin and then ascends to the apex of the axilla (see **Fig. 5**F).

In general, rare revision surgery has a consistent narrow band of additional skin excision along the longitudinal scar to treat recurrent excess skin laxity. In a recent patient who gained 9 kg (20 pounds) after her L brachioplasty, VASERlipo was applied for the removal of 300 mL of fat from each arm for a considerable improvement in appearance 2 years after her original surgery (**Fig. 6**). The harvested fat was used to increase the volume of her spiral flap–reshaped breasts. VASERlipo has proved in several instances to

reduce adipose bulk and redistribute fat after weight gain after major body contouring surgery.

DISCUSSION

The L brachioplasty with liposuction can be applied to a variety of moderate to severe defor-mities of the upper arm. The routine use of excision site liposuction has eliminated significant damage to the neurovasculature. Troublesome intraopera-tive blood loss and injury to important superficial nerves are not issues. Prolonged edema, seromas, and lymphoceles do not occur. The undulating full-length arm scars are as inconspicuous as possible. Resolution of scar hypertrophy may continue for 5 years.

The scars are not seen from in front or posteriorly when the arms are at or near the chest. A crossing axillary scar does not migrate distally onto the arm as in the Lookwood T anchor brachioplasty.[3] The

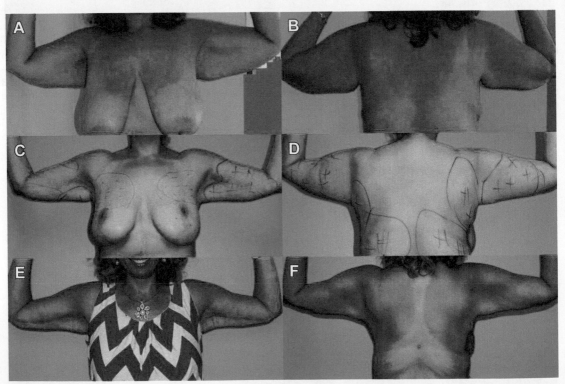

Fig. 6. Frontal and posterior views of the use of VASERlipo to revise L brachioplasty arms after weight gain. (*A, B*) Before L brachioplasty after a 32-kg (70 pound) weight loss in a 48-year-old woman. (*C, D*) Three years after her L brachioplasties her weight was 9 kg (20 pounds) more than before her prior procedure. Her arms are smaller but uncomfortably too large with no muscular definition. Her back is heavy and poorly defined. The superior poles of the breasts are flat. Preoperative marking for VASERlipo throughout the arms and back are seen. Lipoaugmen-tation is planned for the superior breasts. At the operation, 600 mL of fat emulsion were removed from each arm and 3200 mL from her back. Each superior breast pole was filled with 150 mL aspirated from her arms. (*E, F*) Seven weeks after VASERlipo, she returns to the office in a sleeveless summer dress, pleased with her considerably ligh-ter and more attractive arms and back. She also likes her fuller breasts. The tan pattern of her back attests to her approval of the improvement there. Her smaller arms are well shaped to reveal underlying musculature. Likewise, her back skin tightly reveals underlying large muscle form. Her upper torso and arms are more feminine.

scars are not depressed as may happen along the bicipital groove.[5] There is no webbing across the axilla, dog ears, or unsightly Z-plasties. The posterior border of the arm has a subtle convexity. Alternative posterior elliptical excisions[4] tend to eliminate posterior aesthetic convexity, and leave an objectionable visible scar posteriorly when the arms are to the side.

Moderate deformity seems to be fully corrected, leaving excellent definition of muscle masses. VASERlipo and possibly augmentation are useful adjuncts, and in the mild to moderate deformity in the young, is the only treatment that is necessary. Despite tight closures, severe deformity has about 20% recurrence. Patients should be alerted to this possibility and advised as to considerations of secondary skin resection and/or further liposuction.

REFERENCES

1. Hurwitz DJ, Holland SW. The L brachioplasty: an innovative approach to excess tissue of the upper arm, axilla and lateral chest. Plast Reconstr Surg 2006;117(2):403–11.
2. Hurwitz DJ, Jerrod K. L-brachioplasty: an adaptable technique for moderate to severe excess skin and fat of the arms. Aesthet Surg J 2010;30: 620–9.
3. Lockwood T. Brachioplasty with superficial fascial system. Plast Reconstr Surg 1995;96(4):912–20.
4. Aly A, Soliman S, Cram A, et al. Brachioplasty in the massive weight loss patient. Clin Plast Surg 2008; 35:141–7.
5. Rubin JP, Michaels J. Correction of arm ptosis with medial bicipital scar. In: Strauch B, Herman C, editors. Encyclopedia of body sculpting after massive weight loss. New York: Theime; 2010. p. 163–71.
6. Avelar J. Regional distribution and behavior of the subcutaneous tissue concerning selection and indication for liposuction. Aesthetic Plast Surg 1989;13: 155–65.
7. Hoyos A, Perez M. Arm dynamic definition by sculpture and fat grafting. Aesthet Surg J 2012;32(8): 974–87.
8. Hurwitz DJ, Smith D. Treatment of overweight patients by radiofrequency assisted liposuction (RFAL) for aesthetic reshaping and skin tightening. Aesthetic Plast Surg 2012;36:62–71.

Brachioplasty with Limited Scar

Lawrence S. Reed, MD

KEYWORDS

• Brachioplasty • Transaxillary • Hidden scar • Short scar • Minimal incision • Aesthetic surgery

KEY POINTS

- Good for many cases of brachial dermatolipodystrophy. The vertical height from the mid-humerus to the most dependent portion of the mid-upper arm (with the arm at 90° to the body) should be no greater than 12 cm. For excessive upper arm dermatolipodystrophy, the traditional method should be used.
- The tailor-tack method should always be used intraoperatively to confirm the accuracy of the preoperative markings. This should be done after any liposuction is performed. Corrections or modifications can be made at this time. The tailor-tack closure should always be checked with the patient in the upright position and the arm at a 90° angle to the lateral chest.
- A superficial plane should be used for the resection of the involved area, taking only a thin layer of fat with the resected specimen.
- The elbows should not be raised above the level of the shoulders until 3.5 weeks postoperatively.
- During preoperative marking, the transverse axis width of the incision (in the axillary fold) should stop at 1.5 to 2 cm medial to the visible portion of the axillary crease on the anterior and posterior shoulder. This helps to prevent the final scar from extending into visible areas.
- Undesirable anterior axillary and postaxillary fullness can also be corrected during this procedure.
- 12% of patients need some form of revisional surgery performed at 1 year or later, most commonly for scar correction.

INTRODUCTION

The American Society for Aesthetic Plastic Surgery (ASAPS) Statistics for 2012 show that there has been a more than 800% increase in the number of brachioplasties performed in the last 15 years. Most of these patients had traditional brachioplasty, which produces predictably good results. The problem, however, is that the resulting linear scar that courses in some fashion from the axilla to the elbow can be visible when wearing sleeveless apparel. Many patients forego the operation because of the nature and visibility of the scarring.

Numerous techniques for surgical management of upper extremity contour deformities have been described since the first article published about aesthetic brachioplasty in 1954 by Correa-Iturrasspe and Fernandez.[1] The traditional brachioplasty has stood the test of time and is still indicated for those patients with massive weight loss and excessive skin laxity.

I have been performing transaxillary brachioplasty (minimal incision brachioplasty [MIB]) for more than 30 years. In this procedure the scar is confined to the hidden area of the axilla. Inspiration for the MIB came from the seminal work of Pollack and colleagues[2] who in 1972 introduced his revolutionary approach to the treatment of axillary hidradenitis suppurativa, which included wide excision of the involved axillary tissue with direct closure of the defect. Before this bold approach the wounds were either allowed to heal by secondary intention or skin grafted, which was followed by 3 weeks in airplane splinting.

I had the opportunity to use the Pollack technique on a large number of patients and many of

Department of Surgery, Weill Cornell Medical College, 445 East 69th Street, New York, NY 10065, USA
E-mail address: lsreed@aol.com

Clin Plastic Surg 41 (2014) 753–763
http://dx.doi.org/10.1016/j.cps.2014.06.009
0094-1298/14/$ – see front matter © 2014 Elsevier Inc. All rights reserved.

the patients commented on how their arms looked aesthetically more pleasing. This unexpected feedback encouraged me to further explore the use of the Pollack technique for aesthetic improvement of the upper arm. I use the MIB on more than 95% of the patients I see with brachiodermatolipodistrophy. There have been numerous refinements in my technique for the past 30 years as I applied the technique to an ever widening spectrum of patients. Other authors have published articles on variations of this approach that are also modifications of Pollack's original work.[3–9]

I am frequently asked how the MIB can produce such good results without the transverse excision of upper arm skin seen in the traditional brachioplasty. The answer is best demonstrated graphically using the woven bamboo finger trap (**Fig. 1**). When one end is fixed, pulling on the opposite end causes the entire tube to narrow. Moving the skin forcibly toward the axilla produces the same effect.

PATIENT SELECTION

Most of the patients I see with upper arm dermatolipodystrophy are women whose ages range from the early 40s to the mid-60s. They generally present with moderate to severe excess skin and adipose tissue of the upper arms, and feel they can no longer wear sleeveless garments. Most are not patients who have undergone massive weight loss or bariatric surgery. The MIB is applicable to most patients that I examine. For the others, the traditional approach is offered. I have used the MIB technique on several patients who exceeded the parameters for being a successful candidate. These particular patients are those who are willing to accept a lesser improvement rather than having a very visible scar on the inner arm. There is always the option of resorting secondarily to the traditional approach if they are not pleased with the

outcome. I have had to do this on only two occasions.

In deciding which approach to use, I have found that if the distance as measured from the mid-humerous to the bottom of the hanging skin, with the arm at 90° to the lateral chest, is greater than 12 cm then the traditional approach should be considered. This is specifically valid if the problem is one of predominantly excess skin. Those patients, however, who demonstrate significant lipodystrophy are frequently candidates for the MIB approach because the vertical skin height is decreased by the liposuction as the skin contacts. Another exception is seen in those patients in whom vertical height is only greater than 12 cm in the upper third of the arm near the axilla, a not infrequent presentation. They do very well with the MIB approach.

A comprehensive consultation is critical to successful patient selection. Patients are shown the exact location of the axillary scar, which as is true for most body sculpture scars is visible and takes approximately 1.5 to 2 years to heal completely. This is even truer for the axillary scars, which are subjected to constant motion and friction. The terms "microscopic," "hairline," and "fades away" are never used. Prospective patients are also informed that about 12% to 15% of patients need some revisional surgery at 1 year. Most commonly secondary surgery is undertaken for scar revision (85% of the time) but it is also performed for removal of anterior and posterior shoulder dog ears, correction of secondary skin laxity, bow-stringing, and loss of the axillary hollow. Patients are informed that they are not allowed to raise their elbows above their shoulder level for 3.5 weeks, although movement of the forearms and some upper arm movement are permitted.

Another caution applies to those patients whose problem is predominantly crepey skin of the upper arms. This is not improved by the MIB and although the excess skin and fat are removed

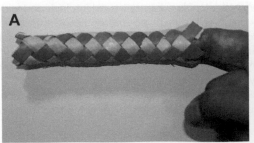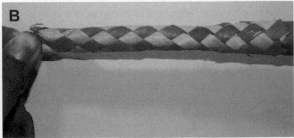

Fig. 1. The bamboo finger trap aptly demonstrates the principle of the transaxillary brachioplasty in which traction in the axilla narrows the circumference of the upper arm. (*A*) Finger trap with no traction on it. (*B*) Traction on one end of finger trap narrows its entire circumference. (*From* Reed LS. Limited scar brachioplasty. In: Rubin JP, Jewell ML, Richter DF, et al, editors. Body contouring and liposuction. Philadelphia: Elsevier; 2013; with permission.)

and good contour established, the crepey appearance remains. For these patients, the traditional brachioplasty may produce a better correction.

Finally, women who have had mastectomies and/or radiation therapy are still, if other patient selection criteria are met, candidates for the MIB. The resection is very superficial and the lymphatic system is not appreciably disturbed. I have done the MIB on several postmastectomy and postradiation therapy patients without any problems.

PREOPERATIVE PREPARATION

Presurgical workups are age and health dependant. Standard preoperative laboratory and diagnostic studies are performed along with venous thromboembolism risk assessment. The patients are instructed not to shave their axillary hair for at least 48 hours before surgery.

SURGICAL TECHNIQUE
Markings

Marking (**Fig. 2**) is performed in the holding area with the patient in the upright position. With arms against the sides, mark the anterior and posterior shoulders at the junction between the axillary and shoulder skin. The final scar should usually not be visible beyond these markings. The entire scar should be confined to the axilla (see **Fig. 2**).

Draw a line between these two marks transversely through the apex of the axillary hollow. This line should stop 1.5 to 2 cm medial to the anterior and posterior axillary crease/shoulder junction markings. This is the first step in avoiding a final scar that extends into the visible area of the shoulder (**Fig. 3**). Next draw a line that bisects the transverse line from the central inner arm, through the center of the transverse line to the lateral chest area (see **Fig. 3**).

Establish the longitudinal length of excision using the pinch technique. First, move the skin of the triceps area forcibly toward the transverse axillary line until a desirable contour improvement is achieved and mark the skin of the upper arm at this point. Next move the lateral chest skin forcibly toward the transverse axillary line thereby accounting for the skin laxity of the lateral chest. This correction is critical to fix and stabilize the upper arm correction (**Fig. 4**).

Now connect these four points as an ovoid shape. Normally this area of planned resection runs from 5 to 8 cm transversely to 10 to 14 cm longitudinally (**Fig. 5**).

Mark the areas that require liposuction. These should include, if indicated, the area of

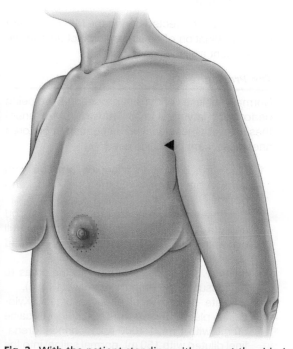
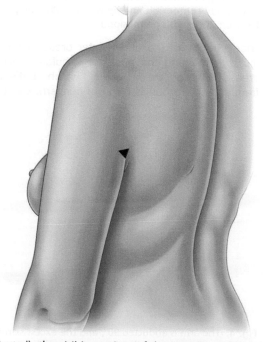

Fig. 2. With the patient standing with arms at the side (adducted), the visible portions of the anterior and posterior axillary folds are marked with a triangle. This mark is used to determine the transverse diameter of the planned exposure, which extends 1 to 1.5 cm medial to the point of each triangle. (*From* Reed LS. Limited scar brachioplasty. In: Rubin JP, Jewell ML, Richter DF, et al, editors. Body contouring and liposuction. Philadelphia: Elsevier; 2013; with permission.)

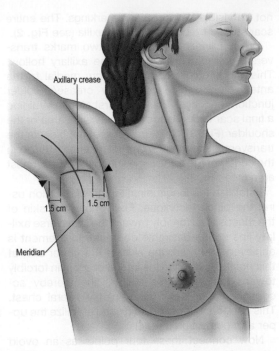

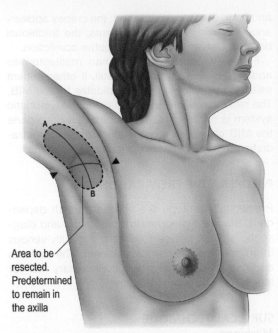

Fig. 3. The arm is sufficiently abducted to mark the axillary hollow or crease apex. This line is then shortened so that it stops about 1.5 cm before hitting the axillary fold marks. The line is bisected and carried up the arm and down the chest wall to mark the meridian of the axilla. (*From* Reed LS. Limited scar brachioplasty. In: Rubin JP, Jewell ML, Richter DF, et al, editors. Body contouring and liposuction. Philadelphia: Elsevier; 2013; with permission.)

lipodystrophy of the upper outer breast/anterior axillary area and the posterior shoulder/axillary area. Both of these areas, which patients frequently point out as being of concern, can be

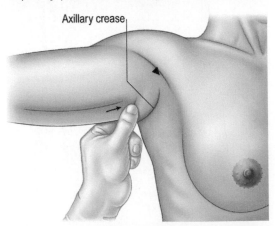

Fig. 4. The arm is abducted 90°, and the excess skin of the triceps area is forcefully advanced toward the axillary crease and marked as point A (as in **Fig. 5**). (*From* Reed LS. Limited scar brachioplasty. In: Rubin JP, Jewell ML, Richter DF, et al, editors. Body contouring and liposuction. Philadelphia: Elsevier; 2013; with permission.)

Fig. 5. The skin of the chest wall is next similarly advanced toward the axillary crease with force adequate to balance the tension (point B). The points are connected to make an oval area of proposed resection. (*From* Reed LS. Limited scar brachioplasty. In: Rubin JP, Jewell ML, Richter DF, et al, editors. Body contouring and liposuction. Philadelphia: Elsevier; 2013; with permission.)

improved and corrected during the MIB procedure by a combination of selective liposuction and the subsequent axillary skin tightening.

The Procedure

Normally, unless concurrent procedures are being performed, laryngeal mask airway (LMA) anesthesia or, at times, local with sedation (monitored anesthesia care [MAC]) is used.

1. Place the patient in a supine position with arms comfortably outstretched on arm boards.
2. Circumferentially prepare arms and chest and apply appropriate dressings that permit full circumferential access to the arms and shoulders.
3. Infiltrate tumescent solution into the areas to be liposuctioned (approximately 1:1 ratio).
4. Infiltrate diluted local anesthesia (1% Xylocaine plain 50 mL and 0.25% Marcaine 50 mL with 1 mL 1:1000 epinephrine [adrenaline] diluted with 150 mL normal saline) into the areas of premarked surgical resection.
5. Liposuction the selected areas of both arms.
6. Use the tailor-tack method to check the accuracy of the preoperative markings. It is

important to perform the tailor-tack procedure with the patient in the upright position and the arm at 90° to the lateral chest. Make any revisions necessary in the preoperative markings. Check for undue tension resulting in bands and also for any abnormal folds or rotations in the skin of the arm. Adjust the position and placement of the tailor-tack sutures to correct any undesirable findings. After the necessary adjustments have been made, remark the planned surgical excision site. Placing several lines perpendicular to the final planned incision line facilitates closure (**Fig. 6**).

7. Remove the tailor-tack sutures or Adairs and with the patient in the recumbent position, excise the involved area with just a thin layer of underlying fat attached to remove the apocrine glands (**Fig. 7**).

8. After hemostasis, clean the area with 5% Betadine and mark the apex of the axillary crease or hollow (**Fig. 8**).

9. Wound closure
   a. For the first layer use 1-0 Vicryl from deep dermis, through the fibrous tissue of the axillary fold and through the deep dermis on the opposite side (**Fig. 9**).
   b. A two-layered closure using number 2 14 × 14 Quill suture.
   c. Skin closure with a running vertical mattress of 3-0 Prolene.

10. Keep the scar confined to the axilla: In many cases the closure of the surgical site can cause the final scar to extend into the visible portions of the anterior or posterior shoulder, or both. This should be addressed at the time of closure using the purse string technique:

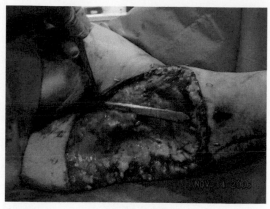

Fig. 7. Intraoperative view of axillary area of resection measuring 17 × 9 cm. (*From* Reed LS. Limited scar brachioplasty. In: Rubin JP, Jewell ML, Richter DF, et al, editors. Body contouring and liposuction. Philadelphia: Elsevier; 2013; with permission.)

   a. Undermine the area where the scar extends to the visible shoulder and defat, if necessary (**Fig. 10**).
   b. Use a 2-0 7 × 7 Quill suture anchored to the axillary fold base and passed subdermally through the elongated portion of the incision site as a purse string suture to bring the visible portion of the incision back into the axillary area. This leaves some bunching and a dog ear. This configuration is largely resolved in 3 to 6 months (**Figs. 11** and **12**).
   c. After the purse string correction, complete the closure in the standard fashion (**Fig. 13**).

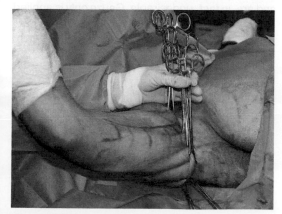

Fig. 6. Final determination of the amount of tissue to be removed is made during surgery, using the tailor-tack method. (*From* Reed LS. Limited scar brachioplasty. In: Rubin JP, Jewell ML, Richter DF, et al, editors. Body contouring and liposuction. Philadelphia: Elsevier; 2013; with permission.)

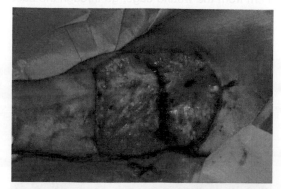

Fig. 8. This intraoperative view demonstrates the amount of tissue removed and the remarking of the axillary crease with methylene blue. Note the presence of subcutaneous fat remaining on the axillary fascia. (*From* Reed LS. Limited scar brachioplasty. In: Rubin JP, Jewell ML, Richter DF, et al, editors. Body contouring and liposuction. Philadelphia: Elsevier; 2013; with permission.)

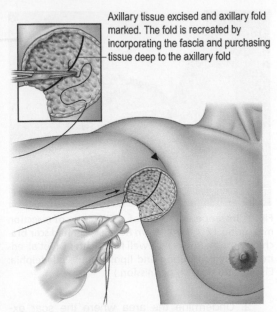

Axillary tissue excised and axillary fold marked. The fold is recreated by incorporating the fascia and purchasing tissue deep to the axillary fold

Fig. 9. After the axillary tissue is excised, the axillary crease is marked again. The fold is recreated during closure, incorporating the fascia into each stitch, using 1-0 Vicryl. (*From* Reed LS. Limited scar brachioplasty. In: Rubin JP, Jewell ML, Richter DF, et al, editors. Body contouring and liposuction. Philadelphia: Elsevier; 2013; with permission.)

11. Selective use of bolster dressings: In those cases where it is believed that the axillary fold may be difficult to recreate or there is obvious tension, a bolster dressing should be used as was described by Pollack and coworkers.[2] A rolled up ABD pad works very well.

Before beginning closure of the surgical site, place 1-0 nylon retention sutures. Beginning 3 cm from the wound edge, go through the base

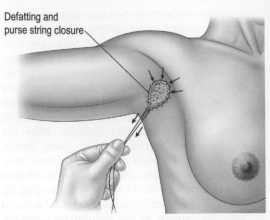

Defatting and purse string closure

Fig. 11. After the incision is defatted at its ends in the subdermal plane, it is closed with a purse string stitch, using 2-0 Quill suture, thus pulling the wound edges further back into the axilla. This bunched tissue usually settles in 3 to 6 months. (*From* Reed LS. Limited scar brachioplasty. In: Rubin JP, Jewell ML, Richter DF, et al, editors. Body contouring and liposuction. Philadelphia: Elsevier; 2013; with permission.)

of the site exiting 3 cm back from the opposite wound edge. Normally three or four of these sutures suffice. After the wound closure is completed these sutures are used to snug the bolster dressing into place. The bolster dressing is normally left in place from 2 to 4 days. The bolster dressings may cause slight discomfort but are well tolerated and help to secure the axillary incision, which is exposed to constant unavoidable motion (**Fig. 14**).

I use bolster dressings on most of my cases. Drains are never used. Bacitracin or other compatible ointments are applied to the wounds, assuming bolster dressings are not used. Neither arm wraps nor surgical arm dressings are used and are, in fact, undesirable. Gauze only is applied.

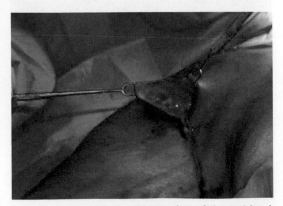

Fig. 10. The extended visible portion of the incision is first undermined and then defatted to the dermis before executing the purse string closure. (*From* Reed LS. Limited scar brachioplasty. In: Rubin JP, Jewell ML, Richter DF, et al, editors. Body contouring and liposuction. Philadelphia: Elsevier; 2013; with permission.)

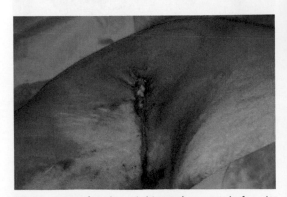

Fig. 12. Area of gathered skin at the wound after the purse string suture closure. This area usually settles out after 3 to 6 months. (*From* Reed LS. Limited scar brachioplasty. In: Rubin JP, Jewell ML, Richter DF, et al, editors. Body contouring and liposuction. Philadelphia: Elsevier; 2013; with permission.)

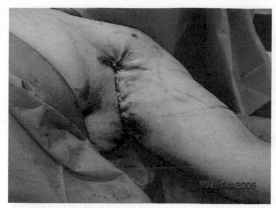

Fig. 13. View of final closure with purse string correction of elongated anterior axillary incision. (*From* Reed LS. Limited scar brachioplasty. In: Rubin JP, Jewell ML, Richter DF, et al, editors. Body contouring and liposuction. Philadelphia: Elsevier; 2013; with permission.)

OPTIMIZING OUTCOMES

Ideal patients have dermatolipodystrophy that can be corrected by the MIB approach. Those patients whose degree of skin laxity is greater than the established parameters are better served by the traditional brachioplasty.

Careful preoperative markings are important. Always use the tailor-tack method before surgical

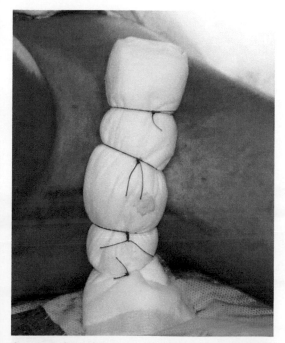

Fig. 14. Bolster dressing in place at end of procedure helps to recreate axillary fold. (*From* Reed LS. Limited scar brachioplasty. In: Rubin JP, Jewell ML, Richter DF, et al, editors. Body contouring and liposuction. Philadelphia: Elsevier; 2013; with permission.)

excision and check it in the upright position and the arm at 90° to the lateral chest. This is the time to make any adjustments that may be warranted.

Do not be timid in planning the amount of tissue to be resected. Remember, you will check the accuracy of your preoperative markings with the tailor-tack method.

There is never a reason to use a T extension incision into the inner upper arm.

If the axillary fold is not well defined or in more fatty arms, a bolster dressing should be used. It may be necessary to defat the area of the axillary fold for better definition using either direct excision or liposuction.

POSTOPERATIVE CARE

No drains or surgical arm dressings are used. A bolster dressing is frequently used. Patients can be reasonably active immediately after surgery but are encouraged to limit arm motion as much as is reasonable or possible. They should not raise their elbows above the height of their shoulders for 3.5 weeks. At this time, they actively start to incrementally raise their arms above their shoulders. Most patients have their arms raised fully upright to the preoperative position of elevation within 5 to 8 weeks. Not one patient was unable to fully raise their arms. Patients may bathe immediately but should keep the surgical sites dry for 48 hours. After this period they wash the surgical areas several times a day with soap and water followed by the application of sanitizer lotion. If bolster dressings are used, the sites must be kept dry until the bolster dressings are removed at 2 to 4 days. At this time the areas can be cleaned. For those patients who have had extensive liposuction, the arms remain swollen for several months, which can cause concern for some patients who cannot see a meaningful result. Most physical and athletic activities can be reintroduced after 3.5 to 4 weeks.

COMPLICATIONS: BASED ON A REVIEW OF 1200 CASES

The most common complication is wound separation, which normally occurs at around 2 weeks and runs from 1.5 to 2.5 cm in diameter. Early on in the evolution of this technique, 12% to 15% of patients would develop some degree of limited separation. All responded to conservative therapy and healed by secondary intention. Now, with the use of the vertical mattress skin closure, the rate of separation is down to 5%. The separations are clearly the result of the constant motion and activity associated with the axillary arm area, and to

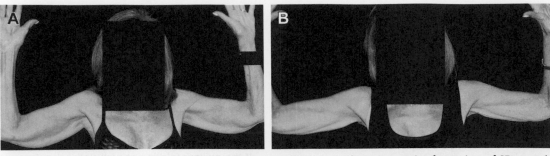

Fig. 15. (*A*) Preoperative front view of 65-year-old patient. (*B*) Six-month postoperative front view of 65-year-old patient.

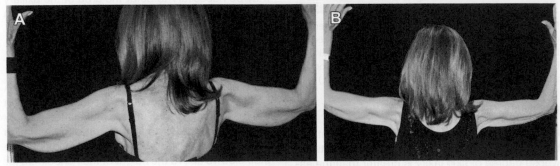

Fig. 16. (*A*) Preoperative back view of 65-year-old patient. (*B*) Six-month postoperative back view of 65-year-old patient.

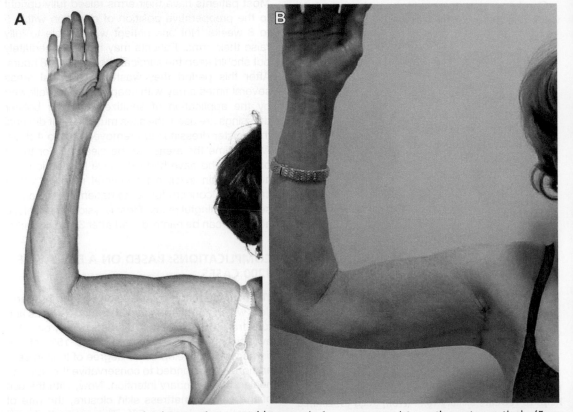

Fig. 17. (*A, B*) Front views of right arm of 63-year-old woman before surgery and 4 months postoperatively. (*From* Reed LS. Limited scar brachioplasty. In: Rubin JP, Jewell ML, Richter DF, et al, editors. Body contouring and liposuction. Philadelphia: Elsevier; 2013; with permission.)

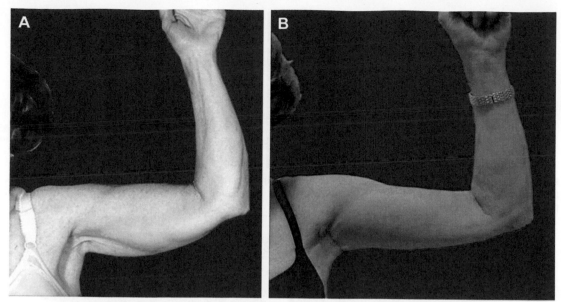

Fig. 18. (*A*, *B*) Front views of left arm of 63-year-old woman before surgery and 4 months postoperatively. (*From* Reed LS. Limited scar brachioplasty. In: Rubin JP, Jewell ML, Richter DF, et al, editors. Body contouring and liposuction. Philadelphia: Elsevier; 2013; with permission.)

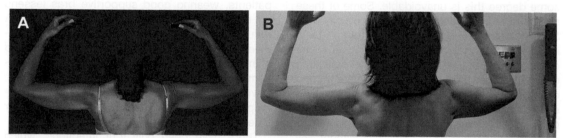

Fig. 19. (*A*, *B*) Back views of 47-year-old woman before surgery and 6 months postoperatively. (*From* Reed LS. Limited scar brachioplasty. In: Rubin JP, Jewell ML, Richter DF, et al, editors. Body contouring and liposuction. Philadelphia: Elsevier; 2013; with permission.)

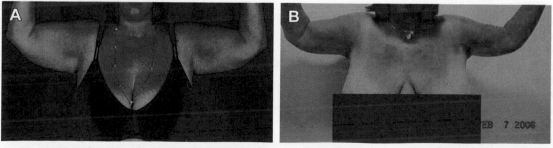

Fig. 20. (*A*, *B*) Front views of 43-year-old woman before surgery and 5 months postoperatively. (*From* Reed LS. Limited scar brachioplasty. In: Rubin JP, Jewell ML, Richter DF, et al, editors. Body contouring and liposuction. Philadelphia: Elsevier; 2013; with permission.)

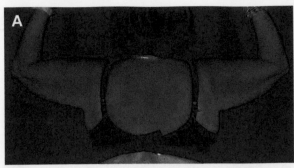
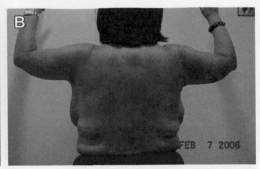

Fig. 21. (*A, B*) Back views of 43-year-old woman before surgery and 5 months postoperatively. (*From* Reed LS. Limited scar brachioplasty. In: Rubin JP, Jewell ML, Richter DF, et al, editors. Body contouring and liposuction. Philadelphia: Elsevier; 2013; with permission.)

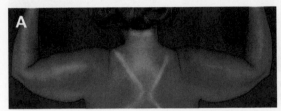
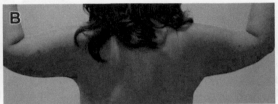

Fig. 22. (*A, B*) Back views of 32-year-old woman before surgery and 11 months postoperatively. (*From* Reed LS. Limited scar brachioplasty. In: Rubin JP, Jewell ML, Richter DF, et al, editors. Body contouring and liposuction. Philadelphia: Elsevier; 2013; with permission.)

some degree this is unavoidable. Some of these separations can become infected, usually with *Staphylococcus*, and the use of Bactroban® facilitates the healing process. For most, wet-to-dry dressings and aggressive wound toilet suffice. In only two cases did I have a complete wound dehiscence resulting from forceful, extreme arm extension occurring within the first 2 weeks of surgery. In both cases, immediate repair was carried out and both went on to heal well without any problems. About 10% to 12% of patients have hypertrophic or unacceptable scarring and these scars are repaired at 1 year. Occasionally, there may be bow-stringing or a bat wing deformity secondary to tension. Although not common, this entity is treated at 1 year with a scar release and Z-plasty or some other scar-lengthening technique. Bolster dressings are always used after this repair for approximately 3 to 5 days. More frequently, however, the bow-stringing or bat wing presentation is not caused by tension but by a separation or distraction of the skin from the base of the wound. One can check for distraction by seeing how easily the distracted skin can be pushed back into the axillary hollow. This presentation is treated by excising the scar and reattaching the skin to the underlying base. A bolster dressing is used for 3 to 5 days. Bow-stringing is not uncommonly seen in women with macromastia or heavy, pendulous breasts. For these

patients, wearing good supportive bras lessens or eradicates the bow-string presentation. A reduction mammoplasty should also be considered. It is important at the initial consultation to identify this problem and discuss the possible outcomes and available options with the patient. Several patients have undergone reduction mammoplasties concurrently with the MIB or at a later time.

There have been only four infections, which responded to antibiotic therapy. There have been no hematomas or seromas. No neurovascular, lymphatic, or musculoskeletal problems have occurred.

SUMMARY

MIB should be considered by every surgeon performing brachioplasties for those cases where a traditional brachioplasty is not mandated. The aesthetic results are equally good and there is no visible inner arm or upper arm scar of any type. Most patients are not happy with the scars from body sculpture surgery but most scars of breasts, abdomen, and buttocks are concealed by appropriate clothing. This is not true for the medial thigh or the upper arm. The rub is that now that the patient has an aesthetically pleasing arm, he or she still will not wear sleeveless garments because of the visibility of the scar. The scar from the MIB procedure is also a typical body sculpture scar but it is hidden from view most of the time (**Figs. 15–22**). Patient satisfaction is very high. What patients do not like is the long time it takes to heal, specifically if there has been extensive liposuction; the limitation of motion early on; and the blunting or diminution of the axillary hollow and definition that can occur. I have had the opportunity over the years to see patients who have had the MIB procedure performed elsewhere and the biggest complaint is that the arm does not look much different. Measure carefully, do not be overwhelmed by the size of the area of resection, tailor-tack the area to confirm the precision of your markings, and go to it. Also, do not sacrifice the result to achieve a better scar. At the end of the day, it is the result on which patients focus. It is worthwhile to note that although the axillary area does not heal as well early on as other areas of the body because it is dark, moist, in constant motion, and with continuous friction, the final scars are among the best, but the process takes more than a year. One interesting note is that in most cases all of the axillary hair-bearing tissue along with the eccrine and apocrine glands is resected and patients always comment about no longer needing deodorant.

REFERENCES

1. Correa-Iturraspe M, Fernandez JC. Dermolipectomia braquial. Prensa Med Argent 1954;41:2432.
2. Pollock WJ, Virnelli FR, Ryn RF. Axillary hidradenitis suppurativa: a simple and effective surgical technique. Plast Reconstr Surg 1972;49:22–7.
3. Teimourian B, Malekzadeh S. Rejuvenation of the upper arm. Plast Reconstr Surg 1998;102:545–51 [discussion: 552–3].
4. Abraham DL. Minibrachioplasty: minimizing scars while maximizing results. Plast Reconstr Surg 2004;114:1631–8.
5. Richards ME. Reassessing minimal incision brachioplasty. Aesthet Surg J 2004;25:175–9.
6. Richards ME. Minimal incision brachioplasty: a first choice option in arm reduction surgery. Aesthet Surg J 2001;21:301–10.
7. Trussler AP, Rohrich RJ. Limited incision medial brachioplasty: technical refinements in upper arm contouring. Plast Reconstr Surg 2008;121:305–7.
8. Reed LS, Hyman JB. Minimal incision brachioplasty: refining transaxillary arm rejuvenation. Aesthet Surg J 2007;27(4):433–41.
9. Reed LS. Limited scar brachioplasty. In: Rubin JP, Jewell ML, Richter DF, et al, editors. Body contouring and liposuction. Elsevier Publications; 2012. p. 35–42.

Circumferential Truncal Contouring
The Belt Lipectomy

Al Aly, MD, FACS[a],*, Melissa Mueller, MD[b]

KEYWORDS

- Body lift • Belt lipectomy • Massive weight loss • Abdominoplasty • Thigh lift • Buttocks lift
- Liposuction • Body contouring

KEY POINTS

- The primary goal of belt lipectomy surgery is to improve the contour of the inferior truncal circumferential unit and to place the resultant scar in natural junctions.
- Excessive intra-abdominal content is a contraindication for belt lipectomy.
- The anterior abdominal resection and contouring should have a higher priority than the back resection.
- The higher the presenting patient's body mass index (BMI), the higher the risk of postoperative complications and the less impressive the results. The converse is also true: the lower the BMI, the lower the risk of complications and the better the results.
- The most common complications are small wound separations and seromas.

INTRODUCTION

As obesity has become an epidemic in the United States, bariatric surgery has rapidly evolved and increased in popularity. The American Society for Metabolic and Bariatric Surgery reports that 36,700 bariatric surgeries were performed in 2000, 171,000 were performed in 2005, and 220,000 were performed in 2009. The increase in obesity and bariatric surgery has led to an increase in the number of patients requesting body contouring after massive weight loss and subsequently the emergence and rapid growth of body contouring.

The term belt lipectomy, first coined by Gonzalez-Ulloa in 1961, describes a combination of procedures designed to enhance the contour and appearance of a patient's abdomen, waist, lower back, buttocks, and thighs. Belt lipectomy combines abdominoplasty, lateral and anterior thigh lift, buttocks lift, and sometimes liposuction, in a manner that coordinates the result to achieve more than can be delivered by any of these procedures individually. Other names that have been

used for circumferential lower truncal procedures include circumferential abdominoplasty, extended abdominoplasty, central body lift, and lower body lift. The authors prefer the term belt lipectomy rather than body lift because both upward lifting and downward pulling forces are applied to truncal areas in the procedure and the term belt is more descriptive of what is removed.

A wide range of patients can benefit from belt lipectomy; patients with massive weight loss, patients with massive weight loss who underwent an anterior-only procedure, patients without massive weight loss in the range of 26 to 29 body mass index (BMI), and normal-weight patients who desire a significant improvement in their lower trunk overall. Discussion in this article is limited to patients with massive weight loss.

PATIENT PRESENTATION

A diverse group of patients can benefit from belt lipectomy and are grouped here into clinically relevant categories.

[a] Cleveland Clinic Abu Dhabi, Abu Dhabi; [b] Department of Plastic Surgery, University of California Irvine, 200 S Manchester Avenue, Suite 650, Orange, CA 92868, USA
* Corresponding author.
E-mail address: mdplastic@aol.com

Clin Plastic Surg 41 (2014) 765–774
http://dx.doi.org/10.1016/j.cps.2014.06.008
0094-1298/14/$ – see front matter © 2014 Elsevier Inc. All rights reserved.

Patients with Massive Weight Loss

Patients with massive weight loss have a wide range of body contours and sizes. Multiple factors contribute to this diversity: the BMI at presentation, the quality of the skin/fat envelope, and the fat deposition pattern. BMI at presentation ranges on a continuum, placing individuals in categories from still significantly obese to those near ideal weight. Whether from bariatric surgery or lifestyle changes, weight loss stabilizes or plateaus at different levels in different individuals and this plateau is not easily altered. The second factor affecting diversity in presentation is the quality of the skin/fat envelope, which includes its thickness and elasticity. An important determinant of skin/fat envelope quality is its translation of pull. Translation of pull is assessed before surgery by pinching the intended area of resection and examining the mobility of surrounding tissues. The third major factor, the fat deposition pattern, describes the genetically controlled amount and location of fat deposition during weight gain and fat loss during weight loss.

Although variable in presentation, patients with massive weight loss share many common body features, particularly an inverted-cone appearance to their inferior trunk with a narrow ribcage and wide pelvic rim. Patients with massive weight loss often lack lateral waist definition because of excess tissue draping, concealing the underlying musculoskeletal anatomy. Many patients have large and distinct hip rolls.

Patients with massive weight loss have pendulous anterior panniculi, typically with 1 to 3 soft tissue rolls. Almost all patients with massive weight loss present with some degree of abdominal wall laxity, caused by rectus muscle diastasis. Some also present with hernias, especially if they have had open bariatric surgery procedures. The mons pubis most often presents with ptosis and lipodystrophy, as well as vertical and horizontal excess. The opening of the vulva in women and the penis base in men are directed downward, rather than the normal anterior inclination.

The buttocks may be overprojected in patients with high BMI, or underprojected in patients with low BMI. Almost all patients lack definition of the buttocks because of a lack of a distinct transition from the lower back to the buttocks. The superior extent of the central buttocks crease may be low and may present with loss of soft tissue overlying the coccyx. The infrabuttocks crease varies greatly with BMI. Patients with high BMI often have an abnormal, horizontally oriented infrabuttocks crease, whereas patients with low BMI may present with crease redundancy.

Back rolls are variable in their presentation and depend on the patient's fat deposition pattern. Some patients present with no back rolls, whereas others present with multiple rolls.

The overall goal of belt lipectomy is to return the patient's inferior truncal contour to within normal range of the general population. Specific goals for the abdomen include elimination of hanging tissue and rolls, creation of a flat contour, restoration of an anterior-facing vulva in women, and restoration of an anterior penile takeoff point in men. Goals for the lateral aspect of the lower trunk include an hourglass figure with narrowing at the waist for women. Goals for the posterior aspect of the lower trunk include reduction or elimination of lower back rolls if present and creation of demarcation between the lower back and the buttocks. If the buttocks are overprojected, this projection should be reduced. If the buttocks are underprojected, definition should be improved and, if needed, projection should be improved. If inferiorly displaced, the superior extent of the buttocks crease should be elevated. Also, the infrabuttocks crease ideally should be returned to a normal semicircular appearance.

Patients with Massive Weight Loss Status Post Anterior-only Resection Surgery

An enlarging subgroup of patients with massive weight loss includes individuals who have previously undergone anterior truncal resections but are disappointed with their lateral and posterior contours, presenting in the form of dog ears and a lack of waist definition. In some of these patients even the anterior resection is inadequate, as shown in **Fig. 1**. The goals of this subgroup of patients are similar to those of patients with massive weight loss who have not undergone prior resection.

PREOPERATIVE EVALUATION

All candidates for belt lipectomy should undergo a complete history and a thorough physical examination.

History

Belt lipectomy should not be performed on patients with significant uncontrolled medical problems or psychiatric disorders. Weight history, exercise routine, and nutritional habits should be specifically documented. Patients must achieve stable weight loss, preferably for a 1-year period, but most experienced postbariatric surgeons are willing to operate if patients have stabilized their weight loss for at least 3 months. Patients with

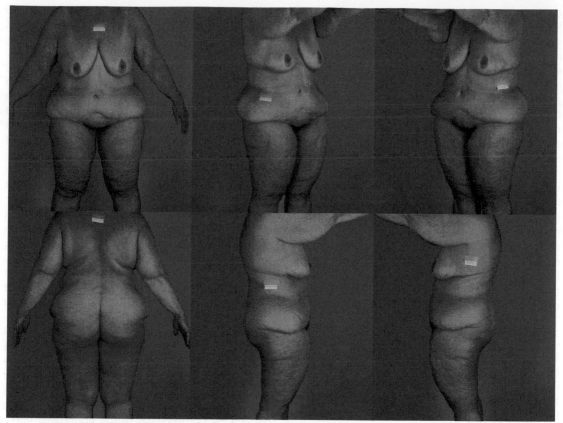

Fig. 1. A 57-year-old woman presents status post an anterior-only procedure; in this case an abdominoplasty. The patient was unhappy with the persistent anterior excess, the lateral dog ears, the lack of waist definition, and the lack of definition of the buttocks.

ongoing weight fluctuation or nonsustainable diet efforts are not ideal operative candidates.

Cardiac, pulmonary, and vascular medical comorbidities should be considered when evaluating a patient's candidacy for belt lipectomy. The possible fluid shifts and changes in intravascular volume during and after a belt lipectomy may place unacceptable stress on a poorly functioning heart. Patients with significant underlying lung disease may not tolerate abdominal wall tightening with rectus fascia plication and may develop pulmonary compromise. With the inherent compromise of blood supply of undermined abdominal tissues during the procedure, conditions associated with decreased vascularity, such as smoking, should also be avoided in most instances.

The thorough medical history taken on all candidates for belt lipectomy should include psychiatric disorders and treatment history. A preoperative psychiatric clearance should be considered given the emotional, physical, and psychological stress involved in recovering from a belt lipectomy. All patients, not only those with psychiatric diagnoses, should be counseled extensively before

surgery given the long recovery and possibility of complications.

Physical Examination

The patient's BMI is determined to help predict results and potential complications. The patient's overall body contour is examined circumferentially, with close attention to the inferior truncal subunit, superior truncal subunit, thighs, and upper arms. The surgeon should search thoroughly for hernias, because incisional, ventral, and umbilical hernias are common in patients with massive weight loss who have undergone open bariatric surgery procedures.

The patient's fat distribution, subcutaneous fat thickness, skin mobility, and skin quality should be examined. In general, skin with a thinner subcutaneous fat layer is more likely to be mobile when resection is attempted.

During abdominal examination, the extent of abdominal wall laxity should be determined and excessive intra-abdominal content should be assessed. Excessive intra-abdominal content is a contraindication to both abdominoplasty and belt lipectomy. The authors find that the best way to determine the extent of intra-abdominal content is to note the patient's abdominal contour in the supine position; if the abdomen is scaphoid, intra-abdominal content is not excessive, which should lead to successful abdominal wall plication. In contrast, if the abdomen in the supine position is convex and protrudes above the ribcage, intra-abdominal content is excessive and not likely to allow a successful abdominal wall plication.

Preoperative evaluation of the mons pubis is important because it is usually one of the patient's main complaints. If the mons pubis is extremely ptotic and redundant, normal contour should neither be expected nor promised. A compromise should be accepted rather than risking over-resection, which can potentially lead to permanent lymphedema of the mons pubis. After complete healing from belt lipectomy, a separate monsplasty can be considered and discussed with the patient.

Testing and Imaging

Because patients with a history of bariatric surgery have a higher likelihood of metabolic abnormalities, the following laboratory tests should be obtained before surgery: complete blood cell count, blood urea nitrogen, creatinine, electrolytes, glucose, urinalysis, liver function, iron, calcium, albumin, prealbumin, total protein, magnesium, and thiamine. Chest radiographs and electrocardiograms should be obtained if indicated.

Markings

The markings are the road map of the surgery and should be tailored for each patient's anatomy and deformity to attain optimal results. The authors prefer markings to be performed in clinic, 1 to 2 days before surgery to allow for accurate photographic documentation and analysis of the markings, which often require adjustments in order to attain the best possible results.

First, the patient's anterior midline is marked. Next, the horizontal mons pubis mark is made with the patient supine and traction placed on the mons pubis to create a more pleasing appearance. With the tissues under tension, the horizontal mark is made 1 to 2 cm superior to the pubic bone extending to the lateral edges of the mons, which results in excision of hair-bearing skin of varying degrees in almost all patients with massive weight loss.

With the patient in the supine position and slightly bent at the waist, traction is placed on the abdominal pannus in a superior medial direction. Next, a line is drawn from the lateral aspect

of the mons pubis mark toward the anterior superior iliac spine (ASIS). The angulation of this mark varies depending on the surgeon's preference. Some surgeons prefer the line to end up below, at, or above the ASIS. Regardless of preference, this mark should be made while elevating the abdominal tissue superomedially to simulate the balance of forces between the inguinal zone of adherence and the pull from abdominal closure after resection, thus allowing better prediction of final scar position.

The abdominal contour typically shows greater deformity and is more visible to the patient, so it should have a higher priority than the posterior contour. The central aspect of the anterior mark is made based on pinching the tissues from the proposed superior mark to the inferior mark, similar to that for a traditional abdominoplasty. However, in most patients with massive weight loss the vertical excess is more extensive and the superior mark is often much higher than the traditional abdominoplasty just above the umbilicus. The lateral extent of the superior abdominal mark, which matches the inferior mark that spans from the lateral edges of the pubic mark to the ASIS, should be fairly flat if the patient is marked in the supine position. Angulating this mark aggressively may result in central flap necrosis caused by compromise of the abdominal flap's intercostal, subcostal, and lumbar vessels.

The markings for posterior resection are made with the patient standing. The back midline is marked. In general, the posterior back excision is more aggressive laterally than centrally because the greatest decent of tissues occurs at the level of posterior axillary line. The resection is thus designed to reverse this deformity. This type of excision allows for greater elevation of the lateral buttocks and lateral thigh regions, which improves lateral contour and the shape of the infrabuttocks crease.

The midline inferior extent of excision is marked first, a little above the midline buttocks crease. Next, the superior extent of the midline back excision is marked using the pinch technique with the patient flexed at the waist, which simulates the patient's position at the conclusion of anterior resection and is important in preventing posterior dehiscence. Next the inferior mark from the midline of the back to the anterior marks is made in a lazy S to reverse the deformity as described earlier. The superior mark, from the midline of the back to the anterior mark, is made by pinching the tissues using the inferior mark as the starting point.

Next, a series of vertical marks are placed to aid with tissue alignment at closure. If anterior and lateral thigh liposuction are needed, those areas are marked. In addition, the patient is placed in all operative positions (supine and both lateral decubitus positions) to assess symmetry and placement of markings.

The inferior marks control scar position anteriorly, which means that the final scar will be considerably closer to the inferior marks because of the zone of adherence located in the inguinal region. In contrast, posteriorly, the superior marks control final scar position. Lower back tissues have stronger zones of adherence and are restricted in their movement, whereas the tissues from the buttocks and lateral thighs are considerably more mobile.

PATIENT POSITIONING AND SURGICAL TECHNIQUE

The circumferential nature of belt lipectomy necessitates intraoperative body position changes. The method described here uses the sequence of supine to lateral/decubitus to lateral decubitus. This sequence prioritizes anterior and lateral resections rather than the posterior resection. Five or 6 people are necessary to reposition the patient safely and efficiently and to ensure that the patient's waist remains flexed at all times to prevent dehiscence. Pressure points are padded; orthopedic body positioners are used to hold patients in the lateral decubitus position with an axillary role and pillows between the knees.

Before surgery, an epidural catheter is placed for postoperative pain management. The authors have not used deep venous thrombosis (DVT)/pulmonary embolus (PE) chemoprophylaxis in more than 15 years but have always used epidural postoperative analgesia. The epidural analgesia in combination with a general anesthetic has been found, in the authors' experience, to essentially eliminate DVT/PE. Sequential compression stockings are placed in the holding room and activated before the induction of general anesthesia. Once in the operating room, the patient is placed in a supine position, general anesthesia is induced, arms are placed just short of 90° angles and padded, and an indwelling urinary bladder catheter is placed. Vertical marks for aligning tissue at closure are marked with methylene blue outside the intended tissue resection. An additional V-shaped mark is made on each side to allow the creation of a temporary dog ear at the end of anterior resection. The patient is then prepped and draped and 2 different colored sutures are placed through the skin of the superior and inferior umbilicus as traction sutures. These sutures are placed deeper within the umbilicus if the stalk needs to be shortened.

The anterior approach begins with a circumbilical incision and dissection down to the rectus fascia,

leaving some adipose tissue on the stalk. The anterior abdominal inferior mark is then incised and dissection is taken down to the level of the Scarpa fascia. The abdominal flap is elevated superiorly, at or just below the Scarpa fascia, up to the level of the umbilicus. Dividing the abdominal flap in the midline from incision to umbilicus facilitates the dissection of a large pannus. In patients with a thin pannus, the dissection is carried up to the costal margins and xyphoid. In patients with a thick pannus, the supraumbilical dissection is limited to the medial edges of the rectus muscle fascia and the flap is thinned by tumescent liposuction.

Abdominal wall plication is performed with a nonpermanent, running, long-lasting barbed suture. If present, hernias are repaired before plication. If the umbilical stalk is part of the hernia sac it may need to be sacrificed. The infraumbilical plication is usually performed before the supraumbilical plication because this is the area of greatest laxity in most patients, especially women. During plication, peak inspiratory pressures should be monitored.

The patient is then flexed at the waist, and the abdominal flap is advanced inferiorly and tailored to the inferior incision. Extensive amounts of anterior abdominal excess often need to be resected in patients with massive weight loss. In the lateral areas of the previously marked V, the temporary dog ear is stapled.

A closed suction drain is placed and brought out through a lateral stab incision. If the patient requires liposuction of the anterior and medial thighs, this is performed either through the open abdominal wound or through appropriate stab incisions. The proper location of the umbilicus is then determined with the abdominal flap temporarily tacked in place. A vertical 1.5-cm to 2-cm incision is made in the midline at the chosen location. The fat deep to the incision is bluntly dissected apart to allow a path for the umbilicus. Three nonpermanent sutures (3-0 Monocryl) are placed at the 3, 6, and 9 o'clock positions at the subcuticular level on both the abdominal flap and the umbilicus, as well as through the surrounding rectus fascia to help invaginate the umbilicus when the sutures are tied. The remainder of the umbilicus is sutured to the abdominal flap with simple, interrupted, nonpermanent, subcuticular sutures. Before abdominal closure, a series of interrupted quilting sutures are placed from the abdominal flap to the rectus fascia to help close dead space and reduce the risk of seroma formation.

The abdominal wound is then closed in multiple layers. First, Scarpa fascia is reapproximated with #1 barbed, nonpermanent, long-lasting, running suture. The next layer is closed with nonpermanent subcuticular staples. The final layer is closed with a running subcuticular 2-0 nonpermanent suture. In addition, tissue glue is applied to the skin to complete the closure.

The patient is then turned to one of the lateral decubitus positions in order to allow maximal resection of the lateral trunk and more direct access to the lateral thighs for liposuction. Once in position, the patient is prepped, draped, and padded over pressure points. The lateral and back marks are reinforced and the vertical marks are tattooed in this position. Just past the midline of the back, a temporary V-shaped dog ear is again marked to allow for the subsequent turn. The lateral thigh is suctioned if necessary.

Unlike the anterior resection, the superior mark is incised first during the back resection, because patients have more inferior than superior laxity in the lateral trunk, so it is best to dissect inferiorly to lift the ptotic buttocks and lateral thighs. Also, the lower back has a tendency to develop seromas, and less dissection in this area is desirable.

The depth at which the inferior flap is elevated is based on the patient's presenting contour. If the patient has overprojected buttocks, as is typical in most patients with high BMI, the dissection is performed at a level just above the muscle fascia, leaving a small amount of fat on the fascia. If the patient has underprojected buttocks, the elevation is performed at the level of the superficial fascia so that as much fat tissue as possible is left behind. In either case, the flap is elevated at least to the level of the proposed inferior line of excision. This dissection can be carried as inferior as is necessary to achieve the desired buttocks contour, which often is down to the level of the midbuttocks.

The inferior flap is then redraped superiorly and tailored accordingly. Tissue is aligned with the help of the vertical skin markings. In the patient who presents with overprojected buttocks, tailoring of the inferiorly based flap should be more aggressive in the fat deep to the superficial fascia to equalize the thickness of subcutaneous fat of the two edges that are brought together. This technique is necessary in order to create a smooth transition between the buttocks and the back given the discrepancy in tissue thickness in these patients. If there are still small discrepancies after closure, liposuction can be performed to create a smooth contour from the waist, through the hip, and down to the lateral thighs and buttocks.

One closed suction drain is placed in the back through a stab incision made laterally, which is eventually routed to the opposite back closure. The back closure is similar to the anterior closure described earlier. Just past the midline, the temporary dog ear is closed with staples to allow for the final turn.

The patient is turned to the other lateral decubitus position, and the other side of the resection is completed in a similar manner. The second side occasionally does not allow tissue resection equal to the first side, so the surgeon should not assume that the same amount can be removed. After the second side is completed, the patient is placed in the supine position with the waist flexed. The patient is then transferred to a hospital bed in the same flexed position.

Management of Abdominal Scars

In patients with upper abdominal surgical scars, such as open cholecystectomy scars, the proposed superior mark should be incised first. These patients are at risk for tissue necrosis inferior to the scar if that tissue is elevated as a typical abdominoplasty flap. Instead, a limited central supraumbilical dissection is performed to allow advancement of the flap to the proposed inferior marks. Next, the blood supply of the tissue inferior to the surgical scar is examined. If viable in appearance, the inferior flap is elevated to the inferior markings and is then tailored to the superior mark. If there is concern for the flap's vascularity, all tissue below the surgical scar is resected and the inferior flap is elevated and tailored to the level of the scar. If this second scenario is necessary, the patient must be made aware that the final scar position is much higher on the abdomen and does not allow alteration of the mons pubis, which then will require an additional procedure.

In patients with midline vertical supraumbilical scars, the scars may be contracted, thus preventing the advancement of the abdominal flap during the tailoring process. The scar is not resected because this may lead to flap necrosis at the inferior aspect where a T would be created during scar excision. In this situation a series of horizontal nicks in the scar may be necessary to release the scar.

POSTPROCEDURAL CARE, REHABILITATION, AND RECOVERY

Several strategies are used to minimize this risk of dehiscence in the immediate postoperative period. First, the operating surgeon oversees the patient's transfer in the operating room to the hospital bed to ensure that the patient maintains the proper flexed position throughout the transfer. Given the circumferential nature of belt lipectomy the patient cannot be overflexed or underflexed, because this would place unacceptable tension on the posterior or anterior closures. Once the patient leaves the operating room, nursing staff are instructed not to move patients until they are fully awake and alert. The patients are instructed before surgery to take charge of their positioning, because only they can sense their opposing wound tensions. With assistance, ambulation is initiated on the day of surgery. A regular diet is also started soon after surgery. The epidural catheter infusion rate is adjusted by the anesthesia team with the goal of maintaining pain relief without interfering with muscle function or regular sensation. The epidural catheter is typically removed early on the second postoperative day and the bladder catheter removed at least 4 hours later. The patient is typically discharged on the second or third postoperative day, once pain control is achieved with oral pain medication.

After discharge, patients continue in a flexed position for the first week after surgery and then begin slow straightening exercises. By 10 to 14 days, most patients can stand fairly straight. Patients are expected to spend as little time in bed as possible. Nonvigorous activity is encouraged for 4 to 6 weeks, whereas strenuous exercise is discouraged for 3 months. Garment compression is most often avoided for a few days to avoid

vascular compromise and flap necrosis. A compression garment is to be worn for up to 6 months. Drains are left in until they are producing less than 40 mL in a 24-hour period. However, the authors have found no particular algorithm for drain management to be effective in preventing seromas. Anterior drain output typically decreases most quickly and this drain is removed in 7 to 10 days, whereas some posterior drains remain after 14 days. If necessary, a sclerosing agent, such as doxycycline, is injected into the drain every 2 to 3 days to decrease the size of the pocket. Once output decreases to 80 mL in 24 hours it is removed and the possible seroma is managed with serial aspirations. The authors often put patients on a mild oral diuretic for 14 to 21 days after the last drain is removed.

OUTCOMES

Final truncal contour is typically achieved by 1 year, with most of the improvement realized over the first 6 months. In general, the lower the BMI at presentation the better the lower truncal contour attained and the less likely the patient

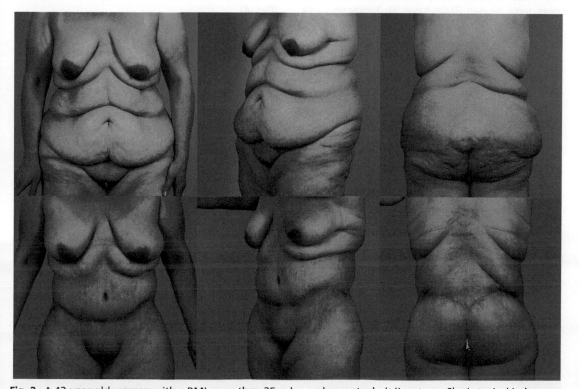

Fig. 2. A 43-year-old woman with a BMI more than 35, who underwent a belt lipectomy. She is typical in her presentation, results, and complications for a patient in this group. Note that her upper abdominal roll was not amenable to elimination through a lower truncal procedure and required an upper body lift. After surgery, she developed a large seroma and dehiscence of her right posterior back incision, which required prolonged treatment to resolve and may require a revision in the long term. Again, this is a typical course for patients in this group of patients with high BMI.

will experience complications. In contrast, the higher the BMI at presentation the less impressive the results and the more likely the patient will experience a complication.

Patients with Massive Weight Loss

BMI is most the important factor in how well patients do after belt lipectomy surgery. The authors have arbitrarily chosen BMI cutoffs to be used as general categories that help the surgeon, and the patient, understand approximately where a patient fits in the spectrum of massive weight loss body contouring results.

BMI Greater than 35

Patients in this subgroup who are still severely obese after massive weight loss achieve significant improvement in inferior truncal contour through belt lipectomy but typically do not achieve a normal contour. These patients also have significant fat deposits in other body areas, which are not addressed with belt lipectomy, and may require additional procedures. These patients with higher BMIs have an increased risk

of complications, most commonly seromas (**Fig. 2**).

BMI of 35 to 30

Patients in this subgroup can attain significant improvement in their inferior truncal contours and may achieve normal body contours. Their complication rate is intermediate between the subgroup with BMIs greater than 35 and the subgroup with BMIs less than 30 (**Fig. 3**).

BMI Less than 30

Patients in this subgroup, who are at or near their ideal body weight, can attain a normal body contour and sometimes can even attain ideal body contour. The closer a patient is to ideal body weight before operation, the better the final contour after belt lipectomy. The remarkable results are possible because the subcutaneous fat layer often allows greater skin mobility. Tissue tension can be distributed further from the area of resection and a larger amount of excess skin can be resected. The complication rate in this subgroup is low compared with the two previous subgroups (**Fig. 4**).

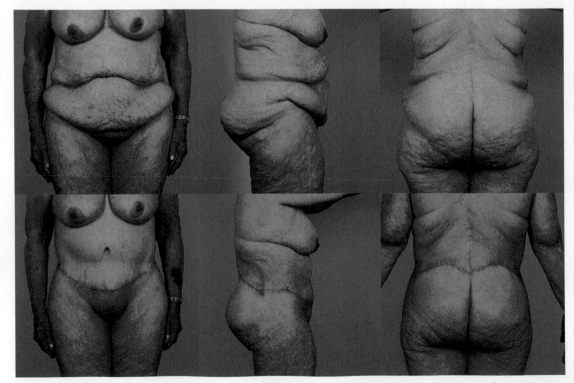

Fig. 3. A 67-year-old woman who underwent a belt lipectomy with a starting BMI in the range of 30 to 35. Note the generalized better level of improvement compared with the patient in **Fig. 2**, but that it is less impressive than the result of the patient in a lower BMI range, shown in **Fig. 4**.

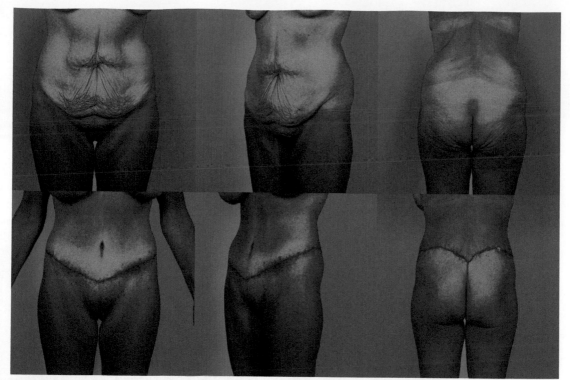

Fig. 4. A 44-year-old woman who underwent a belt lipectomy. She presented initially with a BMI in the lowest category (≤30). Note the generalized better level of improvement compared with the two other subgroups shown in **Figs. 2** and **3**.

Patients with Massive Weight Loss Status Post Anterior-only Resection Surgery

Patients in this subgroup have undergone dermatolipectomy procedures limited to the anterior abdomen. After surgery, these patients are disappointed with their resultant lateral dog ears and desire improvement of the waist, hips, back, and buttocks. Their resultant contour after abdominoplasty or panniculectomy determines whether they are best treated with a partial, modified, or full belt lipectomy (**Fig. 5**).

COMPLICATIONS

Small wound separations are common after belt lipectomy. These separations are most commonly treated with conservative wound care and most often they heal without much evidence.

Seromas are probably the most troublesome aspect of caring for patients after belt lipectomy. Although they occur less often than the small wound separations mentioned earlier, their care requires more work. Although the rate of seromas has decreased in the experience of the authors, they still occur with enough frequency, especially in patients with high BMI, to bother both patients and the physicians on a regular basis. Seromas can be attributed to the large area of dissection and occur most often in the back. The authors' current escalating treatment regimen starts with serial and frequent aspirations, then to the use of sclerosing agents, and finally a small incision is made through the existing scar which has a Penrose drain inserted through to the seroma pocket. This is left in place till the pocket closes around the drain. The Penrose drain is then slowly advanced out. The authors have not had to operate on a seroma in more than 16 years using this regimen.

Dehiscences, defined as separation at superficial fascia level, mostly occurred within the first 24 hours and were caused by mechanical stress on the wounds. To minimize dehiscence it is important to prevent patients from moving until they are completely awake and to instruct them to guide their own ambulation. In addition to mechanical stress on wounds, large seromas can cause breakdown at the wound edge and can lead to dehiscence. Detection and frequent aspiration of seromas helps to reduce this risk.

Infections are infrequent complications after belt lipectomy, but tend to occur in association with

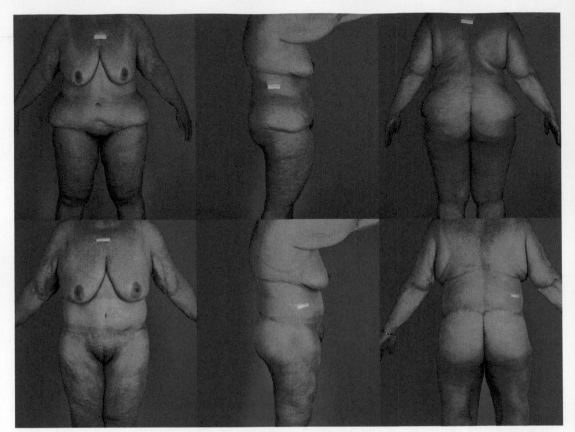

Fig. 5. The same patient shown in **Fig. 1**. She is shown here before and after undergoing a belt lipectomy, as a revision of the anterior-only procedure that was previously undertaken.

seromas. They are managed with appropriate drainage of seromas and appropriate antibiotic therapy. DVT and PE are dangerous complications. Since our first report on belt lipectomy, we have used an epidural catheter infusion for postoperative pain control over a 15-year period and have not experienced any DVT or PE since, despite a high-risk group of patients. We also use sequential compression garments during surgery, and after surgery patients are ambulated within 24 hours, and mostly within 12 hours.

SUGGESTED READINGS

Aly SA, Cram AE. Body lift: belt lipectomy. In: Nahai F, editor. The art of aesthetic surgery: principles &

techniques. St Louis (MO): Quality Medical Publishing; 2011.

Aly A, Cram AR, Chao M, et al. Belt lipectomy for circumferential truncal excess: the University of Iowa experience. Plast Reconstr Surg 2003;111: 398–413.

Aly A. Body contouring after massive weight loss. St Louis (MO): Quality Medical Publishing; 2006.

Van Geertruygen JP, Vandeweyer E, de Fontaine S, et al. Circumferential torsoplasty. Br J Plast Surg 1999;52: 623–8.

Hamrai ST. Circumferential body lift. Aesthet Surg J 1999;19:244–50.

Lockwood TE. Superficial fascial system (SFS) of the trunk and extremities: a new concept. Plast Reconstr Surg 1991;87:1009–18.

Circumferential Body Contouring
The Lower Body Lift

Dirk F. Richter, MD, PhD*, Alexander Stoff, MD, PhD

KEYWORDS

- Lower body lift • Two position circumferential procedure
- Circumferential lower truncal dermatolipectomy • Buttock reshaping • Massive weight loss
- Transposition-Gluteoplasty

KEY POINTS

- Lower body lift (circumferential lower truncal dermatolipectomy, CLTD): Modification of the lower body lift procedure as an alternative to the belt lipectomy.
- Perioperative optimization: Standardized perioperative requirements and settings are highlighted and described in detail.
- Technical details: The correct choice of technique is the key to a higher patient satisfaction. Massive-weight-loss patients are far more tolerant of longer scars, allowing a generally high acceptance of, for example, the fleur-de-lis excision pattern.
- Gluteal enhancement: The loss of gluteal volume is a frequent consequence of weight loss. For specific cases the transposition-gluteoplasty is incorporated, which allows a gluteal reshaping with autologous tissue.
- Procedure combination: The combination of liposuction and lower body lift can be performed for additional contouring of the abdomen, the flank, and gluteal region. For selected cases the harvested fat tissue may be transferred for additional improvement of gluteal volume and shape.

INTRODUCTION

The overweight and massively obese population is growing continuously every year. With the success and increasing number of bariatric procedures, the authors have registered a yearly increase of body contouring procedures. In addition, owing to the rising experience in this field of plastic surgery, these procedures have wider ranges of indications, including patients after massive weight loss, patients with primarily cosmetic indications (aging process), or patients who seek correction of contour deformities after previous liposuction. Coincidentally, the requirements and demands

for such operations are continually increasing. In addition to the typical problem areas such as the abdomen, the mons pubis, and hip region, patients frequently present with growing attention to the aesthetic restoration of the gluteal area.

The variety of gluteal deformities after weight loss results in a wide range of patient complaints and discomfort. Some patients complain of an enlarged buttock, some of a deficient gluteal volume with gluteal flattening (platypygia), and yet others suffer from cellulite or a lengthening of the infragluteal fold. However, patients primarily seek an enhancement of the gluteal shape and projection.

The authors have nothing to disclose.
Department for Plastic and Reconstructive Surgery, Dreifaltigkeits-Hospital, Bonner Strasse 84, Wesseling 50389, Germany
* Corresponding author.
E-mail address: Dr.Dirk.Richter@t-online.de

Clin Plastic Surg 41 (2014) 775–788
http://dx.doi.org/10.1016/j.cps.2014.07.004
0094-1298/14/$ – see front matter © 2014 Published by Elsevier Inc

A well-shaped buttock is characterized by several factors: it is more rounded than angular, the intergluteal fold is short rather than long, and the feminine gluteal cleavage has a superior and inferior buttock separation. Dividing the buttocks into an upper, middle, and lower section, the ideal maximum projection lies between the upper and middle third. The infragluteal fold should run in a round rather than horizontal curve with a minimal crease, ideally without any droop. The side view should illustrate an S-shaped contour in relation to the back and thigh, as a smooth inward sweep of the inferior back and waist area.[1] To meet these ideal characteristics, several techniques are available to plastic surgeons. In the late 1960s surgeons performed gluteal augmentation with existing breast implants. Today various gluteal implants are accessible, which can be implanted epifascially, subfascially, or submuscularly. Nowadays gluteal contouring is most frequently performed through liposuction, particularly by sculpturing the adjoining regions such as the hips, flanks, and saddlebag deformities, achieving excellent results without any direct buttock approach.

During the past decade, buttock augmentation by autologous fat grafting has gained wider acceptance and success. Many different techniques such as macrografting or micrografting are available for contour improvement of the gluteal region, solely or in combination with liposculpturing.[2]

These techniques, however, are not suitable for patients after massive weight loss. These patients suffer from atonic skin quality with a high degree of laxity and, consequently, with the indisputable requirement of tissue resection. These severe deformities have caused a continuous development of various lifting procedures, such as the pioneering circumferential lower body lift described by Ted Lockwood in 1993.[3–6] Further developments of these procedures in combination with autologous tissue augmentation, such as the deepithelialized gluteal flaps for buttock reshaping, enable an improvement in the postoperative results. In 2005, Sozer and colleagues[7] reported of a series of 20 deepithelialized turnover dermal fat flaps for buttock augmentation in bariatric and aesthetic patients undergoing lower body lifts. After more than 200 cases, the technique has evolved to include a split portion of the gluteus maximus muscle, resulting in a better blood supply to the flap, more caudal reach, and a dramatic decrease in fatty necrosis.[8]

In this context, the authors have established a technique of gluteal fat tissue transpositioning (transposition-gluteoplasty) during modification of the lower body lift (circumferential lower trunk dermatolipectomy [CLTD]), which has been shown to be a reliable alternative for enhancement of the gluteal projection and shape.

PATIENT SELECTION AND SCREENING

A precise physical examination and assessment of patients' medical history during the first consultation is mandatory for every patient. The authors recommend a repeat of evaluation before surgery, if it is performed after a delay since the first consultation. The assessment of medical history includes: the current weight; initial and current body mass index or, in future, the A body mass index; the weight history with weight fluctuations and constancy periods; the frequency of exercises; former bariatric procedures; nutritional disorders; medication; the number of pregnancies and children; history of cesarean section, abdominal surgeries, and abdominal hernias; gastrointestinal, cardiac, and pulmonary history; and smoking history. Previous liposuction in the abdominal area has to be asked after from patients, because they might conceal this before treatment. Patients must present a stable weight for at least 6 to 12 months preoperatively; required weight loss should be completed before the surgery.

The clinical examination is the essential part of every medical history assessment. The examination of the lower trunk should include an accurate palpation of the abdominal, lateral thigh, and gluteal adipose tissue in patients while in upright, prone, supine, and lateral position. This approach enables the examiner to assess the tissue conditions in regard of volume and mobility by pinching and metrically measuring. It is crucial to consider the existent adipose tissue at the lateral and posterior lower gluteal and proximal thigh region. Unfortunately, untreated distinct masses of local adipose tissue in these regions will assuredly limit the gluteal improvement, because downward tractions will consequently displace gluteal tissue in the caudal direction. Skin quality with the presence of striae must be evaluated, explaining to the patient that supraumbilical striae will not be resected in abdominoplasty procedures (except for fleur-de-lis procedures). Furthermore, any existing lower and upper abdominal pannus has to be assessed and measured, documenting any existing eczema or consequent hyperpigmentation. Any preexisting scar (subcostal, midline, horizontal) in the abdominal and gluteal area must be documented in writing and photographically, as they can impair the blood supply of the tissue flap. The status of the abdominal muscles must be assessed and any existing rectus diastasis, incisional, epigastric, or umbilical hernia excluded, in specific cases, by supportive computed tomography or magnetic resonance imaging. In cases of elevated intra-abdominal pressure, the abdominal wall elevates above the costal margin and the level of the iliac crest in supine position. Abdominoplasty procedures with fascial tightening should be performed cautiously in such cases.[9,10]

The authors highly recommend preparing a photographic documentation of preoperative and postoperative conditions, consisting of different views (anterior, oblique, lateral, and posterior). Postoperative photo documentation can be made at 3, 9, and 12 months. In individual cases it is recommended that the clinician add photographic documentation of various arm and thigh positions, tissue characteristics with relaxed and contracted muscles, the patient in sitting position to demonstrate redundant upper abdominal laxity and tissue excess, and views of the patient holding up and pinching excess tissue in the specific region. For a classification of the different deformities, the Pittsburgh Rating Scale is helpful for patient demonstration and selection of the adequate operative approach.[11] However, the authors have experienced wider indications for the combined technique of liposuction and excisional procedures in all body regions.[9,10]

Detailed information should be given to patients regarding the operative procedure, alternative techniques, the general and operation-related risks and benefits is an essential part of preoperative documentation. Besides standard and individualized consent forms, which have to be reviewed and signed by the patient at the earliest opportunity and at latest 24 hours before the operation, the authors recommend an audio-visual demonstration of intraoperative details, preoperative and postoperative results, and possible complications. Patients should be informed about their postoperative care including their expected level of activity; they have to understand the limitations of the surgical result in cases of existing variables of bone structure, fat distribution, and any existing scars.[9,12,13]

Recent studies evaluated differences in collagen and elastin contents in the abdominal skin of patients without weight loss in a comparison with those with bariatric weight loss, showing impairment in skin quality in the bariatric group.[14] This fact should be made clear to every patient to limit their postoperative expectations. Patients with multiple striae must be informed that secondary relaxation in their specific case may require a repetitive skin-tightening procedure.

During clinical examination of the abdominal region, the following parameters should be acquired:

- Abdominal tissue excess
- Abdominal skin quality (striae?)

- Umbilical stalk deformity
- Number of skin folds and their continuity to the flanks
- Skin quality
- Adipose tissue volume and mobility
- Abdominal muscle tone
- Mons pubis region

During clinical examination of the gluteal region the following parameters should be acquired:

- Gluteal height
- Gluteal width
- Maximum height of projection
- Round shape versus rectangular shape
- Skin quality
- Adipose tissue volume and mobility
- Gluteal muscle tone
- Back folds
- Vertebral status (eg, scoliosis)

In their massive-weight-loss patient group the authors have established a classification for surgical planning of the gluteal region, which can be simply divided into 3 groups (**Fig. 1**):

1. Large buttocks with excess amount of gluteal adipose tissue
2. Normal-sized buttocks with ptosis and skin redundancy
3. Flattened, hypoplastic buttocks with ptosis and skin redundancy

The adipose tissue in the upper third of the gluteal region has an excess lobular and lamellar structure with a ratio of 1:2 in females and 1:1 in males, whereas the lower third presents a 1:1 ratio in both sexes (**Fig. 2**).[12]

Patients who belong to group 1 may present with residual overweight. To reduce gluteal adipose tissue, preparation is performed below the superficial fascia to eliminate larger amounts of lobular and lamellar adipose tissue. In patients with a group 2 deformity, an epifascial preparation is maintained with preservation of the entire superficial fascia. In this regard the authors refrain from an extensive adipose tissue resection, maintaining the lobular adipose tissue. In cases of deflated and flattened buttocks of group 3 deformities, the authors stringently refrain from any adipose tissue reduction and perform preparation at a superficial subcutaneous level. In contrast to the technique of subfascial dissection described by Lockwood, the authors generally remain above the superficial fascia, which is a constant and strong structure, separating the lamellar and lobular adipose tissue. The gluteal superficial fascia provides comparable features such as the

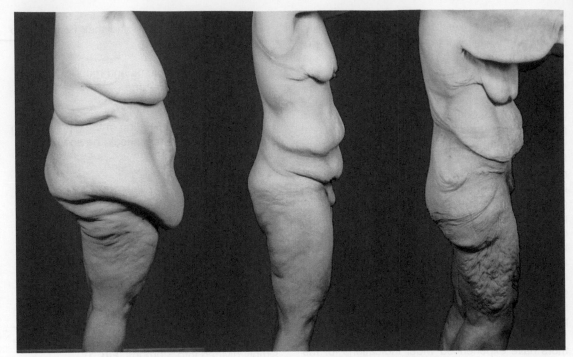

Fig. 1. Patients with group 1 (*left*), group 2 (*middle*), and group 3 (*right*) gluteal deformity.

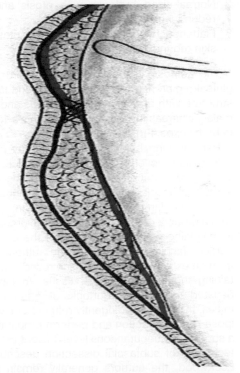

Fig. 2. Relations of lobular (*yellow*) and lamellar (*orange*) adipose structure at the lateral thigh, here in female patients with a 1:2 ratio. The red line indicates the plane of surgical preparation, from initially epifascial to epimuscular at the distal lateral thigh.

fascial superficial muscular aponeurotic syndrome (SMAS) during facelift surgery, for example, the reduction of tension on the skin level and the opportunity to provide a multivectoral remodeling on different tissue levels.[12]

TREATMENT GOALS AND PLANNED OUTCOMES

Circumferential tightening procedures have the goal of restoring and improving the body shape, including the abdominal, flank, and gluteal regions. The abdominal region can be reshaped through preparation steps derived from a standard abdominoplasty, a lipoabdominoplasty, or fleur-de-lis abdominoplasty. The main goals are maximal skin and fat tissue reduction with contouring of the abdominal wall. The flanks are mainly restored by vertical tissue resection; additionally in fleur-de-lis procedures the waist circumference may be reduced by horizontal tissue resection. In the gluteal region there are different approaches available, depending on the patient's preoperative conditions. The available options are gluteal tissue reduction by direct excision or gluteal autoaugmentation in cases of volume and shape deficiency. In both cases, the goal of the body lift procedure is a restoration of gluteal volume and gluteal reshaping in relation to the surrounding regions (**Fig. 3**).

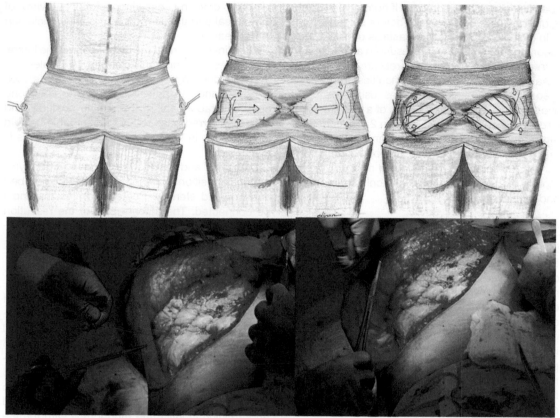

Fig. 3. Schematic (*above*) and intraoperative (*below*) presentation of the gluteal autoaugmentation (transposition-gluteoplasty), which includes subfascial gluteal adipose tissue preservation and entire epifascial mobilization (*left*), 2-dimensional fascial and adipose tissue transpositioning using nonresorbable sutures in single-knot technique (*middle*), and maximization of tissue accumulation at the upper gluteal third (*right*). (*From* Richter DF, Stoff A, Velasco FJ, et al. Circumferential lower truncal dermato-lipectomy. Clin Plast Surg 2008;35:(1):58; with permission from Elsevier Saunders.)

PREOPERATIVE PLANNING AND PREPARATION

Smokers are instructed to quit smoking at least 6 weeks before the surgery. Patients should take antiseptic showers in the evening and morning before the surgery, and the skin folds and the umbilicus should be cleaned thoroughly with antiseptic solutions.

Because postoperative blood transfusion may be necessary, patients have to be informed preoperatively, as this requires a blood typing and informed consent. Anticoagulant drugs and supplements must be avoided 14 days before surgery. In all cases, bowel purgation is advised the night before surgery. In patients with a large hernia, they may be restricted to a fluid diet for 24 hours before surgery.

Patients must be informed about the intraoperative procedures including any change of position, with the risks of postoperative complications, antithrombotic arrangements, Foley catheter, drains and garment placement, and patient-controlled analgesia. Moreover, they must be instructed about the postoperative course including thromboembolism prevention, respiratory exercises, early mobilization, avoidance of high abdominal pressure, the estimated time point for drain and suture removal, and the minimum time required off work and away from exercise.

Patients should avoid any skin irritation or inflammation in the area of the abdominal fold and umbilicus. An inspection of these areas during consultation, and immediately before the operation, is strongly advisable. Prophylaxis for pulmonary embolism and deep vein thrombosis is an essential consideration, especially in smokers and patients taking birth control medications or hormone replacement therapy.[15] The authors initialize heparin therapy in all patients the evening before surgery or, at latest, 2 hours before the surgical procedure. Patients are informed that this specific risk will be decreased if hormonal therapy is discontinued 3 to 4 weeks before surgery.

In cases of a preexisting diastasis or hernia, the reconstruction of the fascia results in an additional increase of intra-abdominal pressure, which may be a source of respiratory difficulties. Therefore, preoperative breathing exercises (using an incentive spirometer) and the wearing of a compression girdle are advised, beginning 1 to 2 weeks before the surgery. A cold, dry cough or any kind of respiratory infection should lead to postponement of surgery, because fits of coughing may provoke a rupture of the fascial sutures with consequent secondary bleeding.[9,12,16]

Markings

Markings are performed in upright standing position. First, the patient is asked to pull up the entire central lower abdominal tissue in a symmetric manner. Meanwhile, after the midline has been drawn, a distance of 6 cm to the upper vulvar commissure is marked. At this height, while the patient is maximally pulling up the entire abdominal tissue with a maximum pull at the lateral aspects, an almost horizontal lower incision line is marked to both flanks, followed by the upper horizontal incision line above the height of the umbilicus. Next, the patient turns and the posterior markings are performed. The upper incision line is marked, generally starting at the highest point of the gluteal cleft and running upward in a round curved shape to the lateral end of the anterior upper incision line. In patients with a short intergluteal cleft, the starting point of the upper incision line may be set a few centimeters higher in the posterior midline. Finally, the lower incision line is assessed and marked by pinching, and is connected to the lower anterior incision line.

In patients with abdominal fleur-de-lis resection, the horizontal resection pattern is marked first. Both vertical incision lines run in a curved manner and should measure an equal distance to the midline. The upper horizontal incision line is marked next, always starting below the height of the umbilicus.

PATIENT POSITIONING

After orotracheal intubation and bladder catheterization, the patient is transferred to the operating room in supine position. Here the patient is turned to the prone position, ideally from the first operating table to a second. It is advisable to use prepared soft cushions for a secure, pressure-reduced, and symmetrical positioning. The entire region of the lower back, the hips, the gluteal region, and the dorsal thigh region are draped with a sterile covering, ensuring a total overview of the gluteal and the surrounding regions, including the gluteal fold.

After final closure of the gluteal region the lateral skin excess is temporarily closed with staples and a sterile dressing. The primary covering is then removed and the patient is turned to a second operating table back in the supine position, and then transferred back to the original table using a sterile cover. In this way a change of the tables is avoidable.

Dressings and staples are removed after symmetrical positioning, and the patient is draped and covered sterilely. Posterior drains may now be connected. The anterior part of the resection is now continued, using either the standard horizontal or fleur-de-lis excision pattern.[9,12]

PROCEDURAL APPROACH

The lower body lift (CLTD) is routinely performed by 2 surgeons, optionally with 1 or 2 medical assistants. The leading surgeon performs the initial markings and their intraoperative verification, and supervises the entire procedure. Tissue preparation, dissection, and wound closure are performed simultaneously on both sides. After surgical scrub and consequent draping, the area of resection and undermining is infiltrated moderately with tumescent solution (1 liter of Ringer solution including 1 mg epinephrin), until the desired turgor is achieved.

The initial skin incision (using a cold blade or alternatively the Colorado microdissection needle) is made along the superior marking line and is continued down to the level of the underlying superficial fascia, which separates the superficial lamellar from the subfascial lobular fat. Next, the dissection is continued caudally just above the robust white superficial fascia. The preservation of fascia to the deep gluteal fat as the "gluteal SMAS" is conceptionally similar to the facial SMAS used in facelifts or abdominal Scarpa fascia. In the lateral gluteal half, the superficial fascia is then incised at the height of the inferior resection line before flap mobilization is continued caudally and bluntly on an epimuscular level down to the gluteal fold. The preservation of superficial fascia to the inferior skin flap allows a reconstruction of the fascial continuity on wound closure. For this maneuver, it is essential to maximally release the lateral gluteal tissue adhesions to the gluteal skin flap as far anterior to the anterior axillary line and caudally to height of the gluteal fold. Further dissection is then continued to the lateral thigh, where the preparation level is above the aponeurosis of the tensor fascia lata muscle. An extended distal mobilization of the lateral thigh may be carried out bluntly, using the Lockwood underminer.

For reduction of wound tension, the entire superior wound edge may additionally be mobilized for further release from the gluteal and back adipose tissue. This mobilization should be performed cautiously, preserving any emerging perforators.

With completion of dissection, the waist and gluteal adipose tissue should be widely mobilized and ideally covered by a stable superficial fascia. For the purpose of autologous gluteal augmentation, 3 to 4 1-0 nonabsorbable braided threads are sutured from lateral to medial before knotting, ideally grasping stable fascia and consequently displacing the gluteal and waist adipose tissue medially. For cranial repositioning, 4 to 5 1-0 threads are sutured from caudal to cranial at the medial to central aspect of the buttocks. Here it is crucial to avoid strangulation of adipose tissue during fascial suturing in terms of avoidance of tissue necrosis. By transpositioning and tightening of the gluteal adipose tissue, the gluteal region is lifted cranially with a consequent final skin closure under reduced tension. Furthermore, this maneuver is able to improve the shape of the waist by mobilization of the waist adipose tissue and its medial transpositioning (**Fig. 4**).[9,12]

In severe or secondary cases of gluteal ptosis it may be advisable to strengthen the gluteal tissue reconstruction with an additional mesh, either resorbable, semiresorbable, or nonresorbable.

The stage of resection should always be supervised by the lead surgeon to assure a symmetrical resection. The authors advise the use of bullet forceps for determination of the amount of resection. The marked vector lines are incised from medial to lateral, and incised under maximal tension. The medial, central, and lateral gluteal flaps arising in this way are measured precisely under tension for symmetrical resection, which is subsequently carried out between the clamps.

Temporary wound closure of the gluteal area is performed with bullet forceps, followed by reconstruction of the superficial fascia system (SFS) with absorbable stable 2-0 monofilament or braided sutures. A subcuticular multilayer wound closure is then performed with absorbable 2-0 and 3-0 monofilament suture in an everting manner before intracuticular suturing. Because of the wound length and resulting tissue tension, absorbable 2-0 monofilament suture is advisable. Finally, Steri strips are applied in perpendicular direction for the initial 3 weeks postoperatively. Alternatively, wound closure at the subdermal level may be performed with a single absorbable barbed suture (2-0) in running manner. Skin closure may alternatively be performed with a 2-component skin-closure system.[17] Two suction drains are placed in each gluteal and lateral thigh region. Before patients are turned to the supine position, a temporary closure of the lateral skin excess is performed using a stapler and an occlusive dressing.

Anterior Preparation

The inferior incision is checked and re-marked, adjusting the initial inferior line to the laterally final ending gluteal incision line. It must always be ensured that the umbilical stalk is thoroughly cleaned. Initially, the lower incision line is infiltrated with local anesthetics to reduce postoperative pain and the consecutive risk of an increase in blood pressure. After incision of the lower incision line, preparation is performed down to the Scarpa fascia after ligation of any superficial epigastric vessels. For adequate preparation of the Scarpa fascia, the authors recommend the use of the Colorado Microneedle to ensure a sufficient upward pull of the abdominal flap. By preservation of Scarpa fascia, the subjacent lymphatic vessels are preserved. In general, the authors have found a thin fat layer below the Scarpa fascia.

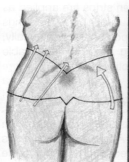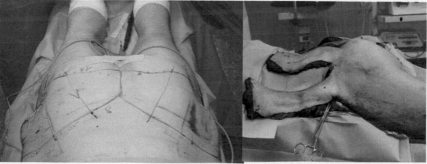

Fig. 4. Schematic (*left*) and intraoperative (*middle*) demonstration of posterior vector lines. Intraoperative lateral view after incision of vectors (*right*). (*From* Richter DF, Stoff A, Velasco FJ, et al. Circumferential lower truncal dermato-lipectomy. Clin Plast Surg 2008;35:(1):62; with permission from Elsevier Saunders.)

The dissection level is performed above the Scarpa fascia, which entails several key advantages: long-lasting swelling can be prevented because the underlying lymphatic vessels are preserved, and the tightening of the SFS craniomedially provides an additional "inner traction" on the deep penetrating fascial system of the thigh (Colles fascia). In this context, the SFS may then be fixed with 1-0 nonabsorbable braided sutures to the anterior rectus fascia.[18] Approximately 3 fingerbreadths below the umbilicus, the Scarpa fascia is dissected and further mobilization of the abdominal flap is performed cranially above the anterior rectus fascia.

At the height of the umbilicus, the abdominal flap is incised in the midline and the umbilical stalk transected square-shaped or circularly, and is completely mobilized from the abdominal flap without any remaining periumbilical fat tissue. Especially in patients after massive weight loss, the umbilical stalk has to be shortened and fixated to the anterior rectus fascia at the height of the stalk base, preferably with stronger absorbable sutures at 3, 6, 9, and 12 o'clock positions. Dissection continues above the anterior rectus fascia up to the xiphoid. The linea alba can easily be identified, as it is distinctively connected to Scarpa fascia. In the area of the costal margin, it is essential to restore the lateral perforators for sufficient flap perfusion. At this point, after finalization of the abdominal flap mobilization, in cases of concomitant rectus diastasis, the plication of the anterior rectus fascia from the xiphoid to the symphysis is accomplished using nonabsorbable or absorbable suture material using any preferred technique. In cases of lower abdominal diastasis, the Scarpa fascia and underlying tissue may be bluntly mobilized to allow for further midline fascial plication. For cases of an asymmetrically located umbilical stalk or for further accentuation of waist tightening with further waist tightening, an additional paramedian plication of the anterior rectus sheath may be facilitated. Because lateral dissection is avoided up to the costal arch for preservation of the lateral perforators, a discontinuous separation of lateral adhesions using the Lockwood underminer may enable further flap mobilization.

During tissue resection, bullet forceps or a Pitanguy tissue demarcator can support the estimation of the upper resection line. Further evaluation of the amount of resection may be facilitated by additional vertical flap incisions and temporary wound closure using bullet forceps. The upper incision line is then marked, and the resection is performed oblique to the wound edge in a 45° angle to enable a more precise adaptation of varyingly thick layers. In selected patients with a pronounced abdominal fat layer, the fatty tissue beneath the Scarpa fascia should be resected in the entire mobilized area. This action may avoid postoperative complications caused by superinfected fat necrosis. In general it is safely practicable to excise the subscarpal fat plane from the abdominal flap, especially in the midline region, for abdominal contour accentuation. After meticulous coagulation, the wound is closed temporarily. The new umbilical position is estimated and marked. Several umbilical incision patterns have been described; the authors prefer the superior based inverted V or U incision. This umbilical section of the abdominal flap is then circumferentially defatted for a circular umbilical depression. After repeated meticulous hemostasis, the Scarpa fascia is sutured down to the anterior rectus fascia with absorbable progressive tension sutures (Baroudi stitches), starting superior to the umbilicus. Alternatively, the supraumbilical subcutaneous tissue may be sutured in the midline to the anterior rectus fascia to accentuate a midline depression for superior aesthetics. After the umbilical stalk is pulled through the new umbilical tunnel, additional progressive tension sutures are placed in the lower flap area.

The patient is then bent into the beach-chair position, and temporary wound closure is performed with bullet forceps starting laterally to medial. In patients with massive weight loss and extensive circular tissue excess in the thigh region, the authors recommend maximal shift of the entire tissue medially. This tissue excess can be pleated at the medial aspect of the proximal thigh and removed at the time of the inner thigh lift.

After the placement of 2 to 3 drains in the abdominal region, the final wound closure is performed for all layers as described. Again, for time reduction in wound closure the use of absorbable barbed sutures and a 2-component skin closure system is routinely advisable.[17] After a final antiseptic wound cleaning, Steri strips are applied as described earlier. These supportive dressings should remain for 3 weeks postoperatively. Finally, a sterile wound dressing and an adjustable compression girdle are applied.

Mons Pubis Reconstruction

Primarily female patients ask for a reconstruction of the mons pubis region. A tissue surplus in this region can be maximally reduced by aligning the lower incision line at 6 cm above the vulvar commissure. In severe cases, a central wedge excision can be performed to reduce the surplus horizontal tissue.

Adjuvant Liposuction

Adipose tissue surplus in the back or upper flank region, which may be detected superior to the resulting scar line, can be reduced by liposuction after wound closure. This adjuvant procedure allows improvements of the gluteal and overall body contour from different perspectives.

Male "Love Handles"

Male patients frequently present with local adipose tissue in the posterior flank region, which may be reduced by liposuction after gluteal wound closure or superiorly, excised in toto during posterior preparation. The authors recommend cautious hemostasis of this localized fat pad during extirpation, because blood supply is ensured by 2 to 3 perforating vessels.[10]

POTENTIAL COMPLICATIONS AND MANAGEMENT

General symptoms after lower body lift procedures include postoperative pain or soreness, numbness of the skin flaps, bruising, general fatigue, and discomfort resulting from increased skin tension for a few weeks postoperatively.

Local complications in all regions include hematoma, seroma, wound infection, fat necrosis, wound dehiscence, paresthesias, and persisting numbness. Seromas are a very common problem in the abdominal region, usually treated with serial punctures and drainage. Persistent seromas may require a secondary surgical procedure. In general, seromas should be detected in time and treated by simple aspiration to avoid a superinfection or any consequent wound separation.

Minor wound dehiscences are common and mostly self-limiting. In the intergluteal cleft region, patients frequently have to deal with wound-healing disorders and their consequent conservative treatments. Wound closure in this specific region is strengthened with nonresorbable simple interrupted sutures to avoid wound separation caused by shearing forces. Because of the use of resorbable sutures for wound closure, the authors regularly see single or multiple local wound-healing disorders throughout the entire wound; however, these occur more often in the gluteal region. Because tension in this region cannot be reduced as sufficiently as in the abdominal region, a consequent wound separation in this area is of higher risk. To improve wound healing, the authors routinely perform wound closure in an everting manner, which reduces wound-healing disorders through reduced interference by suture material on the skin level.

Significant dehiscences may be caused by increased tension or wound-edge necrosis. Appropriate treatment of wound necrosis is initial conservative wound care, until the area of necrosis has demarcated for surgical revision. Additional flap advancement may allow optimal secondary wound closure. Any impairment of the umbilical perfusion should be treated conservatively, as long as the umbilical stalk is adapted on the skin level. Further local complications include dog-ears, hypertrophic or malpositioned scars, and, in the abdominal region, cosmetic problems related to the umbilicus. Most of these issues can be avoided with good preoperative planning and attention to surgical detail. Treatment by liposuction may lead to postoperative contour irregularities and dermal tethering, and further excessive swelling may occur in cases of circular liposuction of the extremities.

Systemic complications include deep vein thrombosis, pulmonary embolism, fat embolism, respiratory compromise resulting from increased intra-abdominal pressure in abdominal cases with fascial tightening, and systemic infections including toxic shock syndrome. All of these complications may be potentially lethal. In general, abdominal tightening procedures have a higher systemic complication rate than any other type of routine cosmetic surgical procedure.[9,10,12,13,19,20]

Unilateral or bilateral soft-tissue relaxation or rupture of the reconstructive gluteal sutures may be revised by a secondary procedure, alternatively with the use of a mesh for tissue support. In cases of general fascial deficiency, a future option may be to apply a mesh support during primary gluteal autoaugmentation.

POSTOPERATIVE CARE

Every patient with a lower body lift procedure receives a single-shot antibiotic therapy intraoperatively; in few cases with preexisting risk factors, the antibiotic therapy may be extended to 5 days. For safety reasons, patients with lower body lift are monitored the initial 24 hours postoperatively on an intensive or intermediate care unit. To ensure an optimal tissue perfusion and appropriate microcirculation, 2500 mL/24 h of Ringer solution is provided during the initial 48 hours postoperatively. Dressings during this period include compression girdles surrounding fluid-collecting compresses. Furthermore, laboratory checks for electrolytes and hemoglobin are performed multiple times during the initial 48 hours and urinary output is monitored. Patients are positioned in the beach-chair position, if available on a soft mattress, with electronically adjustable positions. Low molecular weight heparin and compression stockings are administered for thrombosis prophylaxis. Immediately postoperatively, patients are instructed to move their feet consistently without crossing the legs, followed by early mobilization on the first postoperative day and instructions to obtain deep-breathing exercises for prevention from pneumonia. All patients receive pain treatment during the initial 48 hours using an individualized patient-controlled analgesia pump. Drains are removed with drainage less than 30 mL per 24 hours. The urinary catheter is removed after 2 to 3 days postoperatively.

In cases of reimbursement by a statutory or private health insurance, the average duration of hospitalization after lower body lift in the authors' institution is 6 days. If the procedure is privately financed by the patient, the hospital stay is included in the total costs and lasts 3 to 4 days on average. This time is generally required for full mobilization of the patient and removal of all drains. The immediately postoperative compression therapy is intended to reduce shearing forces for support of the adhesion between different reconstructed tissue layers. In this context, drains are left in place for a minimum of 4 days postoperatively in terms of negative intracavitary pressure. Before patients are discharged, a compression garment is individually adapted for 8 weeks postoperatively.

For reduction of superficial wound tension, Steri strips are applied perpendicularly on the wound for the initial 3 weeks postoperatively. Any suture or wound-closure material is removed at latest 3 weeks postoperatively. For at least 3 months postoperatively, patients are advised to cover all scars with silicon sheets or apply various available scar-reducing skin lotions for improved scar formation.[9,12]

Sporting activities should be omitted for 8 weeks postoperatively. Patients should be advised to avoid saunas and tanning beds.

OUTCOMES

In male patients the postoperative results regarding scar course and appearance in addition to body contour enhancement are usually promising, with stable results continuing for years. Salient points are a very low scar course from the anterior and posterior view, a maximal reduction of the abdominal tissue surplus, favorably avoiding the vertical midline scar from fleur-de-lis, and a maximal reduction of the localized adipose tissue of the lateral and posterior flank region ("love handles"). Thus, in patients after massive weight loss the vertical midline scar may not be

avoidable. In general the authors have observed a stronger skin quality in male patients after weight loss, with a lower rate of secondary relaxation, probably because the rate of patients with conservative weight reduction is higher in the male population (Dirk F. Richter, Unpublished data, 2014).

Female patients, especially after weight loss, have their main focus on the improvement of the abdominal region including the mons pubis. In this regard, the authors have observed high patient satisfaction after fleur-de-lis tightening of the abdominal region, because this procedure enables a tissue reduction to a maximal amount. Because the subcutaneous fat tissue layer in the central upper abdomen is completely excised, the remaining abdominal subcutaneous tissue is maximally thinned out, with consequent maximal aesthetic improvement of the abdominal and waist contour. To avoid a tissue mismatch of the mons pubis region in relation to abdomen, a sufficient reduction is advisable by either liposuction, direct excision, or a wedge excision pattern. The second main focus of female patients is on gluteal reshaping. Because every patient presents with different preoperative conditions, an individual therapy has to be selected. As most patients present with sufficient gluteal fat tissue, the reconstruction by transpositioning of the tissues enables a stable reshaping of the buttocks (**Figs. 5–10**).

Maximal Point of Gluteal Projection

During the first postoperative weeks, patients usually present with a maximal gluteal projection at the upper third of the buttocks. This intentional overcorrection of gluteal projection at this height will be compromised during the first 6 to 8 weeks postoperatively. A surplus of adipose tissue in the area of the lateral and dorsal thigh region may negatively affect the gluteal contour, because any additional downward traction may impair the gluteal projection. Therefore, the authors recommend an extensive reduction of this specific redundant adipose tissue through liposuction as a staged procedure before or during the gluteal procedure. The harvested fat tissue may be prepared and used for additional micrografting in the gluteal region.

Scar Appearance

The authors favor an arch-shaped scar course, which commences at the superior end of the intergluteal cleft and proceeds to the upper lateral gluteal border. The central back region is characterized by a strong midline zone of adherence, which consequently disables any significant skin and soft-tissue sagging. This aspect must be

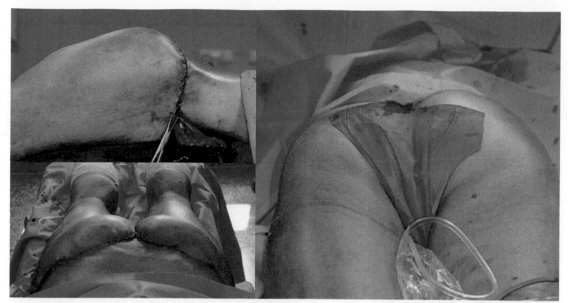

Fig. 5. Intraoperative view of the transposition-gluteoplasty from right lateral and superior view. Demonstration of the overcorrection with maximal projection at the upper third (*left*). Difference in projection after finalization of the right side (*right*). (*From* Richter DF, Stoff A, Velasco FJ, et al. Circumferential lower truncal dermatolipectomy. Clin Plast Surg 2008;35:(1):67; with permission from Elsevier Saunders.)

taken into account, because a more superior scar ending in the dorsal midline may result in a prolonged intergluteal cleft with aesthetic limitations. Furthermore, the arch-shaped scar course accentuates a round-shaped buttock and respects the borders of the gluteal aesthetic unit.

Transition Vectors

Owing to a larger body circumference at the height of the inferior compared with the superior incision line, more tissue has to be moved medially in the lower gluteal area. This fact becomes more apparent when a fleur-de-lis abdominoplasty is

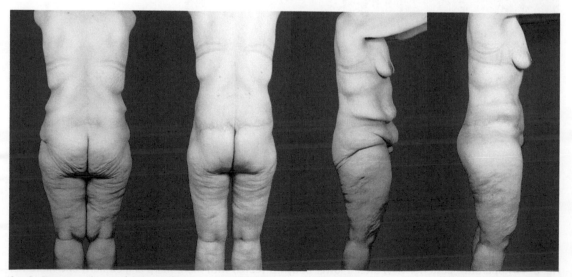

Fig. 6. Preoperative and 24-month postoperative posterior (*left*) and right lateral views (*right*) of a 34-year-old patient after lower body lift (circumferential lower truncal dermatolipectomy [CLTD]). The gluteal reconstruction presents with a stable projection at the upper middle third of the buttock. Her weight at the time of surgery was 85 kg, she lost 90 kg through gastric bypass, and her weight 24 months postoperatively was stable at 84 kg. The weight of tissue resection was 2255 g.

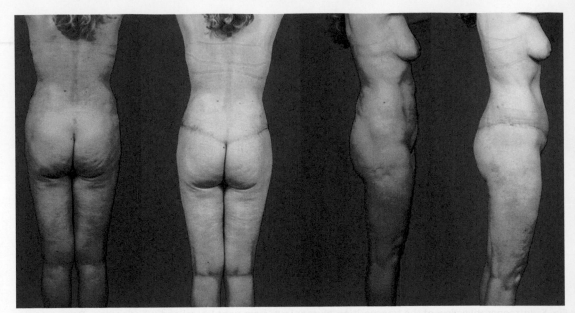

Fig. 7. A 55-year-old patient after multiple liposuction procedures at the gluteal and thigh regions. Preoperative and 4-month postoperative posterior (*left*) and right lateral views (*right*) after lower body lift procedure with sufficient gluteal enhancement. Note the ideal scar course with consequent round-shaped buttocks. Her weight at the time of surgery and 4 months postoperatively was 58 kg. The weight of resected tissue was 620 g.

performed in the anterior part with reduction of the superior circumference. For this reason, the authors symmetrically mark 3 vectors per side, which enables a medial transposition of the lower gluteal tissue with tissue accumulation at the medial buttock, which may further accentuate the gluteal projection.[9,12] This maneuver may induce a slender waist and improve the entire gluteal shape. In cases of extensive tissue surplus in the lateral and anterior thigh region, the authors recommend shifting the entire skin and soft-tissue envelope medially, resulting in skin congestion in the medial

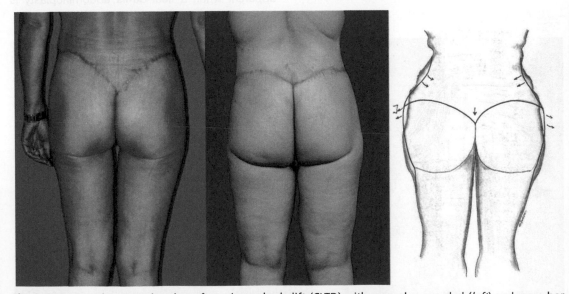

Fig. 8. Postoperative posterior view after a lower body lift (CLTD) with more sharp-angled (*left*) and more horizontal scar course (*middle*). The sharp-angled scar course gives the buttock a more rounded shape without elongation of the intergluteal cleft, whereas the more superior and more horizontal scar course may lead to an unaesthetic prolonged intergluteal cleft with a more square-shaped buttock. (*Right*) Schematic demonstration of contouring effects by optimal scar positioning. (*From* Richter DF, Stoff A, Velasco FJ, et al. Circumferential lower truncal dermato-lipectomy. Clin Plast Surg 2008;35:(1):60; with permission from Elsevier Saunders.)

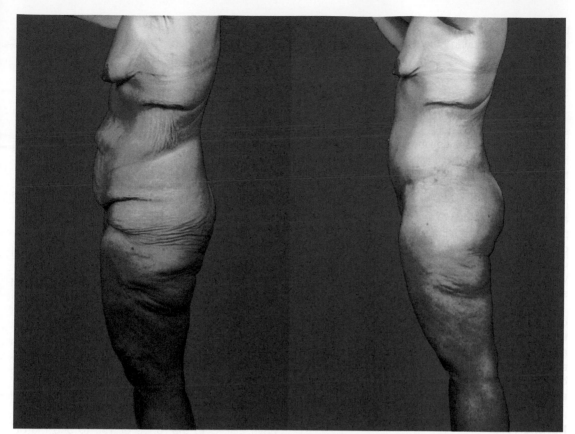

Fig. 9. Preoperative left lateral (*left*) and 18 months postoperative left lateral view (*right*) of a 39-year-old patient after lower body lift (CLTD) and simultaneous liposuction in the adjoining regions of the dorsum for optimal contour improvement and accentuation of the waist/buttock transition. Her weight at the time of surgery was 74 kg, she lost 66 kg through gastric bypass, and her weight 18 months postoperatively was stable at 72 kg. The weight of tissue resection was 2364 g.

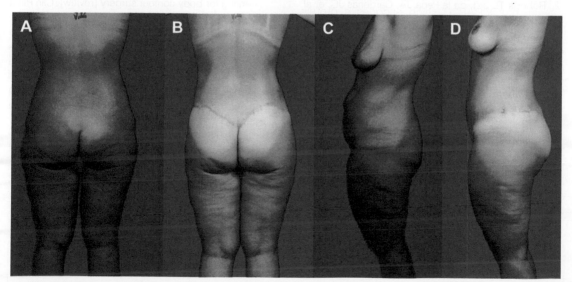

Fig. 10. Preoperative (*A, C*), and 14 months postoperative (*B, D*) posterior and left lateral view of a 36-year-old patient after a lower body lift (CLTD) and mammoplasty. Besides the circumferential tightening, the transposition-gluteoplasty apparently improved the gluteal contour and projection with a stable result after 14 months. Her weight at the time of surgery was 60 kg, she lost 53 kg through diet and sport, and her weight 14 months postoperatively was stable at 57 kg. The weight of tissue resection was 1323 g.

thigh and groin region. This tissue surplus may then be excised during the second stage of inner thigh lift.

SUMMARY

The lower body lift (CLTD) presents an extremely effective procedure for body rejuvenation and body contouring. Besides the advantages and enhancements attainable in the abdominal region, the overall body and gluteal shape can be significantly improved. The gluteal autoaugmentaton (transposition-gluteoplasty) presents an effective and reliable method for gluteal augmentation in terms of transpositioning of the subfascial lateral gluteal, lateral thigh, and hip adipose tissue. It can be integrated into every body lift procedure, without any inconsiderable amount of time extension or additional expenditure.

If clinical routine is ensured, the lower body lift can be safely performed with reduced operating time and, consequently, fewer complications, in addition to high patient satisfaction and optimized aesthetic outcome. However, these expectations depend on the patient's preoperative conditions and tissue characteristics.

REFERENCES

1. Roberts TL 3rd, Weinfeld AB, Bruner TW, et al. Universal and ethnic ideals of beautiful buttocks are best obtained by autologous micro fat grafting and liposuction. Clin Plast Surg 2006;33(3):371–94.
2. Roberts TL 3rd, de la Pena JA, Cardenas JC, et al. Cosmetic surgery of the buttocks region. Aesthet Surg J 2003;23(5):381–7.
3. Lockwood TE. Superficial fascial system (SFS) of the trunk and extremities: a new concept. Plast Reconstr Surg 1991;87(6):1009–18.
4. Lockwood TE. Lower body lift with superficial fascial system suspension. Plast Reconstr Surg 1993;92(6): 1112–22.
5. Lockwood TE. The role of excisional lifting in body contour surgery. Clin Plast Surg 1996;23(4):695–712.
6. Lockwood TE. Maximizing aesthetics in lateral-tension abdominoplasty and body lifts. Clin Plast Surg 2004;31(4):523–37.
7. Sozer SO, Agullo FJ, Wolf C. Autoprosthesis buttock augmentation during lower body lift. Aesthetic Plast Surg 2005;29:133–7 [discussion: 138–40].
8. Sozer SO, Agullo FJ, Palladino H. Split gluteal muscle flap for autoprosthesis buttock augmentation. Plast Reconstr Surg 2012;129(3):766–76.
9. Richter DF, Stoff A. Liposuction and circumferential lower truncal dermatolipectomy. In: Rubin P, Jewell M, Richter DF, et al, editors. Body contouring and liposuction. 1st edition. St Louis (MO): Elsevier, Saunders; 2012. p. 385–402.
10. Stoff A, Richter DF. Abdominoplasty and body contouring. In: Farhadieh R, Bulstrode N, Cugno S, editors. Plastic and reconstructive surgery. United Kingdom: Wiley; 2014.
11. Song AY, Jean RD, Hurwitz DJ, et al. A classification of contour deformities after bariatric weight loss: the Pittsburgh rating scale. Plast Reconstr Surg 2006; 116(5):1535–44.
12. Richter DF, Stoff A, Velasco FJ, et al. Circumferential lower truncal dermato-lipectomy. Clin Plast Surg 2008;35(1):53–71.
13. Hunstad JP, Repta R. Atlas of abdominoplasty. Philadelphia: Saunders Elsevier; 2009.
14. Orpheu SC, Coltro PS, Scopel GP, et al. Collagen and elastic content of abdominal skin after surgical weight loss. Obes Surg 2010;20(4):480–6.
15. Krueger JK, Rohrich RJ. Clearing the smoke: the scientific rationale for tobacco abstention with plastic surgery [review]. Plast Reconstr Surg 2001;108(4): 1063–73 [discussion: 1074–7].
16. Rubin JP, Nguyen V, Schwentker A. Perioperative management of the post-gastric-bypass patient presenting for body contour surgery [review]. Clin Plast Surg 2004;31(4):601–10, vi.
17. Richter DF, Stoff A, Blondeel PN, et al. A comparison of a new skin closure device and intradermal sutures in the closure of full thickness surgical incisions. Plast Reconstr Surg 2012;130(4):843–50.
18. Richter DF, Stoff A. The Scarpa lift - a novel technique for minimal invasive medial thigh lifts. Obes Surg 2011;21(12):1975–80.
19. Richter DF, Stoff A. Abdominoplasty procedures. In: Neligan P, editor. Plastic surgery. 3rd edition. Philadelphia: Elsevier, Saunders; 2012. p. 530–58.
20. Aly AS. Body contouring after massive weight loss. St Louis (MO): Quality Medical Publishing; 2006.

Noninvasive and Minimally Invasive Techniques in Body Contouring

Paul N. Afrooz, MD[a], Jason N. Pozner, MD[d],
Barry E. DiBernardo, MD[b,c],*

KEYWORDS

- Body contouring • MInimally invasive • Noninvasive

KEY POINTS

- The strong patient demand for safer, less invasive body contouring procedures will inevitably drive technology toward more effective modalities that minimize downtime and recovery, while improving results.
- The future of body contouring will likely stratify patients into more distinct categories, such as those requiring aggressive surgical excision, minimally invasive liposuction techniques with adjunctive energy-delivering modalities or mesotherapy, and noninvasive techniques achieving volume reduction and skin tightening through additional energy-delivering modalities.
- Currently, the most ideal candidates for these types of procedures are those who are accepting of a mild to moderate result.

MINIMALLY INVASIVE MODALITIES
Introduction

Surgical body contouring procedures have several inherent drawbacks, including hospitalization, anesthetic use, pain, swelling, and prolonged recovery. It is for these reasons that body contouring through noninvasive means has become one of the most alluring areas in aesthetic surgery. Patient expectations and demands have driven the field toward safer, less-invasive procedures with less discomfort, fewer side effects, and a shorter recovery.

The future of body contouring will most likely involve completely noninvasive procedures for mild cases, minimally invasive procedures for moderate cases, and invasive procedures reserved for massive weight loss and larger patients.

In this article the current minimally invasive and noninvasive modalities for body contouring are reviewed.

ADJUNCTIVE MODALITIES IN LIPOSUCTION

After the modern reinvention of liposuction more than 30 years ago, liposuction was performed as an inpatient procedure, often requiring blood transfusion postoperatively.[1] The introduction of the tumescent technique has significantly optimized the outcomes and safety profile of liposuction procedures and has subsequently become the gold standard in body contouring procedures.[1–6] Furthermore, refinement of body site-specific cannulas and the use of manual syringe suction for autologous transfer and fine contouring have optimized liposuction techniques and improved outcomes.[3] Adjunctive energy-delivering modalities, such as laser-assisted liposuction (LAL) and ultrasound-assisted liposuction (UAL), have shown promise in facilitating fat removal, reducing procedure duration, surgeon strain, patient recovery time, and postoperative pain.[1–3,6]

[a] Department of Plastic Surgery, University of Pittsburgh Medical Center, Pittsburgh, PA 15213, USA; [b] Department of Surgery, Division of Plastic Surgery, University of Medicine and Dentistry of New Jersey, Newark, New Jersey; [c] New Jersey Plastic Surgery, Montclair, New Jersey; [d] Cleveland Clinic Florida, Department of Plastic Surgery, Weston, Florida
* Corresponding author.
E-mail address: BerdMd@verizon.net

Clin Plastic Surg 41 (2014) 789–804
http://dx.doi.org/10.1016/j.cps.2014.07.006
0094-1298/14/$ – see front matter © 2014 Elsevier Inc. All rights reserved.

Laser-Assisted Liposuction (LAL)

LAL uses a small fiber (300 to 1000 μm) delivered through a narrow cannula of approximately 1 mm to deliver energy to tissues. The distinct advance in laser delivery has allowed for the delivery of laser energy under, rather than through, the skin. This approach allows more energy to be placed directly at the target instead of passing through epidermis and dermis, with simultaneous cooling mechanisms for protection of the surface from intense heat. With the safety mechanism defined and delineated, the advantage of the laser is the proven efficacy in skin tightening. An additional advantage of LAL is the ability to treat scarring, dimpling, and cellulite in the superficial layers with the small cannula. This small cannula reduces the risk of contour irregularities seen with larger cannulas. Some disadvantages include the higher cost of equipment, the need for precise temperature measurement, and the potential for burns or blisters without this monitoring. Previous disadvantages were related to duration of the procedure; however, as technology progresses, additional wavelengths have been proven to be 40 times more efficient in fat disruption while maintaining similar cannula size.

Preoperative preparation

Patients are evaluated for potential fat reduction and skin laxity improvement. When treating specific areas, these areas of adiposity are marked in a standard fashion, in addition to 5 × 5 cm squares representing the areas of skin laxity targeted for energy application. Approximately 50 to 100 mL of tumescent fluid is administered per 5 × 5 cm sector (**Fig. 1**). This procedure is routinely performed with oral and local anesthesia only, but may be supplemented with intravenous (IV) sedation, epidural block, or general anesthesia.[1,7]

It is essential to manage patient expectations during the initial consultation. Patients must understand that the skin tightening effect hinges on several variables, including age, genetics, and skin condition from environmental factors, such as smoking and sun exposure.

Surgical technique

The laser system (Triplex; Cynosure, Westford, MA, USA) allows individual as well as sequential emission of 1064-nm, 1320-nm, and 1440-nm wavelengths. Energy is delivered to the subdermal tissue through a 600-μm or 1000-μm fiber threaded through a 1-mm microcannula that extends 2 to 3 mm beyond the distal end of the microcannula. When the microcannula is inserted into the tissue, the laser is activated and the microcannula is moved slowly and evenly through the deep fat layer with a 1064-nm to 1440-nm combination, or the superficial subdermal layer with a 1064-nm to 1320-nm combination (**Fig. 2**). For ideal absorption and performance, wavelength combinations are used for preferential target affinity of fat and water, respectively.

Using the biplanar technique, adipose cells are disrupted, resulting in a more liquefied material that can be removed through a smaller cannula. This smaller cannula refines the removal, particularly close to the surface, thereby reducing potential contour irregularity that can be seen with larger instrumentation. To achieve increased skin elasticity and tightening, surface temperature goals of 40°C to 42°C superficially, and deep temperature goals of 45°C to 47°C are delineated. The lower temperature goal is used for darker skin colors.

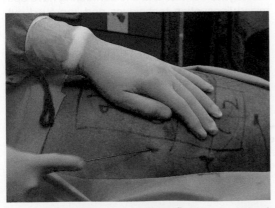

Fig. 1. Application of tumescent fluid 50 to 100 mL per sector.

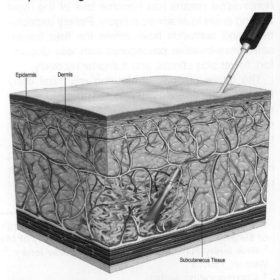

Fig. 2. Diagrammatic representation of placement of deep laser energy for adipocyte and fibrous disruption.

Achieving and maintaining these temperature goals uniformly is essential to achieving optimal efficacy.

Safe energy delivery is monitored via an accelerometer delivery system (Smart Sense; Cynosure) attached to the laser handpiece, used to minimize the occurrence of localized thermal damage during treatment. The handpiece contains a motion-sensing feedback chip that provides constant information of cannula movement to the laser device. Slower movement of the handpiece triggers a reduction in laser power. If the handpiece stops, energy delivery ceases within 0.2 seconds. This safety feature prevents excess accumulation of energy in a given area.[1] Temperature safety is measured with a thermastore probe at the tip of the cannula, which is set for a safe range according to the above-mentioned parameters. When the threshold is reached, the laser automatically stops firing.[7]

A 2-layer/2-step technique is used in which the deep fat layers (1–3 cm below the epidermis) within the premarked squares are treated first (see **Fig. 2**). Insertion of the microcannula is facilitated with the use of 1-mm incisions made with a number 11 blade for appropriate access to the treatment area. The superficial subdermal layer (0.5 cm below the epidermis) is treated in the second step of the 2-layer technique (**Fig. 3**). Aspiration is performed with a standard 3-mm suction cannula to remove any remaining fat, disrupted cells, and free fat oils.[7] Clinical examples are shown in **Figs. 4–6**.

Optimization of this procedure hinges on proper delivery of energy while maintaining an appropriate safety margin. Inadequate tightening can often be the result of insufficient temperature attainment necessary to achieve the desired

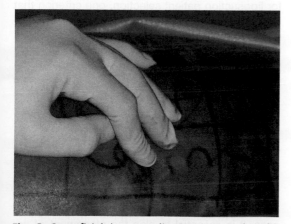

Fig. 3. Superficial laser application just under the dermis, with visualization of helium neon guiding beam.

effect. Too much energy applied in one area can result in excessive heat build-up and fat necrosis. If too much heat is applied superficially, the result will be skin blistering, burns, or pigmentation changes. If used properly, the built-in safety mechanisms will help control temperature and avoid harmful buildup of heat.[7]

Postoperative care

Firm pressure dressings are applied to the wounds on completion of the aspiration, and compression garments are worn for 3 to 4 weeks postoperatively. Dependent incisions are left open for drainage, and oral antibiotic prophylaxis is administered.[1,7,8]

Skin and tissue firmness is examined 1 week postoperatively. Excessive swelling or dense edema is treated with the use of the Triactive Device (Cynosure) or equivalent massage, edema reduction, and lymphatic drainage enhancement for 3 weeks postoperatively. Patients are reminded of the time necessary for skin changes to occur during the dynamic fibroblast stimulation period (90 days). If further enhancement of skin is desired after 3 months, acceptable external skin devices can be applied, and additional treatments in adjacent areas can be performed after tissue effects have subsided.[7]

Complications and management

Complications of LAL include blisters, end hits, burns, blowholes, prolonged edema, heat/pressure problems, neurapraxia, permanent nerve damage, contour irregularity, minor asymmetries, and insufficient effect.[1,8] If performed properly, the occurrence of these complications is rare.

Summary

Previous work has led to an improvement in the safety and an enhancement of the cosmetic results of LAL. By reducing blood loss, minimizing complications, and promoting skin tightening, LAL has proven to be a safe and effective body contouring procedure in appropriate candidates. Future applications of fiber-deliverable energy will aim to address the superficial irregularities of the skin, such as dimpling, scars, and cellulite.[1,7,9]

Ultrasound-Assisted Liposuction (UAL)

Ultrasonic energy was first applied to body contouring surgery in the late 1980s by Scuderi and coworkers[10] and later popularized by Zocchi,[11] who introduced the technique to the United States in 1993. The third-generation VASER system (Sound Surgical Technologies, Louisville, CO, USA) was introduced in 2001 and is currently the most commonly used UAL technology.[12–14]

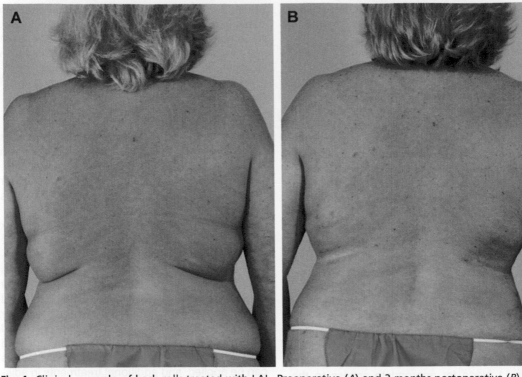

Fig. 4. Clinical example of back rolls treated with LAL. Preoperative (*A*) and 3 months postoperative (*B*).

Ultrasound interacts with tissue by 3 basic mechanisms: thermal, mechanical, and cavitation.[7,12,15–18] The thermal effect is initiated by the heat generated from the rapidly vibrating ultrasonic probe.[19] The mechanical effect is created when the rapidly vibrating tip of the ultrasonic probe contacts tissue.[20] Cavitation is the tissue interaction most responsible for causing fat emulsification with current UAL devices. When the wetting solution is dispersed within the tissues, small microbubbles are lodged within the fat tissue matrix, which then implode and collapse with the application of ultrasound. This process separates fat cells within the fat tissue matrix, which subsequently mix with the tumescent solution by means of acoustic streaming to create an emulsion. This emulsion is subsequently harvested by means of a suction cannula.[7,12,16–18]

Preoperative preparation

Even though UAL has expanded the parameters for liposuction patient selection, one criterion that remains unchanged is the patient's candidacy to undergo an elective surgical procedure. Once this has been established, preoperative preparation may proceed.

Preoperative markings are performed in the standing position. There are 5 distinct anatomic areas that should be avoided in patients undergoing UAL. These areas, termed the "zones of adherence," include the gluteal crease, the lower lateral thigh area of the iliotibial tract, posterior distal thigh above the popliteal crease, midmedial thigh area, and lateral gluteal depression area. Violation of these areas often leads to iatrogenic contour deformities. During the preoperative marking process, it is essential to plan the placement of access incisions carefully. UAL requires a greater number of slightly longer access incisions to

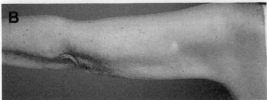

Fig. 5. Clinical example of brachial fat removal and skin tightening from laser. Preoperative (*A*) and 3 months postoperative (*B*).

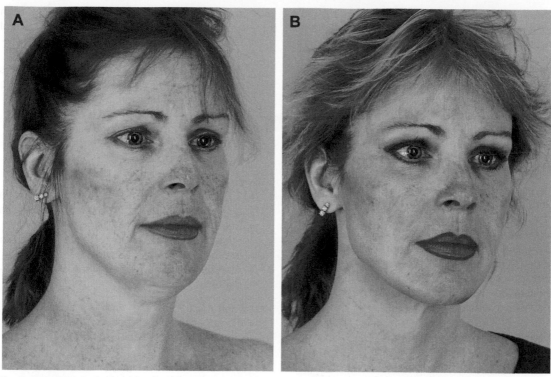

Fig. 6. (*A, B*) Clinical example of neck treatment with LAL in a 48-year-old patient, 3 months postoperative. Note slight muscle bands evident.

accommodate the skin protectors and to avoid placing torque on the ultrasonic probe over curved anatomic areas.[12]

VASER probe selection must consider the characteristics of localized fat in the region to be treated. The characteristics of fat cells in different regions of the body differ with respect to collagen structure and septi among the fat cells, as described by de Souza Pinto and colleagues.[18] Knowledge of these differences is essential for probe selection to achieve optimal outcomes.

Penetration of tissue is influenced by probe diameter and the number of grooves at the tip. For a probe of a given diameter, more grooves emulsify fat tissue more efficiently. However, they do not penetrate fibrous tissues easily because of vibratory energy that is transferred to the sides of the probe as opposed to the front surface. Fibrous tissues are better addressed with probes with fewer grooves. Smaller-diameter probes also penetrate fibrous tissue more easily. The 3.7-mm probes achieve rapid debulking and contouring of medium to large volumes of soft to fibrous tissues. The number of grooves at the tip of the probe will vary according to the fibrous nature of the anatomic area. For treating smaller, soft to extremely fibrous localized fat deposits in sensitive areas, fine contouring is achieved with 2.9-mm probes.[18]

In general, continuous mode should be used for fibrous tissue, faster fragmentation, and times when tissue emulsification is not readily achieved in VASER mode. VASER mode is more suited for delicate work, finer sculpting, or softer tissues. The device must be adjusted such that the probe moves smoothly through tissue.[18]

Experience and practice have delineated application times. In general, 1 minute of application time may be used per 100 mL of infused solution in VASER or continuous mode. Loss of resistance to probe movement in all intended areas can be considered the surgical endpoint. Following emulsification, aspiration can be performed with suction-assisted or power-assisted liposuction.[18]

Surgical technique

The prone position provides good access to the back, flanks, lateral thighs, and superior posterior thighs. General endotracheal anesthesia is preferred for patients requiring prone positioning and for large volume aspirations. Many surgeons also prefer the lateral decubitus position, which requires one additional patient repositioning. Despite additional repositioning, some authors maintain that the lateral decubitus position offers better access with less trauma and is particularly helpful for evacuating large volumes from the flanks and back with the goal of creating more aesthetic waistlines. Supine positioning offers access to the abdomen, anterior and medial thighs, knees, calves, arms ankles, breasts, and face.[12]

Maintaining core body temperature is best accomplished by running IV fluids through a fluid warmer in addition to the use of forced warm air by means of a Bair Hugger (Arizent Inc, Eden Paris, MN, USA). The access incisions are placed in previously marked areas using a number 11 blade and must be long enough to accommodate the fluid-infiltrating cannula. The rate of flow is controlled on the infusion pump according to the anatomic area. Generally, a wetting solution is prepared with 1 mL of epinephrine added to 1 L Ringer's lactate at room temperature (1:1,000,000 dilution).[12] In cases not using general anesthesia, lidocaine may be added to the wetting solution. The dose of lidocaine should not exceed 35 mg/kg, although some authors routinely use doses exceeding 50 mg/kg while maintaining a safety margin.[21]

Treatment recommendations
Posterior trunk
- 3.7-mm 2-ring probe at 80% energy level in continuous mode for most of the back[12]
- 3.7-mm one-ring probe at 80% energy level in continuous mode for tight fibrous back rolls
- Posterior trunk areas require slightly longer ultrasound application, usually between 12 and 14 minutes on average
- Aspiration is accomplished with a small-diameter cannula

Abdomen
- 3.7-mm 3-ring ultrasonic probe is used at an energy setting of 80% in VASER mode
- Continuous mode is used for the area above the costal margin
- Average ultrasound time is 8 to 9 minutes
- Aspiration is accomplished with a small-diameter cannula

Extremities and buttocks
- 3.7-mm 3-ring ultrasonic probe is used at an energy setting of 70% in VASER mode for the superior medial thigh
- Around the knees and superior posterior thigh, a short 3-mm 3-ring probe is used in 80% VASER mode
- Depending on how fibrous the subcutaneous layer may be, the anterior and lateral thigh areas are also performed with the 3.7-mm 3-ring probe in 80% VASER or continuous mode
- Average ultrasound time is approximately 3 minutes for both knees, 5 minutes for both

superior medial thighs, 8 minutes for both anterior thighs, 6 to 7 minutes for both lateral thighs, and 4 minutes for both superior posterior thighs
- For the axillary area, a 3-mm, 3-ring probe is inserted into the subcutaneous space through a small access incision in the axillary fold
- The energy setting is 70% VASER mode, applied for approximately 2 minutes per arm
- Aspiration is performed through a small-diameter cannula

Gynecomastia
- 3.7-mm one-ring probe or the gynecomastia arrow probe can be used efficiently in this area
- Energy levels are set at 80% to 90% at continuous mode at an average of 3 to 4 minutes per breast
- Aspiration is performed through a small-diameter cannula

Face and neck
- Three access incisions are recommended: one behind each earlobe and one in the submental crease
- Smaller-diameter, highly precise instrumentation is used for facial UAL
- Ultrasound is applied by a 2.4-mm 3-ring ultrasonic probe at 50% to 60% energy levels in VASER mode for approximately 2 to 3 minutes
- Aspiration is performed with a fine cannula

HIV-associated cervicodorsal lipodystrophy
- 3.7-mm one- or 2-ring probe is used depending on the fibrous nature of the area
- The energy setting is 80% continuous mode and the time will vary according to the volume of fat being treated
- Aspiration is performed with a fine cannula

Optimizing outcomes
- Apply the least amount of ultrasound energy necessary to obtain fat emulsification
- The clinical endpoint of ultrasound application is loss of tissue resistance against the probe
- Incision placement must be planned appropriately to facilitate access to the treatment area while avoiding torque on the ultrasonic probe
- Small-diameter cannulae provide the greatest precision, particularly in the aspiration of superficial fat
- Liberal use of wetting solution dispersed evenly through the fat maximizes efficiency of ultrasonic cavitation, minimizes blood loss, and provides added protection against thermal effects of UAL

- Circumferential contouring provides a more harmonious result than local fat extraction
- Postoperative use of foam compression garments, lymphatic drainage massage, and skin-moisturizing regimens can optimize UAL outcomes and decrease recovery times

Postoperative care

Following large-volume UAL procedures, close monitoring of fluid replacement and urine output is required. Postoperatively, most patients with large volume aspirations continue to leak fluid through the incisions for 24 to 36 hours. A significant volume of the infiltrating solution does get absorbed during the first 12 hours following major UAL and this must be considered when planning fluid replacement. Oral intake of fluids is permitted on waking. Early ambulation is encouraged, and patients are discharged on the first postoperative day. Foam and compression garments can be applied to most UAL patients in the immediate postoperative period. Lymphatic drainage and skin moisturizing regimens are helpful as soon as the patient can tolerate them.[12]

Complications and management

The most common complications of liposuction procedures are under-extraction, over-extraction, or irregular contour. In general, these complications are prevented by the use of intraoperative flow sheets documenting infusion and aspiration volumes for each anatomic area. Under-extraction is usually corrected by revisionary extraction, whereas overcorrection may require fat grafting. Paresthesias, edema, and ecchymosis are usually self-limiting. The vibrating ultrasonic probe generates heat, which could lead to thermal injury, particularly around the incision site. The use of skin protectors is essential, along with the use of a wet towel adjacent to the incision to provide added protection. The most important factor in preventing skin burns is avoiding torque on the probes.[12,22]

Seromas are the result of too much ultrasonic energy applied to the tissues either as a result of increased generator settings or prolonged application.[12,22] It is seldom necessary to use energy settings greater than 80% applied for 1 to 1.5 min/100 mL of wetting solution to a particular area to achieve proper tissue fragmentation and emulsification.[12]

NONINVASIVE MODALITIES
Cryolipolysis

Cryolipolysis refers to a noninvasive technology that uses precisely controlled cooling to selectively target and eliminate adipocytes without damage to surrounding tissues.[7,23] Cryolipolysis is performed using the Zeltiq Breeze system as part of the CoolSculpting procedure (Zeltiq Aesthetics, Pleasanton, CA, USA).

The mechanism of action of cryolipolysis is not fully understood. However, evidence suggests the onset of an inflammatory reaction within the adipose tissue in response to cold exposure.[24] Adipocytes respond differently to cooling than other cell types. Precisely controlled cooling causes lipid crystallization and triggers apoptosis in adipocytes, whereas in non-lipid-storing cells, lipids are left undamaged. Lipids released by apoptotic fat cells are removed gradually through the lymphatic system, thereby reducing tissue volume.[23,25]

Preprocedure preparation

Proper evaluation of adiposity is performed with the patient standing, such that local adiposity is subject to gravity. One can assess how much fat will be drawn into the applicator opening by mimicking the applicator opening using a C-shaped cup technique (**Fig. 7**). For best results, a minimum of 2.5 cm of fat should be drawn into the cup.[7]

Before treatment, the clinician should mark the center point of each bulge with an "X" using the templates provided by Zeltiq. If a large section of fat is to be treated, several marks may be required and placed such that there is slight overlap of the applicator when treating adjacent marked areas.[7]

A gel pad provides thermal contact between the patient's skin and the applicator and should be placed over the center of the treatment site. The applicator should be placed directly on the gel pad over the "X" making sure that the gel pad extends beyond the edges of the panels in the applicator cup (**Fig. 8**).[7]

Technique

The treatment regimen is selected from the instrument's touch screen console. Some regimens

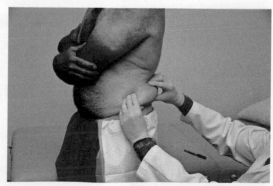

Fig. 7. Assessing a patient's fat using a C-shaped cup technique.

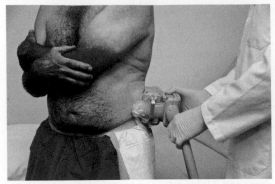

Fig. 8. Proper placement of the gel pad and applicator on a patient.

include a short massage session, which enhances the selective injury to the adipocytes.

Once the applicator is properly placed and the patient is comfortably positioned, the clinician may begin the cooling cycle. Vacuum pressure is used to draw the target tissue into the applicator for optimal cooling.[7]

Optimizing outcomes

Proper patient selection for cryolipolysis is essential to achieving successful outcomes. For optimal results, patients should be at or near their ideal body weight with good skin tone and minimal

laxity. Ideal candidates have distinct pockets of fat that are resistant to diet and exercise.[7]

A 20% reduction in the thickness of the fat layer is typically achieved with each treatment (**Figs. 9** and **10**).[26] Although results are visible with a single procedure, multiple procedures may be recommended to achieve the aesthetic goals. Although results may be observed as early as 3 weeks following treatment, final results are visible in 2 to 4 months.[7]

Postprocedure care

Following the procedure, the treated areas may feel cold and firm with a red and raised appearance. These effects are transient and usually resolve within a few minutes to hours. Bruising, soreness, tenderness, cramping, and tingling may occur, but usually resolve within a few days to weeks.

Complications and management

Very rarely, some patients may experience significant pain following cryolipolysis. This pain is self-limiting and usually resolves within 2 to 3 weeks.

Summary

Cryolipolysis is a novel, safe, and effective option for patients who desire a noninvasive procedure to reduce distinct areas of adiposity, such as fat in bulges, rolls, or other small areas that are

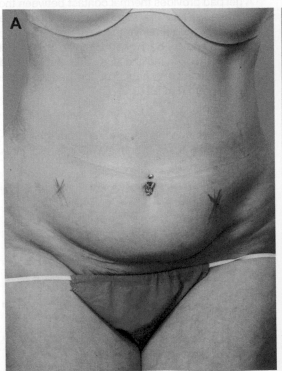
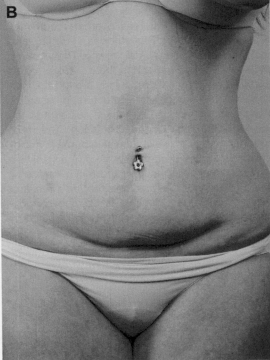

Fig. 9. Before (A) and 2 months after (B) CoolSculpting™, front view.

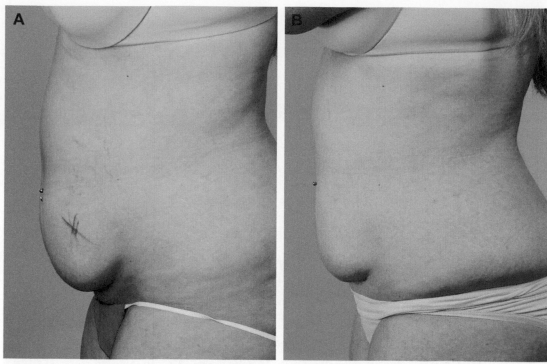

Fig. 10. Before (*A*) and 2 months after (*B*) CoolSculpting, profile view. Ultrashape® device.

resistant to diet and exercise. Although reduction in local adiposity can be achieved, cryolipolysis does not have an effect on tightening collagen within the skin or deeper layers.

High-Intensity Focused Ultrasound

High-intensity focused ultrasound (HIFU) body contouring devices Ultrashape and Liposonix are novel technologies that result in noninvasive adipocyte death leading to noninvasive volume reduction and body contouring. These devices are different with respect to the frequency of the ultrasound waves used to target fat. The UltraShape device operates at 0.2 MHz and has a proposed cavitation effect within adipocytes. The Lipsonix device operates at 2 MHz and has a proposed thermal mechanism, whereby adipocytes are destroyed through heat. Both procedures lead to adipocyte death. Lipids subsequently released are removed gradually through the lymphatic system, thereby reducing tissue volume.[7,27,28]

Preprocedure preparation

Patient assessment should be performed in the standing position so that the fat is subject to gravity. The clinician should assess the fat thickness, because a minimum of 1.5 cm of fat is generally needed for efficacy, although advances in this technology may allow smaller volumes to be

treated. The areas to be treated are marked in a standard fashion.

Technique

Most patients are able to undergo treatment without the need for analgesics or sedation. The transducer is placed on the skin, which is lubricated with oil to enhance conduction. The operator follows a pattern on the device screen, which ensures that the target area receives even treatment without overlap. The transducer dwells for 1 second per area while delivering the ultrasonic energy, and the tracking system keeps track of the area treated. The usual treatment protocol calls for 3 sessions, 2 weeks apart, with radiofrequency (RF) treatments at the same time and during the untreated weeks.[7]

Optimizing outcomes

Patient expectations must be addressed preoperatively, and there must be an understanding that these devices are less efficacious than liposuction. Most patients will see results, but results are highly variable. Results may be observed as early as 3 weeks posttreatment, but final outcomes are visible in 2 to 4 months (**Figs. 11** and **12**).

After procedure care

There are no posttreatment limitations following HIFU, and patients may resume all activities

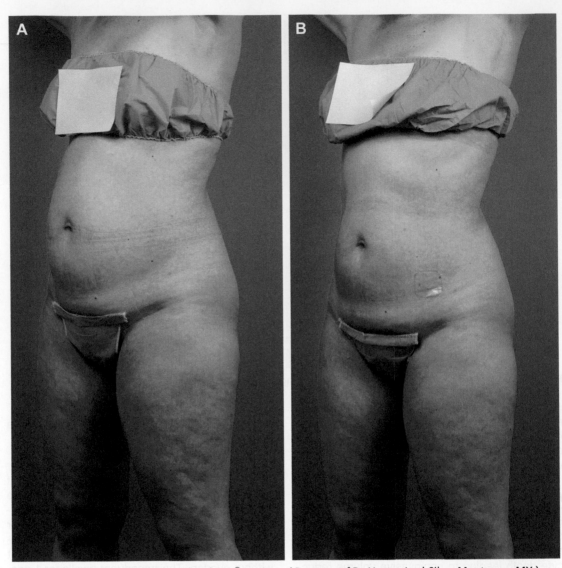

Fig. 11. Before (*A*) and after (*B*) 3 Ultrashape® sessions. (*Courtesy of* Dr Hector Leal-Silva, Monterrey, MX.)

immediately. The treated areas may be slightly ecchymotic and edematous; however, these changes resolve within a few days. Sensory changes may also occur but usually resolve in a few days to weeks.

Complications
In rare cases, a burn may occur with treatment.

Low-Level Laser Therapy

Low-level laser therapy (LLLT) is characterized as treatment with a dose rate that causes no immediate detectable increase in tissue temperature and no macroscopically visible changes in tissue structure.[29,30] The Zerona (Erchonia) is a low-level laser device that emits a wavelength at 635 nm and has

shown efficacy as an effective therapeutic strategy for circumferential reduction of the waist, hips, and thighs.[31]

The mechanism of action of LLLT remains somewhat controversial, but it is thought that the 635-nm low level Zerona laser penetrates the first few millimeters of fat and creates a temporary pore in the adipocyte cell membrane through which lipids are released.[29] Lipids are subsequently released into the interstitial space, gradually removed by the lymphatic system, and tissue volume is subsequently reduced.

The Zerona laser is a device with 5 rotating independent diode laser heads each emitting 17 mW of 635 nm of laser light. It was the first noninvasive aesthetic device to receive US Food and Drug

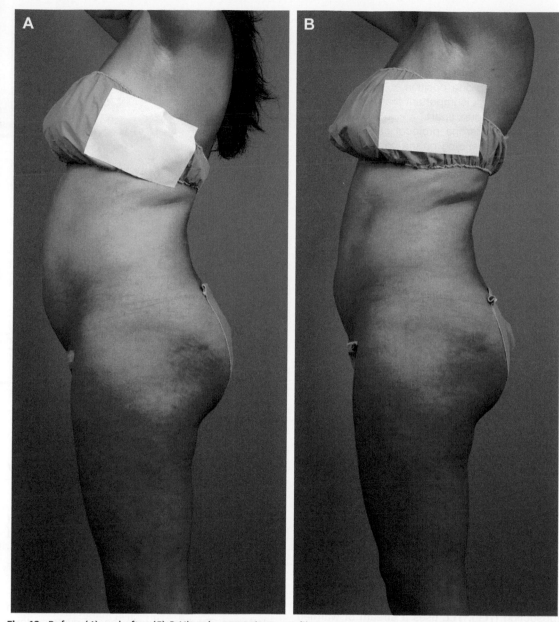

Fig. 12. Before (*A*) and after (*B*) 3 Ultrashape sessions, profile.

Administration (FDA) market clearance in the United States for circumferential reduction of the waist, hips, and thighs following completion of a placebo-controlled, randomized, double-blind, multisite clinical investigation evaluating 67 participants.[32] Results of this study showed an average reduction of 3.51 inches across patients' waist, hips, and thighs in as little as 2 weeks.[32,33]

Preprocedure preparation

Patient assessment should be performed in the standing position so that the fat is subject to gravity. The areas to be treated are marked.

Between treatments, patients are asked to walk 30 minutes per day, drink 1 L of water, and take a supplement called Curva that contains niacin among other homeopathic substances, which are designed to increase lymphatic flow. Smoking and alcohol cessation should be encouraged.

Technique

The commercial Zerona unit has an array of diodes, which are adjusted to within 6 inches of the patient's body. The patient is treated for 20 minutes in the waist, hips, and thighs in both the supine and the prone positions. The center diode is positioned 4 to 12 inches above the abdomen centered in the midline, and the 4 remaining diodes are positioned above the lateral abdomen and thigh regions. The diodes are repositioned in a similar fashion in the prone position.[32] To optimize the transitory pore, it is important that treatments are conducted 48 hours apart.

The current Zerona protocol calls for 6 to 12 treatments, depending on the habitus of the patient. On average, patients undergoing Zerona treatment receive a total of 9 treatments every 48 hours over a period of 2 weeks. It is possible to combine Zerona with other more focal, ablative, fat reduction technologies to enhance general slimming and local fat reduction.

Complications

Complications with LLLT can include thermal skin injury. However, complications are rare and mainly include patient dissatisfaction due to unrealistic expectations.[31]

Summary

LLLT is a unique technology in the noninvasive body-contouring armamentarium. Volume reduction without inducing cell death is achieved, thus representing a truly noninvasive modality leaving well-selected patients very satisfied with their treatment. Future goals aim to optimize treatment protocols.

Tissue Liquefaction Lipoplasty

Tissue liquefaction technology for body contouring and lipoplasty was approved by the FDA in 2010 (**Fig. 13**). In 2013, this technology was approved by the FDA for fat harvest during autologous transfer. Based on an innovation in cataract surgery that has been in use since 2003,[34] this new category of lipoplasty uses a process of targeted liquefaction of adipose tissue called tissue liquefaction liposuction (TLL). TLL uses a stream of warmed (37–55°C), low pressurized (300–1100 psi), pulsed saline that is emitted inside of the distal end of the liposuction cannula, remaining inside the cannula until it is aspirated. This saline stream is not injected into the subcutaneous space. Rather, subcutaneous fat and nonfat tissue are drawn into the cannula through the side aperture or aperatures and are impacted by the saline stream within the interior lumen of the cannula (**Figs. 14** and **15**). This stream causes a targeted phase transition of fat from a solid to a liquid, while nonfat tissue remains intact. The mechanical and thermal energies within the saline stream are low-level energies and work synergistically to achieve the minimum threshold of energy required to liquefy

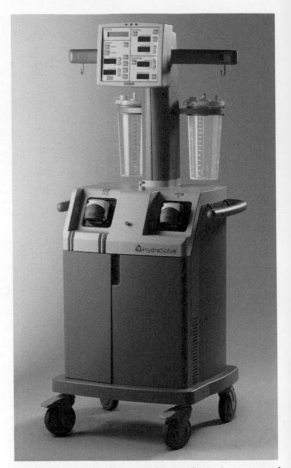

Fig. 13. Base unit of HydraSolve machine. (*Courtesy of* Hydrasolve, Tustin, CA; with permission.)

fat tissue, while remaining below the threshold of energy to liquefy nonfat tissues, such as blood vessels, nerves, and connective tissue (Christopher P. Godek MSA. Tissue Liquefaction Lipoplasty, 2014).

Tissue liquefaction technology is unique and differs from traditional water-assisted liposuction platforms. Traditional water-based systems tend to use high-pressure water jet saline streams often delivered externally from the distal end of the cannula. The external stream of these systems has a tendency to create soft tissue distortion as well as disruption of nonfat tissues within the subcutaneous space. The saline delivered with TLL remains entirely within the cannula, and therefore,

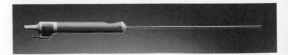

Fig. 14. Cannula for HydraSolve machine. (*Courtesy of* Hydrasolve, Tustin, CA; with permission.)

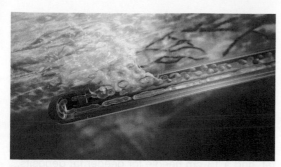

Fig. 15. Schematic diagram of subcutaneous fat and nonfat tissues drawn into the cannula through the side apertures, which are then impacted by the saline stream within the interior lumen of the cannula. This stream causes a targeted phase transition of fat from a solid to a liquid, while nonfat tissue remains intact. (*Courtesy of* Hydrasolve, Tustin, CA; with permission.)

no soft tissue distortion and minimal disruption of the surrounding connective tissue network occur.

Early clinical results with TLL have been quite favorable. Patients experience less bruising, swelling, and pain postoperatively in comparison with both suction-assisted lipoplasty and UAL. This is thought to be due to the tissue selectivity of TLL. Furthermore, TLL is a single-staged procedure that does not require placement of skin protection ports. The unique flow characteristics of the pulsed, heated saline allow the liquefied fat to travel continuously through the aspiration tubing without clogging or vapor locks. In comparison with the traditional stroke rate, TLL extracts fat most efficiently when the cannula thrust rate is slowed to approximately one-half to one-third of the traditional rate. This rate facilitates a more efficient and precise process with less surgeon fatigue. Although saline is used by TLL for fat extraction, tumescent fluid is still recommended.

TLL has been shown to be clinically successful in harvesting fat for autologous fat grafting. In a nude rat model, human fat extracted by TLL was shown to be comparable to traditional, syringe-aspirated fat.[35] Microscopic studies of fat harvested by TLL demonstrate 97% viability (Data on File, Adipose tissue cell viability of four fat arvesting modalities. Andrew Technologies LLC, 2011). The lipoaspirate is a suspension composed of small clusters of adipose tissue containing approximately 100 to 400 adipocytes per functional unit (Data on File, Comparison of lipoaspirate clump size between Hydrasolve and syringe fat harvesting methods. Andrew Technologies, 2011). Early clinical applications in body and facial fat grafting have been successful. Some potential advantages of fat harvested by TLL include less blood and oil contamination as well as less fibrous tissue within the lipoaspirate compared with

traditional methods of fat harvest. In theory, fewer contaminants may lead to reduced inflammation and improved fat graft survival.

Radiofrequency (RF)

Radiofrequency (RF) devices have recently been marketed for fat reduction and body contouring, although there is no direct FDA approval for fat reduction. RF use in body contouring is based on data that demonstrated a 60% loss of adipocyte viability following heating of adipose tissue to 45°C with RF energy. Limitations of RF devices include the lack of uniformity and consistency in tissue heating, and pain and discomfort with skin heating.

Vanquish (BTL Aesthetics, Boston, MA, USA) is a new device that offers selective RF using multipolar technology that emits an electromagnetic field over a large area that specifically targets the deep tissue layer wherein the energy is optimally absorbed. Vanquish uses a proprietary frequency that is delivered wirelessly and falls under the ISM band that is reserved internationally for the use of RF energy for industrial, scientific, and medical purposes. This technology was designed to emit energy based on differential electromagnetic impedances of tissues within the body. Tissue with higher impedance has higher resistance to the flow of the electromagnetic field, thereby increasing the temperature in that tissue relative to the surrounding tissue with lower impedance.

The frequencies used by Vanquish are best suited for the impedance of adipocytes in the deep tissue layer. The device selectively heats adipose tissue, so the depth of penetration varies based on the thickness of adipose tissue as well as the distance between the applicator and the body. The closer the applicator is to the body, the more superficial the penetration. Conversely, the further the applicator is from the body, the deeper the penetration. To achieve heat efficacy in the fat layer, the applicator should be placed such that the applicator is not touching the skin, but is spaced approximately 10 mm away from the skin surface. (Christopher P. Godek MSA. Tissue liquefaction lipoplasty. 2014.)

This device was initially tested in animals followed by human clinical trials.[36] Forty-one subjects aged 18 to 68 received four 30-min abdominal and flank treatments at weekly intervals. Thirty-five patients completed the study. There were no adverse events reported, and 89% of patients reported that the treatment was comfortable or very comfortable. A decrease in abdominal circumference was achieved in 32 of 35 patients (91.4%). This decrease in circumference ranged from 1 to 13 cm with an average of

4.93 cm. Seventy-one percent of patients reported to be satisfied or very satisfied with the results.[37] Ongoing studies are examining longer treatments and shorter treatment intervals.

Mesotherapy

Mesotherapy refers to the injection of various agents into the subcutaneous tissue to promote adipose tissue reduction. Agents can include a combination of homeopathic and pharmaceutical medication, plant extracts, and vitamins that are injected into the mesoderm layer targeting the adipose fat cells, dermal vasculature, and connective tissue septae.[27,38]

Formulations

The selection of medications, herbal extracts, and medicines is generally at the discretion of the practitioner. It is important to choose medications based on treatment goals, and the formula for each patient will differ based on these goals. Treatment of fat alone will use medication for lipolysis, vasodilation, and perfusion, while treatments for cellulite will also include dissolution of septae and banding. Agents used must be isotonic, biocompatible, and sterile, with a pH between 5 and 7. Theophylline tends to be the drug of choice for lipolysis in Europe, whereas in the Americas it is usually phosphatidylcholine.[39]

Preparation for mesotherapy

Proper selection of patients for mesotherapy is paramount for successful treatment and patient satisfaction. Patients with body mass index (BMI) greater than 30 are not ideal candidates for mesotherapy and will likely be dissatisfied with inadequate results.

Consultation with the patient should include a thorough medical history and physical examination of the areas to be treated. The patient's cellulite should be evaluated and classified according to the degree of severity. Areas to be treated and BMI should be measured and recorded. Weekly documentation should be maintained throughout therapy.[38]

Injections

Once the formula is selected, the frequency and technique of treatment are determined. Mechanical or manual injection techniques can be used. Mechanical injection is more precise, delivering an exact amount of medication to the desired depth with each injection.

The number of treatments and frequency are determined by the severity of the patient's symptoms and response to therapy. In general, treatments are usually given at least 1 week apart, but this interval can be increased if the patient has lingering swelling or reactions to the medications used. To be most effective, the time between treatments should not usually be longer than 4 weeks. Most patients will begin to see results after the third treatment.

Needle selection is based on the selection of fat and cellulite in relation to the fat in the mesoderm layer. A size 0.4-cm needle is used for cellulite and scar reduction, a 0.6-cm needle for superficial fat, and a 13-cm needle for deeper fat deposits.

Proper technique for mesotherapy injections includes appropriate spacing with a gridlike pattern between injections, 1.5 cm apart.[38]

Nappage technique can also be used for scarring, particularly if it is a result of surgery or liposuction. A 0.4-cm needle can be used to pierce the scar 0.1 cm apart along the length of the scar to break the fibrous bands in the dermis and subcutaneous layer. Lidocaine is usually added to the formula for pain relief. Collagenase and hyaluronidase are also essential additives.[38]

Side effects and treatment

Most side effects of mesotherapy occur from the trauma of injection, which may cause transient redness at the injection sites. Patients may complain of site tenderness or pruritis, which usually dissipates within 10 minutes of the treatment. Some patients may develop transient urticaria that is usually self-limiting. Arnica gel application to the skin following treatment may prevent these complications.

The most common side effect of mesotherapy is bruising, which usually lasts for several days and is also self-limiting. For large bruises, ice and heat therapy protocols can be used. Compounds such as arnica montana, and bromelain can be taken before and after treatments as a preventative measure.

After several treatments, there may be clusters of small blood vessels originating from the needle injection site. This neovascular response usually occurs distal to the knee. Treatment should be discontinued indefinitely in this instance as this change may not resolve. Vascular lasers or Intense Pulsed Light (IPL) may be necessary to address this neovascular response.

Allergic reaction such as wheal and flare may develop in response to some of the components of the medication. If a reaction occurs, patch-testing should be done after 1 week. Benadryl and topical cortisone creams typically alleviate this reaction; however, if it persists or becomes painful, a Medrol Dosepak should be prescribed.[40]

Other adverse reactions reported are cutaneous granulomas, atypical mycobaterial infections, lichenoid eruptions, ulcerations, and exacerbation of psoriasis. These complications can be avoided by seeking physicians well-trained in mesotherapy with proper use of sterile technique and sterile conditions.[41]

Summary

Although mesotherapy has attracted wide acceptance among the medical community in Europe and South America, the absence of double-blind studies hinders the widespread acceptance among the US medical community. Nevertheless, those practitioners who have been properly trained have consistently observed successful results in their patients.[38]

SUMMARY

The strong patient demand for safer, less invasive body contouring procedures will inevitably drive technology toward more effective modalities that minimize downtime and recovery, while improving results. The future of body contouring will likely stratify patients into more distinct categories, such as those requiring aggressive surgical excision, minimally invasive liposuction techniques with adjunctive energy-delivering modalities or mesotherapy, and noninvasive techniques achieving volume reduction and skin tightening through additional energy-delivering modalities.

With proven safety and efficacy, the future of minimally invasive and noninvasive body contouring is very promising. However, judicious patient selection cannot be overemphasized, and these procedures should not be overpromoted. Currently, the most ideal candidates for these types of procedures are those who are accepting of a mild to moderate result.

By incorporating these technologies into a plastic surgery practice, the ability to offer a multifaceted approach to body contouring will ultimately lead to greater patient and physician satisfaction, and is undoubtedly an emerging model of minimally invasive and noninvasive body contouring surgery.

REFERENCES

1. Goldman A, Gotkin RH. Laser-assisted liposuction. Clin Plast Surg 2009;36(2):241–53, vii; [discussion: 255–60].
2. Parlette EC, Kaminer ME. Laser-assisted liposuction: here's the skinny. Semin Cutan Med Surg 2008;27(4):259–63.
3. Mann MW, Palm MD, Sengelmann RD. New advances in liposuction technology. Semin Cutan Med Surg 2008;27(1):72–82.
4. Klein JA. Anesthesia for liposuction in dermatologic surgery. J Dermatol Surg Oncol 1988;14(10):1124–32.
5. Klein JA. Tumescent technique for local anesthesia improves safety in large-volume liposuction. Plast Reconstr Surg 1993;92(6):1085–98 [discussion: 1099–100].
6. Heymans O, Castus P, Grandjean FX, et al. Liposuction: review of the techniques, innovations and applications. Acta Chir Belg 2006;106(6):647–53.
7. DiBernardo BE, Pozner JN. Principles of new invasive modalities. In: Rubin JP, Jewell M, Richter DF, et al, editors. Body contouring and liposuction. Philadelphia: Elsevier Saunders; 2013. p. 534–42.
8. DiBernardo BE. Recognition and management of complications of fat and cellulite treatments. In: Katz BE, Sadick NS, editors. Recognition and management of complications of fat and cellulite treatments in body contouring. Philadelphia: Elsevier Saunders; 2010. p. 183–92.
9. DiBernardo BE. Treatment of cellulite using a 1440-nm pulsed laser with one-year follow-up. Aesthet Surg J 2011;31(3):328–41.
10. Scuderi N, Devita R, D'Andrea F, et al. Nuove prospettive nella liposuzione la lipoemulsificazone. Giorn Chir Plast Ricostr ed Estetica 1987;2(1):33–9.
11. Zocchi ML. Clinical aspects of ultrasonic liposculpture. Perspect Plast Surg 1993;7:153–74.
12. Garcia O Jr. Ultrasonic liposuction. In: Rubin JP, Jewell M, Richter DF, et al, editors. Body contouring and liposuction. Philadelphia: Elsevier Saunders; 2013. p. 543–58.
13. Zocchi ML. Metodo di trattamento del tessuto adipose con energia ultrasonic. Rome, Italy: Congresso dell Societa Italiana di Medicina Estetica; April 1988.
14. Zocchi ML. New prospective in liposculpturing: the ultrasonic energy. Zurich, Switzerland: Proceedings of the 10th ISAPS Congress; 1989.
15. Coleman III WP BH, Narins RS, et al. Update from the ultrasonic liposuction task force of the American Society for Dermatological Surgery. Dermatol Surg 1997;23:211–4.
16. Graf R, Auersvald A, Damasio RC, et al. Ultrasound-assisted liposuction: an analysis of 348 cases. Aesthetic Plast Surg 2003;27(2):146–53.
17. Lawrence N, Coleman WP 3rd. The biologic basis of ultrasonic liposuction. Dermatol Surg 1997;23(12):1197–200.
18. de Souza Pinto EB, Abdala PC, Maciel CM, et al. Liposuction and VASER. Clin Plast Surg 2006;33(1):107–15, vii.
19. Cimino WW, Bond LJ. Physics of ultrasonic surgery using tissue fragmentation: part I. Ultrasound Med Biol 1996;22(1):89–100.
20. Bond LJ, Cimino WW. Physics of ultrasonic surgery using tissue fragmentation: part II. Ultrasound Med Biol 1996;22(1):101–17.

21. de Jong RH, Grazer FM. Titanic tumescent anesthesia. Dermatol Surg 1998;24(6):689–91.

22. Jewell ML, Fodor PB, de Souza Pinto EB, et al. Clinical application of VASER–assisted lipoplasty: a pilot clinical study. Aesthet Surg J 2002;22(2):131–46.

23. Manstein D, Laubach H, Watanabe K, et al. Selective cryolysis: a novel method of non-invasive fat removal. Lasers Surg Med 2008;40(9):595–604.

24. Avram MM, Harry RS. Cryolipolysis for subcutaneous fat layer reduction. Lasers Surg Med 2009; 41(10):703–8.

25. Zelickson B, Egbert BM, Preciado J, et al. Cryolipolysis for noninvasive fat cell destruction: initial results from a pig model. Dermatol Surg 2009;35(10): 1462–70.

26. Rosales-Berber I, Diliz-Perez E, Allison J. Accumulative abdomen fat layer reduction from multiple Zeltiq cryolipolysis procedures. American Society for Laser Medicine and Surgery 2010 Annual Meeting. Phoenix (Arizona): 2010.

27. Jewell ML, Solish NJ, Desilets CS. Noninvasive body sculpting technologies with an emphasis on high-intensity focused ultrasound. Aesthetic Plast Surg 2011;35(5):901–12.

28. Jewell ML, Jewell JL. High intensity focused ultrasound and non-invasive body contouring. Body contouring and liposuction. Philadelphia: Elsevier Saunders; 2013. p. 559–71.

29. Neira R, Arroyave J, Ramirez H, et al. Fat liquefaction: effect of low-level laser energy on adipose tissue. Plast Reconstr Surg 2002;110(3):912–22 [discussion: 923–5].

30. Brown SA, Rohrich RJ, Kenkel J, et al. Effect of low-level laser therapy on abdominal adipocytes before lipoplasty procedures. Plast Reconstr Surg 2004; 113(6):1796–804 [discussion: 1805–6].

31. Mulholland RS, Paul MD, Chalfoun C. Noninvasive body contouring with radiofrequency, ultrasound, cryolipolysis, and low-level laser therapy. Clin Plast Surg 2011;38(3):503–20, vii–viii.

32. Jackson RF, Dedo DD, Roche GC, et al. Low-level laser therapy as a non-invasive approach for body contouring: a randomized, controlled study. Lasers Surg Med 2009;41(10):799–809.

33. Avci P, Nyame TT, Gupta GK, et al. Low-level laser therapy for fat layer reduction: a comprehensive review. Lasers Surg Med 2013;45(6):349–57.

34. Mackool RJ, Brint SF. AquaLase: a new technology for cataract extraction. Curr Opin Ophthalmol 2004;15(1):40–3.

35. Davis K, Rasko Y, Oni G, et al. Comparison of adipocyte viability and fat graft survival in an animal model using a new tissue liquefaction liposuction device vs standard Coleman method for harvesting. Aesthet Surg J 2013;33(8):1175–85.

36. Weiss R, Weiss M, Beasley K, et al. Operator independent focused high frequency ISM band for fat reduction: porcine model. Lasers Surg Med 2013; 45(4):235–9.

37. Fajkosova K, Machovcova A, Onder M, et al. Selective radiofrequency therapy as a non-invasive approach for contactless body contouring and circumferential reduction. J Drugs Dermatol 2014;13(3):291–6.

38. Neil S, Sadick MS. Mesotherapy for body contouring and cellulite. In: Rubin JP, Jewell M, Richter DF, et al, editors. Body contouring and liposuction. Philadelphia: Elsevier Saunders; 2013. p. 572–9.

39. Rittes PG. The use of phosphatidylcholine for correction of localized fat deposits. Aesthetic Plast Surg 2003;27(4):315–8.

40. Urbani CE. Urticarial reaction to ethylenediamine in aminophylline following mesotherapy. Contact Dermatitis 1994;31(3):198–9.

41. Gokdemir G, Kucukunal A, Sakiz D. Cutaneous granulomatous reaction from mesotherapy. Dermatol Surg 2009;35(2):291–3.

Prevention and Management of Complications in Body Contouring Surgery

Jeffrey A. Gusenoff, MD

KEYWORDS

- Complications • Body contour • Infection • Hematoma • Seroma • Dehiscence
- Delayed wound healing • Plastic surgery

KEY POINTS

- Avoid complications before they occur with careful preoperative patient selection, screening, consent, and management of patient expectations.
- Perioperative chemoprophylaxis and antibiotic use can help prevent major complications in body contouring.
- Intraoperative details such as patient positioning, operating room temperature, fluid status, and communication with the operating room team can avoid intraoperative complications.
- Most complications are minor, and can be managed conservatively.
- Wound dehiscence, if identified early, can be treated quickly with minimal long-term sequelae and improved scar quality.
- Seroma often resolves with serial aspirations; however, patients must be seen frequently.
- Recurrent skin laxity is common in body contouring after massive weight loss. Revisions can often be delayed until second-stage procedures are performed.

INTRODUCTION

Body contouring after massive weight loss has increased in popularity over the past 10 years, with more than 40,000 procedures performed annually.[1] Many of these cases are caused by weight loss after bariatric surgery. After weight loss, deformities are severe and often involve more than one body area. Many patients choose to have multiple procedures, and may increase the risk of complications.[2] Several studies have documented higher complication rates in patients who have body contouring after massive weight loss, with complications being even higher in those who have lost weight via bariatric surgery.[3–11]

Complications in body contouring surgery after bariatric surgery are common and approach 50% in most of these studies. In self–weight loss patients, the rate of complications is slightly lower, at around 30%, but still high. How complications are defined in the literature is inconsistent, and thus the true rate of complications in this population is uncertain. However, most of these complications are minor wound healing problems that can be managed conservatively and rarely require return to the operating room. Many of these complications are preventable or at least of lesser severity with careful preoperative, intraoperative, and postoperative planning and monitoring.

Disclosures: The author has nothing to disclose.
Life After Weight Loss Program, Department of Plastic Surgery, UPMC Plastic Surgery Center, University of Pittsburgh, 3380 Boulevard of the Allies, Suite 180, Pittsburgh, PA 15213, USA
E-mail address: gusenoffja@upmc.edu

Clin Plastic Surg 41 (2014) 805–818
http://dx.doi.org/10.1016/j.cps.2014.06.006
0094-1298/14/$ – see front matter © 2014 Elsevier Inc. All rights reserved.

PREOPERATIVE EVALUATION

A careful preoperative evaluation is the best way to avoid long-term complications. Understanding the patient's weight loss history can give insight into any potential problems that may be encountered and help determine surgical candidacy. Care should be taken to ask how patients lost their weight, what was their maximum weight before weight loss, current weight, and lowest weight. Patients should be asked about any weight fluctuation over the past month or 3 months. After bariatric surgery, most patients reach a nadir and then plateau at a slightly higher weight.[12] Identifying how patients are progressing in their weight loss is important for predicting long-term results and satisfaction. Patients should ideally be at least a year out from their bariatric procedure and weight stable for 3 months.[6,13–15]

Several studies have suggested a body mass index (BMI) cutoff (eg, 32 kg/m^2 or 35 kg/m^2) at which patients should not be operated on; however, these guidelines are suggestions and not supported by significant outcomes data.[16,17] Although complications do increase with increasing BMI, there is no set cutoff point because all patients present with different body morphologies and should be evaluated individually. Some women presenting for breast contouring may have significant gynoid morphology with most of their weight in their thighs, which does not exclude them from a breast procedure. Some postbariatric patients may have a large pannus that is disproportionate to the rest of their body.

Nutritional status can also be assessed before surgery and helps to avert postoperative complications. Bariatric procedures such as the Roux-en-Y gastric bypass have malabsorptive and restrictive components.[18–20] Many patients have aversions to animal proteins after this procedure, and they may have reduced intake of protein overall. Careful preoperative assessment by a dietitian can calculate protein intake. Goals should be around 70 to 100 g a day around the time of surgery to avoid wound healing problems. Patients who present after surgery with wounds that do not heal should be assessed for nutritional deficiencies. Preoperative albumin and prealbumin studies may be helpful in patients who report low-protein diets or frequent episodes of dumping syndrome. Patients having gastric bypass are prone to iron deficiency anemia, folate, calcium, and B$_{12}$ deficiencies. Patients who are not on routine supplementation may need to be tested or revisit with their bariatric surgeons.

A careful medical history should be performed to assess for medical comorbidities that existed before weight loss and may still be present after weight loss.[21] A single past medical history often lists many medical issues that have since resolved with weight loss, such as diabetes, sleep apnea, and hypertension. Common medical conditions that often do not resolve as frequently include arthritis, anxiety, and depression. Preoperative clearances may be required for any outstanding medical conditions. Smokers are referred to their primary care physicians for assistance with smoking cessation. All patients are tested for smoking with a urine cotinine test a few weeks before surgery. Anyone with a positive test is not booked for surgery and must wait 3 months until a negative test is obtained. Patients are made aware of the increased risk of wound healing problems and infection with smoking.[22,23] Any current medications that could interfere with surgery, such as aspirin-containing drugs, anticoagulants, steroids, or immunosuppressive agents, are assessed. Herbal medications are also reviewed because many are associated with bleeding risks.[24]

A past surgical history is obtained to identify anything that may increase the risk of complications, such as prior cancer surgery, history of nonhealing wounds or infections, scars on the abdomen, and prior plastic surgery such as liposuction to the areas to be treated. Large open cholecystectomy scars are important to identify early because they may change the surgeon's plan with regard to scar placement or the degree of undermining that can be performed in a given area.[25,26]

PERIOPERATIVE INTERVENTIONS

Before surgery, it is critical to be aware of several important patient safety issues. Avoiding thromboembolic events with sequential compression devices or chemoprophylaxis may be indicated depending on the type of procedure, duration of procedure, and patient risk factors. Risk of thromboembolic events has been described as being as high as 9.7% in the literature, with most articles citing risk below 3%.[16,27–30] Caprini risk scores can be calculated before surgery to determine the need for a particular thromboembolic prevention protocol.[31,32] Various treatment methods for chemoprophylaxis exist, including the use of subcutaneous heparin before surgery, or the use of low-molecular-weight heparin the morning after surgery. There are few data in the body contouring literature to support a particular recommendation. Patients with a history of deep venous thrombosis or pulmonary embolism may benefit from the use of a temporary inferior vena cava filter.

Patients undergoing large body contouring procedures are at risk for hypothermia. Hypothermia in body contouring has been associated with increased seroma, bleeding, and need for transfusion.[33] Markings for large body contouring procedures involving multiple body areas can take 30 minutes or longer with the patient completely exposed. Photographs of the markings may also be taken. Warming blankets should be used before marking and throughout the operative procedure. Warming pads on the operating table, warming blankets, fluid warmers, and warm prep solution can aid in maintaining body core temperatures. The room temperature for body contouring procedures should be maintained at 21°C (70° Fahrenheit). For complex cases in which both lower body and upper body procedures are being performed, sterile so-called Bair Hugger sandwiches can be made and then removed at certain times during the procedure. To achieve this, the patient is fully prepped for all areas using warmed prep solution. A sterile sheet is placed on the upper or lower body, then the Bair Hugger is placed, then another sterile sheet is placed making the warmer sandwich. This sandwich is removed before beginning that part of the operation and a new Bair Hugger is placed on the area that was recently completed.

Patient positioning in surgery is important to optimize patient safety.[34] During long procedures or procedures with position changes, care should be taken to pad the extremities with foam, protect the eyes, and use appropriate axillary or shoulder rolls. Superficial nerves should be padded, especially the arms and legs. Hands should be in a neutral resting position and not supinated on the arm boards. Postoperative neuropraxia can result from poor arm positioning or arms being abducted more than 90° during the procedure. Neuropraxia can also be caused by leaning on the patient during the procedure, pressure from foot plates at the bottom of the bed to prevent the patient from sliding off, or external pressure on the peroneal nerve at the head of the fibula when the patient is in a frog-legged position. Treatment of neuropraxia is conservative at first. Consultation with a neurologist can aid in reassuring the patient. Additional nerve conduction studies may be necessary if improvement does not occur over the next several months. Resolution is usually slow and patient reassurance is critical and often difficult.

Maintaining close communication with the anesthesia team during the procedure can avoid complications. For multiple-procedure cases, the fluid status should be assessed frequently. Use of colloid during the resuscitation can aid in reducing fluid volumes in cases in which extremity edema may cause problems with wound closure, such as in brachioplasty. Periodic evaluation of blood pressure can help in optimizing hemostasis during

surgery. Core temperature should be monitored frequently to prevent hypothermia. Operating on one body area at a time and moving from one area to the next is the safest way to progress through surgery so that, if anesthesia has any concerns and the operation needs to end, there are not several partially completed operative areas, which may be disconcerting to the patient.

COMMON COMPLICATIONS IN BODY CONTOURING
Infection

Prevention
Perioperative antibiotic use has become an important tool in preventing postoperative infections. Many institutions provide their own recommendations. Often they involve the use of a safe, cost-effective agent that offers a spectrum of action that covers most of the probable intraoperative contaminants for the given surgical case. First-generation or second-generation cephalosporins satisfy these criteria for most body contouring procedures. Vancomycin is not recommended for routine use because of the potential for development of antibiotic resistance, but is acceptable for patients allergic to β-lactams. Fluoroquinolones and clindamycin can be used in selected situations. Current recommendations are for use within 1 hour of surgical start, and up to 2 hours ahead of time for vancomycin or clindamycin because of increased infusion time. Antibiotics are typically discontinued 24 hours after surgery, and 48 hours for cardiac surgery, even if drains and tubes are still in place. Guidelines for body contouring procedures with large tissue flaps and multiple drains have not been established; however, prospective studies in plastic surgery show significant reductions in infection with the use of preoperative versus no preoperative antibiotics.[35]

If shaving is required before surgery, it is recommended to use clippers rather than a razor to reduce the risk of infection. Patients can be advised to shave their pubic areas several days before surgery. Cleansing with chlorhexidine or antibacterial soap for 2 days before surgery is also advised. Foley catheters should be removed within 24 to 48 hours after surgery.

Diagnosis
Infection is usually evident 7 or more days after surgery. Often the first sign is erythema, pain, or induration around a localized site. A cellulitis may develop and should be marked to determine whether it is spreading. More aggressive infections may appear sooner and may occur in diabetics or immunocompromised hosts. Erythema may

spread and patients may experience fevers and chills. Drainage from the incision may be noted or the fluid from the drainage tubes may become turbid. Differential diagnosis can include fungal rashes from prior intertrigo, irritation from binders or garments, foreign body reaction from suture or staples, or contact dermatitis from skin glues.

Management

A suspected cellulitis can be treated empirically with broad-spectrum antibiotics. Because of the high prevalence of methicillin-resistant *Staphylococcus aureus* or oxacillin-resistant *S aureus*, Bactrim is a common first-line drug. If a patient is admitted with systemic symptoms, vancomycin and Zosyn are usually initiated. Infectious disease consultations may be appropriate for infections that do not respond to initial therapy. Aggressive cellulitis that does not respond to antibiotic therapy may require imaging or surgical intervention. If fluctuance is present at the initial evaluation, an incision and drainage is performed. Depending on the comfort of the surgeon and patient, and the degree of infection, an incision and drainage may be performed in the office setting. Wounds after drainage are thoroughly irrigated with half-strength peroxide and then saline. The wound is packed with gauze and local wound care is initiated twice daily. Cultures should be obtained at the time of initial drainage. Some localized abscesses respond well to incision and drainage without the need for any antibiotics. More severe infections may need to be drained in the operating room with significant irrigation and debridement including the use of pulse lavage.

Wound Dehiscence

Prevention

Wound dehiscence is best prevented by avoiding undue tension on incisions. Wound dehiscence is the most common complication in body contouring procedures, with rates as high as 60%.[3,36–44] Acute dehiscence (usually during the hospitalization) is usually technical in nature. Wound closure in layers using the deep fascial layer as described by Lockwood[45] aids in securing the deeper structures so less tension is placed on the skin closure. Some procedures are more prone to wound breakdown or dehiscence, such as the lower body lift incision in which autoaugmentation is performed. This tendency may be caused by prolonged pressure on the buttocks, because lower body lift procedures are often performed first, followed by an abdominal procedure, and then a delay in ambulation during the hospitalization. Thighplasty incisions are prone to wound breakdown at the T point because of the warm, moist,

bacteria-laden groin region. T-point junctions in the thigh as well as on the abdomen or under the breast may experience higher rates of delayed healing. Incisions in the axilla for brachioplasty procedures are also prone to problems caused by motion and moisture. Reducing the amount of undermining and tension on these closures may aid in prevention of dehiscence.

Diagnosis

Acute dehiscence is often noted soon after surgery when patients are either moved in the bed or moving on their own. A drain that does not hold suction after surgery should be considered a wound dehiscence until proved otherwise. Provided the drain is sewn in correctly and the holes are in the patient, there may be an area of the incision that is not closed completely or may have opened during moving of the patient. Often patients note a gush of blood or fluid when the wound opens, mostly likely caused by an underlying seroma or hematoma that may have accumulated under the tissues. Patients may feel a popping or bursting sensation when they move or bend too far. Delayed wound dehiscence is often seen in concert with some degree of tissue necrosis.

Management

Early patient education about dehiscence is an important part of managing the problem. Patients should be advised that, if an acute dehiscence is noted, they should call immediately to be seen and treated. Closure can often be performed immediately in the office or emergency room, without having to return to the operating room, depending on the size of the wound and other factors such as bleeding. If the patient tolerates local anesthetic, the wound can be irrigated with Betadine or chlorhexidine and closed in layers over a Penrose drain (**Fig. 1**). The drain can be removed in a few days. Antibiotics are typically given for 5 to 7 days. Wounds that present in a delayed fashion can be more of a challenge. The key is to get control of the wound. Debridement, either enzymatic or sharp, may be required. Normal saline wet to dry dressings initially can aid in transitioning to other wound modalities such as negative pressure wound therapy (**Fig. 2**). Operative intervention may be necessary for large contaminated wounds that are not amenable to bedside debridement. Wounds may make many months to heal. Early delayed closure may be a good option to speed healing once the tissue inflammation has diminished (**Fig. 3**). Nutritional status should be scrutinized in patients who have difficulty healing.

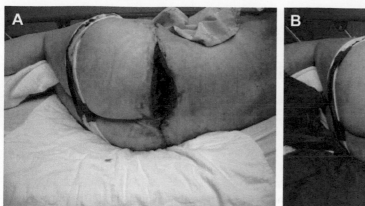
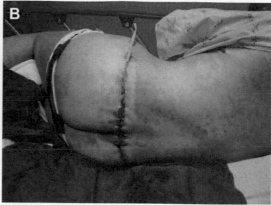

Fig. 1. (*A*) Dehiscence of a lower body lift incision 2 weeks after surgery. (*B*) The wound was cleansed with Betadine and thoroughly irrigated. A Penrose drain was placed at the time of reclosure. Return to the operating room was not required.

Hematoma

Prevention

Hematoma incidence in a large study of patients after body contouring ranged from 4% in women to 15% in men.[46] The best way to prevent a hematoma is with careful hemostasis, using electrocautery, hemoclips, or sutures. The use of tumescent or dilute epinephrine solutions can avoid significant blood loss during surgery. General anesthetics may induce a reduction in blood pressure during surgery. Checking with anesthesia at the time of hemostasis to identify a hypotensive state is important. Restoration of normotension during this time can help avoid a postoperative hematoma. A Valsalva maneuver can also aid in checking for any venous back bleeders or missed arterial

bleeders that may become evident during extubation when the patient is coughing on the endotracheal tube. Abdominal binders may aid in postoperative compression; however, their use as well as the use of drains does not prevent hematoma formation. Hematoma formation is common in patients who are on anticoagulant therapy and are bridged with heparin or low-molecular-weight heparin around the time of surgery. Patients undergoing large body contouring procedures with bridging anticoagulation should be well informed about the risk of bleeding and should be prepared for the need for transfusion or prolonged stay in the intensive care unit. These patients should consider the risk/benefit ratio carefully before proceeding with surgery.

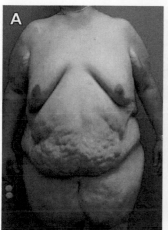
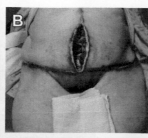
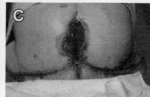
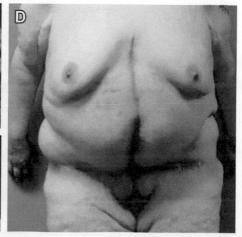

Fig. 2. (*A*) A patient with morbid obesity underwent a T-type panniculectomy and experienced wound dehiscence. (*B*) At 2 weeks after surgery, there was a significant amount of tissue necrosis that required serial debridements and then negative pressure wound therapy. (*C*) Improvement in the wound at 3 months with negative pressure wound therapy. (*D*) Complete wound closure achieved at 6 months after surgery.

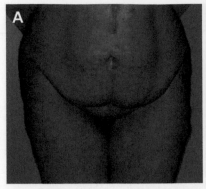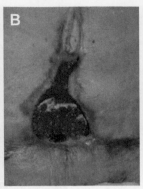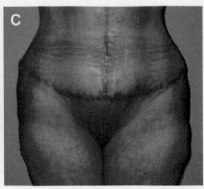

Fig. 3. (*A*) Preoperative photograph of a patient who underwent a T-type abdominoplasty. (*B*) The patient developed wound dehiscence and suture extrusion. (*C*) Once inflammation settled down and a good granulating bed of tissue was present, the patient was taken back to the operating room for a revision of the scar to both speed the recovery and optimize the cosmetic result.

Postoperative prevention of hypertension can also help prevent a postoperative hematoma.

Diagnosis

Hematomas in body contouring are sometimes evident, and sometimes subtle. When evident, drain outputs may be increased, and the patient may be symptomatic with decreased blood pressure, decreased urine output, and tachycardia. Ecchymosis may be present, along with an asymmetric bulge over an area of significant pain (**Fig. 4**). Sentinel bleeding or oozing around the drain site or from the incision soon after surgery that does not improve with direct pressure may be a sign of an impending hematoma. Early ecchymosis, especially in the genital region, is often an early sign of a hematoma as well. Early identification of areas of increased pain should be

investigated by takedown of the dressings. In areas that are wrapped circumferentially, such as the arm, failure to visualize the incision could result in a missed hematoma with significant bullae formation and impending skin loss (**Fig. 5**).

Management

Small hematomas may be managed conservatively. Drains may already be in place and may be dark, indicating the presence of clot. It often takes weeks for the hematoma to liquefy and come out of the drain. Hematomas that take a long time to resolve may also leave permanent contour deformities. Early intervention by incision and drainage may aid in the overall cosmetic result, but may create a temporary wound that needs to be managed conservatively for a period of time.

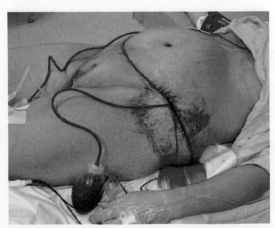

Fig. 4. Postoperative hematoma after abdominoplasty. Abdominal distention, labial swelling, full drainage bulbs, and leaking near the drain site are all indicators of a clinically significant hematoma requiring emergent drainage in the operating room.

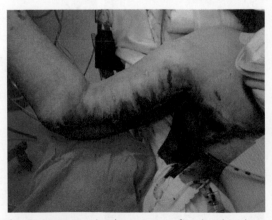

Fig. 5. Postoperative hematoma after brachioplasty. The patient complained of increased pain on the right side versus the left. Dressings were removed and the hematoma was identified. Early operative intervention avoided long-term sequelae of skin loss.

For large or life-threatening hematomas, emergent return to the operating room is critical. A type and screen, if not previously obtained, should be crossed for at least 2 units of packed red blood cells. Fluids should be opened wide and anesthesia should be notified immediately. After evacuation of a large hematoma, bleeders are identified and controlled. Hemostatic agents may be placed in the wound to aid with clotting because the wound bed is often oozy. New drains are placed. Resuscitative measures are improved with communication between the surgeon and anesthesiologist.

Fat Necrosis

Prevention

Fat necrosis occurs in less than 10% of patients undergoing multiple procedures in body contouring.[3] It occurs when the blood supply to the fat is cut off either from sutures or surgical technique. Long, narrow flaps or perforator-based flaps used for autoaugmentation of the breasts or buttocks may be most susceptible to fat necrosis.[47] Care should be taken not to allow blood vessels to retract because bleeding into the tissues can lead to hematomas in the fat that can lead to fat necrosis.

Diagnosis

Hard lumps may be palpable under the incision and are commonly found in the lower abdominal incision or in the breasts. Fat necrosis caused by the use of sutures in the superficial facial system is often felt directly under the incision as a marble-sized mass. If it is within the parenchyma of the breast, it may be larger. If it involves the pedicle under the nipple areola complex, it could even compromise the nipple areola complex.

Treatment

Management is often conservative. Areas of firmness soften over time, but may take several months. If lumps are of concern or painful after a year's time, surgical excision under local anesthesia can be performed. Lumps in the breast that are concerning to a patient should be referred for breast imaging. Ultrasonography can usually determine fat necrosis from other causes. Fine-needle aspiration is an option for concerned patients or for indeterminate ultrasonography interpretations.

Lymphedema

Prevention

Postoperative edema occurs in approximately 0% to 15% of patients after brachioplasty, with rates for sentinel lymph node biopsy at around 3% to 5% and axillary node dissection at 10% to 20%.[48] The rates of postoperative edema in thighplasty range from 0% to 29%, with higher rates associated with injury to the saphenous vein.[49] Many patients undergoing body contouring after massive weight loss have preexisting lower extremity vascular disease from their long-standing obesity.[50] Preventing lymphedema by dissecting carefully in the regions of the groin and axilla can avoid disruption of lymphatics. In the thigh, dissection should be superficial to the saphenous vein and very superficial in the femoral region above the adductor magnus. Dissection around the knee should be superficial as well. In brachioplasty surgery, care should be taken to avoid hollowing out the axilla. In combined mastopexy/brachioplasty procedures, the surgeon should avoid over-resecting the lateral chest wall and axillary areas where lymph nodes reside. In combined abdominoplasty/vertical medial thighplasty procedures, scar placement may be low on the abdomen and femoral lymph nodes may be injured. Some surgeons advocate excision site lipectomy of the thigh with liposuction; however, this is anecdotal and there are no prospective controlled trials investigating whether this reduces lymphatic injury in the long term, especially with rates of lymphatic complications already being low.

Diagnosis

Preoperative diagnosis of lower extremity edema can help with the diagnosis of postoperative edema. Many patients present before surgery with lipedema. Lipedema is often mistaken for lymphedema. There is symmetric swelling of the legs extending from the hips to the ankles with fatty overgrowth. Lymphedema is often asymmetric, but can complicate lipedema in the morbidly obese. The fat hangs over the ankle bones (**Fig. 6**). The cause is unknown and does not improve with diet or exercise. Pain and hypersensitivity are common. Careful examination of the extremities includes documentation of varicosities, venous stasis disease, and edema. Patients may need vascular assessments for deep venous thrombosis, venous insufficiency, or evaluation with a Doppler ultrasonography. Swelling can be anterior or posterior. Socks should be removed because they often cut off at the level of the ankle, so edema of the foot cannot be assessed.

Extremity swelling after surgery is common. Onset may be more noticeable 2 to 3 weeks after surgery as the patient becomes more active. Dependent edema typically resolves within 3 months after surgery. Permanent swelling, lymphedema, is rare and not well documented in the literature.[51] Lymphedema has been associated with the vertical incision technique, hypothyroidism, and male

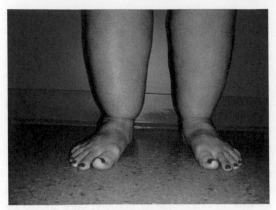

Fig. 6. Lipedema is often confused with lymphedema. Lipedema is common after massive weight loss and results in swelling to the level of the ankles. The dorsum of the foot is spared, whereas in lymphedema swelling extends to the toes. It is important to remove the patient's socks and document the preoperative degree of swelling and asymmetry before surgery to avoid unnecessary examinations afterward for what might have been a preexisting condition.

gender, and is inversely related to a high BMI. This relationship may be caused by difficulty in diagnosing the lymphedema in obese patients.[52]

If swelling is acute (ie <72 hours), a deep vein thrombosis (DVT) should be ruled out. Additional history should document any pain, cramping, dehydration, drugs (such as calcium channel blockers, prednisone, antiinflammatory drugs), systemic illness, or sleep apnea.[53] Physical examination should focus on distribution of the swelling, tenderness, pitting, varicosities, Kaposi-Stemmer sign (the inability to pinch a fold of skin on the dorsum of the foot at the base of the second toe), and skin changes (warty texture vs brown hemosiderin). Laboratory studies may be warranted (complete blood count, urine analysis (UA), electrolytes, creatinine, blood sugar, thyroid-stimulating hormone, albumin). Echocardiogram, electrocardiogram, or chest radiograph may be needed. D-dimers, if normal, rule out a DVT if suspicion is low. If increased, a Doppler ultrasonography scan should be checked.

Management

If patients has a DVT, they should be referred to the emergency department or medical doctor. Enoxaparin 1 mg/kg/dose subcutaneous every 12 hours may be initiated, or a heparin drip may be started along with Coumadin. Several other new blood thinners may be more suitable. For venous insufficiency, elevation and knee-high compression at 30 to 40 mm Hg at the ankle along with intermitted pneumatic compression pumps may be helpful. If swelling is unresolved 4 to

8 weeks after conservative measures, referral to a lymphedema expert is warranted. Treatment usually involves exercise, elevation, manual lymphatic drainage, and intermitted pneumatic compression. Further procedures such as surgery may be an option (eg, excisional, microsurgery). Psychosocial support is important for patients who develop chronic lymphedema (**Fig. 7**).

Seroma

Prevention

Seroma is a common complication in body contouring surgery and has a propensity for developing in certain procedures. The abdomen is the most common site of seroma formation and rates range from 0.1% to 40%.[3,33,39,46,54–58] Other areas of common seroma formation include the distal aspect of the arm in a brachioplasty, distal thigh in the thighplasty, and occasionally the buttocks area of a lower body lift. Seroma formation is less common in breast and bra-line lifts, in which dead space is minimal.

Careful surgical dissection in the proper planes can help prevent seroma formation. Seroma can be prevented in the lower abdomen by maintaining some of the tissue deep to the Scarpa fascia above the abdominal wall up to the level of the umbilicus. At this umbilicus, dissection can transition to be directly on the abdominal wall, preserving the lymphatics in the abdominal flap.[59] Other options to reduce seroma include quilting sutures and fibrin glue.[57,58,60–64] The use of drains can also prevent seroma formation.[63]

Diagnosis

Drains, if used, are typically removed 1 to 2 weeks after a procedure when outputs are less than 30 mL over a 24-hour period. A palpable or visible fluid wave noted after removal of the drains is the easiest way to diagnose a seroma. Ultrasonography or computed tomography scans are also useful tools, but expensive. Therefore, an attempt at needle aspiration may prove more cost-effective than sending the patient for further imaging.

Management

The initial management of a seroma should be conservative, with serial needle aspirations.[65] Once identified, the area to be drained can be numbed with a small amount of local anesthetic and drained using sterile techniques. Patients should be reassessed at 2 weeks or less to assess whether it has reaccumulated. Frequent drainage usually results in decreased aspirations at each visit. If outputs remain high, a seroma catheter can be placed in the office and secured with a suture. This catheter can then be used for injection

Algorithm

Extremity edema: usually limited to 3 months

If > 4-8 weeks, bilateral? Volume overload: consider short course of diuretics

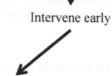

Intervene early

Communicate with lymphedema specialist Usually deal with lymph node issues and permanent problems!

Warn specialist and patient: the patient will be scared

Edema >1 year: a bad sign

Fig. 7. Management algorithm for patients presenting with postoperative lower extremity edema.

of sclerosing agents if necessary. These agents include doxycycline or bleomycin. One formula for sclerosing includes 500 mg of doxycycline in 50 mL of normal saline with 10 mL of 1% lidocaine in a 60-mL syringe. This mixture is injected into the catheter and then the patient is turned every 15 minutes for an hour while the drain is clamped. Interventional radiology may be used for ultrasonography-guided placement of catheters for deeper or more complex fluid collections. If catheter drainage fails to decrease over time with sclerosing, the seroma can be marsupialized and packed so that the wound can heal secondarily. Failure to resolve the seroma with these methods may require a return to the operating room for removal of the seroma cavity. Seromas can be confused with lymphoceles, which are small, firm collections of lymph fluid that continue to reaccumulate despite drainage[66] and may need surgical excision if they do not resolve with time (**Fig. 8**).

Suture Extrusion

Prevention
Suture extrusion is a common complication in body contouring procedures. With multiple

procedures, there is a high likelihood that at least one suture will spit along a suture line. When patients are counseled ahead of time of the risk of a suture extrusion, it is accepted well once it occurs. In the operating room, care should be taken to make sure knots are buried. Avoid the use of permanent braided sutures in areas such as the groin, mons, or axilla, because these can lead to late suture granulomas and extrusion (**Fig. 9**).

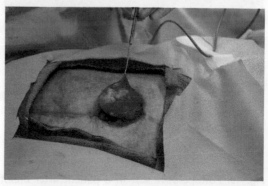

Fig. 8. Lymphocele from a medial thighplasty requiring operative excision. Attempts at recurrent needle aspirations were unsuccessful.

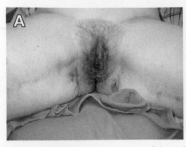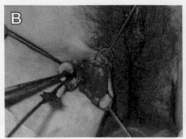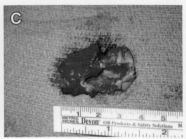

Fig. 9. (*A*) Suture extrusion of braided nylon used in a vertical medial thighplasty procedure. (*B*) The patient developed sinus tracts to both of the sutures used to restore the superficial fascial system of the thigh to Colles fascia. (*C*) Excised sinus tract.

When using barbed sutures, the barbs should not encounter sponges or drapes where fragments of these materials can be dragged into the incision line and may elicit an inflammatory response. Barbed sutures should also be kept at the deep dermal level and it is important not to buttonhole the skin with the suture material.[67,68]

Diagnosis
Suture extrusion is usually identified by the patient as a protruding suture from the suture line, usually with some surrounding erythema or drainage. Impending suture extrusions may appear as blisters on the suture line. For continuous sutures, once one area has become exposed, there is potential for other areas along the suture line to develop delayed suture extrusion as well (**Fig. 10**).

Management
The suture causing the problem should be identified using sterile pickups. Removal of the suture material usually results in rapid healing. Failure to remove the suture material results in a prolonged wound and chronic inflammation until the stitch is completely extruded. Impending suture extrusions may present with blisters on the suture line.

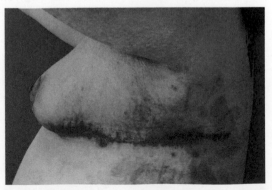

Fig. 10. Postoperative scar in a patient after breast reduction who underwent skin closure with a barbed suture. Multiple skip areas of suture extrusion developed after 1 area became exposed.

These blisters can be managed by observation, or can be ruptured with an 18-gauge needle and then probed with forceps to identify the suture causing the problem. Once the suture is removed, the area can be treated with topic antibiotic and gauze. Chronic sites of granulation tissue can be treated with silver nitrate. For suture granulomas, these sinus tracts may need a more formal excision in the operating room if they are deep or communicate with the rectus plication.

RECURRENT SKIN LAXITY

Recurrent skin laxity is a complex problem after body contouring surgery, especially in patients after massive weight loss, in whom it can be both unpredictable and severe. Patients should be educated about this before surgery so that patient expectations can be managed appropriately. Incorporating the risk of recurrent skin laxity in the surgical consent form creates a reminder to the surgeon to discuss it before surgery. Failure to educate patients beforehand can lead to patient dissatisfaction soon after surgery despite significant improvements in overall contour. Any area of body contouring can be susceptible to recurrent skin laxity (**Fig. 11**).

ASYMMETRY

All patients have some degree of asymmetry at baseline before their body contouring procedures. This asymmetry should be documented both in the medical record and with photographs before surgery. It is helpful to review these photographs as part of the surgical planning to avoid major postoperative asymmetries. The consent process should alert patients to the risk of postoperative asymmetry and that plastic surgery is not an exact science. Some degree of asymmetry should be expected after surgery and setting these expectations ahead of time can avoid significant postoperative dissatisfaction.

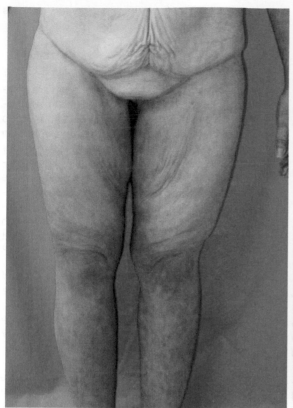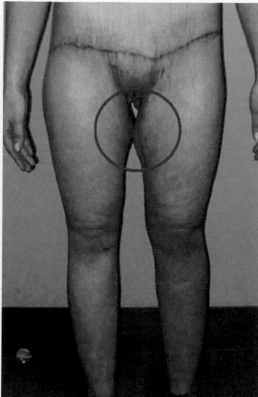

Fig. 11. Recurrent skin laxity in the upper medial thigh after a vertical medial thighplasty procedure.

THE DISAPPOINTED PATIENT

Management of the disappointed patient can take many approaches. First is to listen to the patient and acknowledge the problem. Many small asymmetries, dog ears, or areas of fat necrosis may improve over 6 months to a year. Letting patients know your revision policy before surgery can aid in improving the patient-doctor relationship. Some policies include waiving surgeon's fees, but patients may still be responsible for anesthesia or hospital fees. For patients planning multiple stages of surgery, small revisions can be made at subsequent stages. Careful documentation with preoperative photographs can often ease a patient's dissatisfaction if they can see how great an improvement they have received.

PROCEDURE-SPECIFIC SURGICAL PEARLS
Abdomen

For patients with subcostal scars, be careful not to undermine above the level of the scar, so as to reduce the risk of delayed healing in the triangle of tissue formed by the subcostal scar and the lower abdominal scar.

For Fleur-de-lis or vertical T-type abdomino-plasty procedures, avoid undermining beyond the planned area of resection. Wide undermining to the costal margins may increase the risk of delayed wound healing at the T point.

For restoration of mons ptosis, avoid permanent suture for elevation, which may result in delayed suture extrusion or suture granuloma.

Breasts

To prevent T-point necrosis under the breast, incorporate a small cheat at the inframammary fold incision that can be removed later if the closure is not under tension.

Excision of tissue on the lateral chest wall should be superficial, just deep to the superficial fascial system, to avoid injury to muscle or lymph nodes.

Arms

Dissection in the axilla should be superficial, just under the dermis. Attempts to defat the axilla in a more aggressive manner may lead to removal of lymph nodes and potentially increase the risk of long-term lymphedema in the extremity.

Massage of the axilla after 3 weeks should be encouraged to prevent scar contracture and limited range of motion of the arm.

Care should be taken to avoid dissection near the basilic vein, because injury to the medial antebrachial cutaneous nerve is more likely.

Thighs

In short scar vertical medial thighplasty procedures, it may be hard to get a smooth transition between the middle and lower thirds of the thigh. Patients should be advised before surgery that a dog ear revision may be required in the future (**Fig. 12**).

Permanent suture at the T point in the groin can be left in place for 2 to 3 weeks after surgery and helps prevent wound breakdown.

Buttocks

When autoaugmenting the buttocks, avoid unnecessary excess tension on the closure. It is better to be conservative with the estimated area of resection than to develop significant wound breakdown in this area.

Reinforcing the closure site with permanent suture may aid in preventing dehiscence; however, if

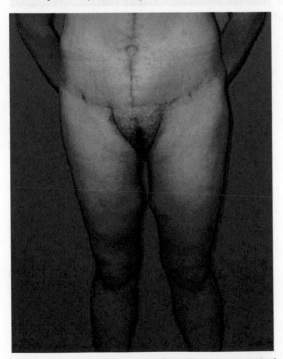

Fig. 12. Dog ear formation after short scar vertical medial thighplasty. Because of the cone shape of the thigh, taking a superior wedge out of the cone may result in a dog ear deformity. Patients are warned about this before surgery and the dog ear is revised at a later date in the office under local anesthesia.

sutures are left in for more than a week, patients can develop significant scarring.

SUMMARY

Complications following body contouring are common and vary significantly, from wound-related issues such as seroma or delayed wound healing to satisfaction-related issues such as recurrent skin laxity. Although many of these issues are minor and can be treated conservatively, the best prevention is early education and counseling of the patient that these complications may occur. Patients will then be more accepting of problems after surgery and easily reassured. Despite the high risk of minor postoperative complications, patient satisfaction with body contouring remains high.

REFERENCES

1. Available at: http://www.plasticsurgery.org/Documents/news-resources/statistics/2013-statistics/body-contouring-massive-weight-loss-stats.pdf. Accessed April 4, 2014.
2. Coon D, Michaels JT, Gusenoff JA, et al. Multiple procedures and staging in the massive weight loss population. Plast Reconstr Surg 2010;125:691–8.
3. Coon D, Gusenoff JA, Kannan N, et al. Body mass and surgical complications in the post-bariatric reconstructive patient: analysis of 511 cases. Ann Surg 2009;249:397–401.
4. Gusenoff JA, Coon D, Rubin JP. Implications of weight loss method in body contouring outcomes. Plast Reconstr Surg 2009;123:373.
5. Hasanbegovic E, Sorensen JA. Complications following body contouring surgery after massive weight loss: a meta-analysis. J Plast Reconstr Aesthet Surg 2014;67:295–301.
6. Greco JA III, Castaldo ET, Nanney LB, et al. The effect of weight loss surgery and body mass index on wound complications after abdominal contouring operations. Ann Plast Surg 2008;61:235–42.
7. Staalesen T, Olsen MF, Elander A. Complications of abdominoplasty after weight loss as a result of bariatric surgery or dieting/postpregancy. J Plast Surg Hand Surg 2012;46:416–20.
8. Davison SP, Clemens MW. Safety first: precautions for the massive weight loss patient. Clin Plast Surg 2008;35:173–83.
9. Fischer JP, Wes AM, Serletti JM, et al. Complications in body contouring procedures: an analysis of 1797 patients from the 2005 to 2010 American College of Surgeons National Surgical Quality Improvement Program databases. Plast Reconstr Surg 2013;132:1411–20.

10. Shermak MA. Pearls and perils of caring for the postbariatric body contouring patient. Plast Reconstr Surg 2012;130:585e–96e.

11. Breiting LB, Lock-Anderson J, Matzen SH. Increased morbidity in patients undergoing abdominoplasty after laparoscopic gastric bypass. Dan Med Bull 2011;58:A4251.

12. Pories WJ, Swanson MS, MacDonald KG, et al. Who would have thought it: an operation proves to be the most effective therapy for adult-onset diabetes mellitus. Ann Surg 1995; 222(3):339–52.

13. Bossert R, Rubin JP. Evaluation of the weight loss patient presenting for plastic surgery consultation. Plast Reconstr Surg 2012;130(6):1361–9.

14. Van der Beek ES, van der Molen AM, van Ramshorst B. Complications after body-contouring surgery in postbariatric patients: the importance of a stable weight close to normal. Obes Facts 2011;4:61–6.

15. Au C, Hazard SW, Dyer A, et al. Correlation of complications of body contouring surgery with increasing body mass index. Aesthet Surg J 2008;28(4):425–9.

16. Nemerofsky RB, Oliak DA, Capella JF. Body lift: an account of 200 consecutive cases in the massive weight loss patient. Plast Reconstr Surg 2006; 117(2):414–30.

17. Colwell AS, Borud LJ. Optimization of patient safety in postbariatric body contouring: a current review. Aesthet Surg J 2008;28:437–42.

18. Agha-Mohammadi S, Hurwitz DJ. Nutritional deficiency of post-bariatric surgery body contouring patients: what every plastic surgeon should know. Plast Reconstr Surg 2008;122:604.

19. Agha-Mohammadi S, Hurwitz DJ. Enhanced recovery after body-contouring surgery: reducing surgical complication rates by optimizing nutrition. Aesthetic Plast Surg 2010;34:617–25.

20. Naghshineh N, O'Brien Coon D, McTigue K, et al. Nutritional assessment of bariatric surgery patients presenting for plastic surgery: a prospective analysis. Plast Reconstr Surg 2010;126:602–10.

21. Shermak MA. Body contouring. Plast Reconstr Surg 2012;129(6):963e–78e.

22. Gravante G, Araco A, Sorge R, et al. Wound infections in post-bariatric patients undergoing body contouring abdominoplasty: the role of smoking. Obes Surg 2007;17:1325–31.

23. Rogliani M, Labardi L, Silvi E, et al. Smokers: risks and complications in abdominal dermatolipectomy. Aesthetic Plast Surg 2006;30:422–4.

24. Heller J, Gabbay JS, Ghadjar K, et al. Top-10 list of herbal and supplemental medicines used by cosmetic patients: what the plastic surgeon needs to know. Plast Reconstr Surg 2006;117:436–45 [discussion: 446–7].

25. Rieger UM, Erba P, Kalbermatten DF, et al. An individualized approach to abdominoplasty in the presence of bilateral subcostal scars after open gastric bypass. Obes Surg 2008;18:863–9.

26. Shermak MA, Mallalieu J, Chang D. Do preexisting abdominal scars threaten wound healing in abdominoplasty? Eplasty 2010;10:e14.

27. Shermak MA, Chang D, Magnuson TH, et al. An outcomes analysis of patients undergoing body contouring surgery after massive weight loss. Plast Reconstr Surg 2006;118(4):1026–31.

28. Aly AS, Cram AE, Chao M, et al. Belt lipectomy for circumferential truncal excess: the University of Iowa experience. Plast Reconstr Surg 2003; 111(1):398–413.

29. Shermak MA, Chang DC, Heller J. Factors impacting thromboembolism after bariatric body contouring surgery. Plast Reconstr Surg 2007;119:1590–6 [discussion: 1597–8].

30. Reish RG, Damjanovic B, Colwell A. Deep venous thrombosis prophylaxis in body contouring surgery: 105 consecutive patients. Ann Plast Surg 2012;69:412–4.

31. Hatef DA, Kenkel JM, Nguyen MQ, et al. Thromboembolic risk assessment and the efficacy of enoxaprin prophylaxis in excisional body contouring surgery. Plast Reconstr Surg 2008;122:269–79.

32. Jeong HS, Miller TJ, Davis K, et al. Application of the Caprini risk assessment model in evaluation of non-venous thromboembolism complications in plastic and reconstructive surgery patients. Aesthet Surg J 2014;34(1):87–95.

33. Coon D, Michaels JT, Gusenoff JA, et al. Hypothermia and complications in postbariatric body contouring. Plast Reconstr Surg 2012;130:443–8.

34. Shermak MA, Shoo B, Deune EG. Prone positioning precautions in plastic surgery. Plast Reconstr Surg 2006;117:1584–8 [discussion: 1589].

35. Buck DW, Mustoe TA. An evidence-based approach to abdominoplasty. Plast Reconstr Surg 2010;126(6):2189–95.

36. Michaels JV, Coon D, Rubin JP. Complications in postbariatric body contouring: postoperative management and treatment. Plast Reconstr Surg 2011; 127:1693.

37. Neaman KC, Hansen JE. Analysis of complications from abdominoplasty: a review of 206 cases at a university hospital. Ann Plast Surg 2007;58(3): 292–8.

38. Arthurs ZM, Cuadrado D, Sohn V, et al. Post-bariatric panniculectomy: pre-panniculectomy body mass index impacts the complication profile. Am J Surg 2007;193(5):567–70 [discussion: 570].

39. Kitzinger HB, Cakl T, Wenger R, et al. Prospective study on complications following a lower body lift after massive weight loss. J Plast Reconstr Aesthet Surg 2013;66:231–8.

40. D'Ettorre M, Gniuli D, Iaconelli A, et al. Wound healing process in post-bariatric patients: an experimental evaluation. Obes Surg 2010;20:1552–8.

41. Hurwitz DJ, Agha-Mohammadi S, Ota K, et al. A clinical review of total body lift surgery. Aesthet Surg J 2008;28:294–303.

42. Light D, Arvanitis GM, Abramson D, et al. Effect of weight loss after bariatric surgery on skin and the extracellular matrix. Plast Reconstr Surg 2010; 125:343–51.

43. Albino FP, Koltz PF, Gusenoff JA. A comparative analysis and systematic review of the wound-healing milieu: implications for body contouring after massive weight loss. Plast Reconstr Surg 2009; 124:1675–82.

44. Strauch B, Herman C, Rohde C, et al. Mid-body contouring in the post-bariatric surgery patient. Plast Reconstr Surg 2006;117:2200–11.

45. Lockwood TE. Superficial fascial system (SFS) of the trunk and extremities: a new concept. Plast Reconstr Surg 1991;87:1009–18.

46. Chong T, Coon D, Toy J, et al. Body contouring in the male weight loss population: assessing gender as a factor in outcomes. Plast Reconstr Surg 2012; 130(2):325e–30e.

47. Hurwitz DJ, Agha-Mohammadi S. Postbariatric surgery breast reshaping: the spiral flap. Ann Plast Surg 2006;56(5):481–6.

48. Migliori FC, Ghiglion M, D'Alessandro G, et al. Brachioplasty after bariatric surgery: personal technique. Obes Surg 2008;18:1165–9.

49. Ellabban MG, Hart NB. Body contouring by combined abdominoplasty and medial vertical thigh reduction: experience of 14 cases. Br J Plast Surg 2004;57:222–7.

50. Katzel EB, Nayar HS, Davenport MP, et al. The influence of preexisting lower extremity edema and venous stasis disease on body contouring outcomes. Ann Plast Surg 2013. [Epub ahead of print].

51. Moreno CH, Neto HJ, Junior AH, et al. Thighplasty after bariatric surgery: evaluation of lymphatic drainage in lower extremities. Obes Surg 2008;18: 1160–4.

52. Shermak MA, Mallalieu J, Chang D. Does thighplasty for upper thigh laxity after massive weight loss require a vertical incision? Aesthet Surg J 2009;29:513–22.

53. Ely JW, Osheroff JA, Chambliss ML, et al. Approach to leg edema of unclear etiology. J Am Board Fam Med 2006;19(2):148–60.

54. Levesque AY, Daniels MA, Polynice A. Outpatient lipoabdominoplasty: review of the literature and practical considerations for safe practice. Aesthet Surg J 2013;33(7):1021–9.

55. Bertheuil N, Thienot S, Huguier V, et al. Medial thighplasty after massive weight loss: are there any risk factors for post-operative complications? Aesthetic Plast Surg 2013;38(1):63–8.

56. Vastine VL, Morgan RF, Williams GS, et al. Wound complications of abdominoplasty in obese patients. Ann Plast Surg 1999;42:34–9.

57. Pollock H, Pollock T. Progressive tension sutures: a technique to reduce local complications in abdominoplasty. Plast Reconstr Surg 2000;105:2583–6.

58. Pollock T, Pollock H. Progressive tension sutures in abdominoplasty: a review of 597 consecutive cases. Aesthet Surg J 2012;32(6):729–42.

59. Pascal JF, Le Louarn C. Remodeling bodylift with high lateral tension. Aesthetic Plast Surg 2002;26:223–30.

60. Schwabegger AH, Ninkovic MM, Anderl H. Fibrin glue to prevent seroma formation. Plast Reconstr Surg 1998;101:1744.

61. Grossman JA, Capraro PA. Long-term experience with the use of fibrin sealant in aesthetic surgery. Aesthet Surg J 2007;27:558–62.

62. Toman N, Buschmann A, Muehlberger T. Fibrin glue and seroma formation following abdominoplasty. Chirurg 2007;78:531–5.

63. Bercial ME, Sabino Nto M, Calil JA, et al. Suction drains, quilting sutures, and fibrin sealant in the prevention of seroma formation in abdominoplasty: which is the best strategy? Aesthetic Plast Surg 2012;36:370–3.

64. Andrades P, Prado A, Danilla S, et al. Progressive tension sutures in the prevention of postabdominoplasty seroma: a prospective, randomized, double-blinded clinical trial. Plast Reconstr Surg 2007;120: 935–46 [discussion: 947–51].

65. Shermak MA, Rotellini-Coltvet LA, Chang D. Seroma development following body contouring surgery for massive weight loss: patient risk factors and treatment strategies. Plast Reconstr Surg 2008;122:280–8.

66. Borud LJ, Cooper JS, Slavin SA. New management algorithm for lymphocele following medial thigh lift. Plast Reconstr Surg 2008;121:1450–5.

67. Shermak MA. The application of barbed sutures in body contouring surgery. Aesthet Surg J 2013;35: 72S–5S.

68. Rubin JP, Hunstad JP, Polynice A, et al. A multicenter randomized controlled trial comparing absorbable barbed sutures versus conventional barbed sutures for dermal closure in open surgical procedures. Aesthet Surg J 2014;34(2):272–83.

Index

Note: Page numbers of article titles are in **boldface** type.

Clin Plastic Surg 41 (2014) 819–822
http://dx.doi.org/10.1016/S0094-1298(14)00119-9
0094-1298/14/$ – see front matter © 2014 Elsevier Inc. All rights reserved.

United States Postal Service

Statement of Ownership, Management, and Circulation
(All Periodicals Publications Except Requestor Publications)

1. Publication Title	2. Publication Number	3. Filing Date
Clinics in Plastic Surgery	0 0 6 - 5 3 0	9/14/14

4. Issue Frequency	5. Number of Issues Published Annually	6. Annual Subscription Price
Jan, Apr, Jul, Oct	4	$490.00

7. Complete Mailing Address of Known Office of Publication (Not printer) (Street, city, county, state, and ZIP+4®)

Elsevier Inc.
360 Park Avenue South
New York, NY 10010-1710

Contact Person
Stephen R. Bushing
Telephone (Include area code)
215-239-3688

8. Complete Mailing Address of Headquarters or General Business Office of Publisher (Not printer)

Elsevier Inc., 360 Park Avenue South, New York, NY 10010-1710

9. Full Names and Complete Mailing Addresses of Publisher, Editor, and Managing Editor (Do not leave blank)

Publisher (Name and complete mailing address)

Linda Belfus, Elsevier, Inc., 1600 John F. Kennedy Blvd. Suite 1800, Philadelphia, PA 19103-2899

Editor (Name and complete mailing address)

Joanne Husovski, Elsevier, Inc., 1600 John F. Kennedy Blvd. Suite 1800, Philadelphia, PA 19103-2899

Managing Editor (Name and complete mailing address)

Adrianne Brigido, Elsevier, Inc., 1600 John F. Kennedy Blvd. Suite 1800, Philadelphia, PA 19103-2899

10. Owner (Do not leave blank. If the publication is owned by a corporation, give the name and address of the corporation immediately followed by the names and addresses of all stockholders owning or holding 1 percent or more of the total amount of stock. If not owned by a corporation, give the names and addresses of the individual owners. If owned by a partnership or other unincorporated firm, give its name and address as well as those of each individual owner. If the publication is published by a nonprofit organization, give its name and address.)

Full Name	Complete Mailing Address
Wholly owned subsidiary of	1600 John F. Kennedy Blvd, Ste. 1800
Reed/Elsevier, US holdings	Philadelphia, PA 19103-2899

11. Known Bondholders, Mortgagees, and Other Security Holders Owning or Holding 1 Percent or More of Total Amount of Bonds, Mortgages, or Other Securities. If none, check box ☐ None

Full Name	Complete Mailing Address
N/A	

12. Tax Status (For completion by nonprofit organizations authorized to mail at nonprofit rates) (Check one)
The purpose, function, and nonprofit status of this organization and the exempt status for federal income tax purposes:
☐ Has Not Changed During Preceding 12 Months
☐ Has Changed During Preceding 12 Months (Publisher must submit explanation of change with this statement)

PS Form 3526, August 2012 (Page 1 of 3 (Instructions Page 3)) PSN 7530-01-000-9931 **PRIVACY NOTICE:** See our Privacy policy in www.usps.com

---

13. Publication Title	14. Issue Date for Circulation Data Below
Clinics in Plastic Surgery	April 2014

15. Extent and Nature of Circulation		Average No. Copies Each Issue During Preceding 12 Months	No. Copies of Single Issue Published Nearest to Filing Date
a. Total Number of Copies (Net press run)		1,080	1,014
b. Paid Circulation (By Mail and Outside the Mail)	(1) Mailed Outside-County Paid Subscriptions Stated on PS Form 3541. (Include paid distribution above nominal rate, advertiser's proof copies, and exchange copies)	583	556
	(2) Mailed In-County Paid Subscriptions Stated on PS Form 3541 (Include paid distribution above nominal rate, advertiser's proof copies, and exchange copies)		
	(3) Paid Distribution Outside the Mails Including Sales Through Dealers and Carriers, Street Vendors, Counter Sales, and Other Paid Distribution Outside USPS®	205	168
	(4) Paid Distribution by Other Classes Mailed Through the USPS (e.g. First-Class Mail®)		
c. Total Paid Distribution (Sum of 15b (1), (2), (3), and (4))	▲	788	724
d. Free or Nominal Rate Distribution (By Mail and Outside the Mail)	(1) Free or Nominal Rate Outside-County Copies Included on PS Form 3541	101	76
	(2) Free or Nominal Rate In-County Copies Included on PS Form 3541		
	(3) Free or Nominal Rate Copies Mailed at Other Classes Through the USPS (e.g. First-Class Mail)		
	(4) Free or Nominal Rate Distribution Outside the Mail (Carriers or other means)		
e. Total Free or Nominal Rate Distribution (Sum of 15d (1), (2), (3) and (4))	▲	101	76
f. Total Distribution (Sum of 15c and 15e)	▲	889	800
g. Copies not Distributed (See instructions to publishers #4 (page #3))	▲	191	214
h. Total (Sum of 15f and g)	▲	1,080	1,014
i. Percent Paid (15c divided by 15f times 100)	▲	88.64%	90.50%

16 Total circulation includes electronic copies. Report circulation on PS Form 3526-X worksheet.

17. Publication of Statement of Ownership
If the publication is a general publication, publication of this statement is required. Will be printed in the October 2014 issue of this publication.

18. Signature and Title of Editor, Publisher, Business Manager, or Owner	Date
Stephen R. Bushing – Inventory Distribution Coordinator	September 14, 2014

I certify that all information furnished on this form is true and complete. I understand that anyone who furnishes false or misleading information on this form or who omits material or information requested on the form may be subject to criminal sanctions (including fines and imprisonment) and/or civil sanctions (including civil penalties).

PS Form 3526, August 2012 (Page 2 of 3)

Printed and bound by CPI Group (UK) Ltd, Croydon, CR0 4YY

03/10/2024

01040374-0014